Medical-Legal and Forensic Aspects of Communication Disorders, Voice Prints, and Speaker Profiling

Dennis C. Tanner, Ph.D.

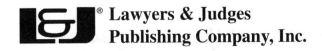
® Lawyers & Judges
Publishing Company, Inc.

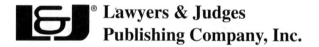 **Lawyers & Judges
Publishing Company, Inc.**

P.O. Box 30040 • Tucson, AZ 85751-0040
(800) 209-7109 • FAX (800) 330-8795
e-mail: sales@lawyersandjudges.com
www.lawyersandjudges.com

Library of Congress Cataloging-in-Publication Data

Tanner, Dennis C., 1949-
   Medical-legal and forensic aspects of communication disorders, voice prints, and speaker profiling / Dennis C. Tanner.
      p. cm.
   ISBN-13: 978-1-933264-13-4 (hardcover : alk. paper)
   ISBN-10: 1-933264-13-6 (hardcover : alk. paper)
   1. Communicative disorders. 2. Voiceprints. 3. Medical jurisprudence. I. Title.
   RC423.T2646 2007
   614'.1--dc22

                    2006100864

ISBN 1-933264-13-6
ISBN 978-1-933264-13-4
Printed in the United States of America
10 9 8 7 6 5 4 3 2 1

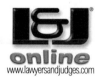

Table of Contents

Part II Medical-Legal and Forensic Aspects of Speech-Language Pathology and Audiology

Chapter 10. Medical-Legal and Forensic Aspects of Communication Disorders Resulting from Traumatic Brain Injury

Part III The Forensic Aspects of Voice Prints

Part IV Speaker Profiling

Preface

I have written *The Medical-Legal and Forensic Aspects of Communication Disorders, Voice Prints, and Speaker Profiling* to be the "go-to" resource for lawyers, judges, and law enforcement personnel. This book expands, explains, and further develops the medical, legal, and forensic concepts addressed in my preceding books: *The Forensic Aspects of Communication Sciences and Disorders* and *The Forensic Aspects of Speech Patterns: Voice Prints, Speaker Profiling, Lie and Intoxication Detection* (with M. Tanner). With the interest shown for these books, I decided to write a four-section, updated, comprehensive, and expanded text that addresses all of the major medical, legal, and forensic issues associated with speech, voice, language, and hearing. To give the reader necessary academic background information, the first section of this book reviews the discipline of communication sciences and disorders and discusses the research methodology used to expand its knowledgebase.

The second section of this book addresses issues related to medical malpractice and other legal areas for all of the major communication disorders, including dysphagia, a swallowing disorder. In this section, there are italicized sources to legal cases involving a particular legal and forensic issue. However, there is no discussion of their outcomes or legal opinions; they are used for illustrative purposes only. Additionally, there are relevant case studies based on my experience as an expert witness. I have taken literary license with some of them to clarify important medical, legal, and forensic concepts.

Part III of this volume examines spectrographic voice identification, the use of voice prints to identify or confirm the identity of a suspect. Since the tragic events of September 11, 2001 and the global war on Islamic fascists, voice prints have taken on more important forensic roles and are being used to verify the authenticity of terrorists' recorded messages. Included in this section is an expanded discussion of the acoustics of speech, a comprehensive review of phonetics, and voice prints showing and describing their salient forensic features.

The most comprehensive addition to this book concerns the evolving art and science of speaker profiling. Several chapters in Part IV address the "facts" that can be concluded and "conjecture" drawn about what a speaker says and how he or she says it. A speaker's accent and dialect provide important socioeconomic information. While not racial profiling, accent and dialect can be used as one method of determining whether a suspect is traveling from a hostile region of the world. Speaker profiling provides information about intoxication giving police officers probable cause for detainment and further investigation. In this section, there is a detailed discussion of speaker profiling during the forensic interview and interrogation including factual and conjectural information gleaned from the speaker's voice, fluency, articulation, and language patterns. A new addition to the concept of speaker profiling concerns persons with communication disorders. Millions of Americans have communication disorders, and in this volume, there is a review of the facts and conjecture about these speakers.

I believe *The Medical-Legal and Forensic Aspects of Communication Disorders, Voice Prints, and Speaker Profiling* addresses the major medical, legal, and forensic issues associated with human communication and its disorders. It is designed to be the most authoritative, comprehensive text on these subjects, and a valuable resource for lawyers, judges, and professionals from law enforcement, homeland security, and intelligence agencies. At least, that was my goal in writing it.

Dennis C. Tanner, Ph.D.
Flagstaff, Arizona

Foreword

As a practicing criminal defense attorney for thirty-two years the one precept outside of "innocent until proven guilty" that I endorse is that in either prosecution or defense positions no matter how seemingly minute, subtle or insignificant, "everything matters." This book puts a fine point on the "everything matters" concept relating to voice, speech, language and hearing by providing details valuable to professionals in the medical, legal, and law enforcement fields who hold the lives of others in their hands on a regular basis. To the untrained or unexposed North American ear, speakers who share a common native language other than English may offer few clues to the subtle differences in speech patterns between regions or cultures. Likewise, speech subtleties in this country vary from region to region and within subcultures of the same area. As the population of the United States becomes more diverse and the global interaction of America expands in commerce, personal travel, and political arenas, the legal system will, assuredly, be affected by the diversity of cultures. The preservation of individual rights protected by the constitution will increasingly require both the art and science of communication in its broadest sense to bring more science to every arena of the legal system. This book acknowledges the art and documents the science of speech-language pathology as a useful tool in voice prints and speaker profiling.

I once defended a case where a defendant shared the same name as another individual identified in the situation. Both were speakers of languages other than English. Each, though speaking a common language, came from different regions of the same country. The case turned on such mundane evidentiary data as the subtleties of a bean soup recipe that varied from region to region within the country. While seemingly boring and insignificant as a courtroom tactic, the effort to distinguish between the two individuals as to the regional differences in their culture, including food preparation, was crucial to a positive resolution for the defendant. Oh, to have had available more scientifically supported information regarding speaker profiling using accent and dialect to detect subtle regional and cultural differences. The content of this text offers a valuable tool to assist attorneys for both defense and plaintiff in sorting the "bean soup" of speech and language evidence in a manner that has a more reliable scientific basis. Such a tool now exists in *Medical-Legal and Forensic Aspects of Communication Disorders, Voice Prints, and Speaker Profiling.*

Dr. Tanner has produced a veritable primer for the novice and an in-depth exposition for the seasoned legal professional regarding both the pragmatic and academic aspects of speech and language disorders and treatment strategies relating to medical malpractice issues. This book provides valuable insight into contributions of the speech-language scientist in addressing the critical clinical events and professional judgments that come to bear in assessing purported responsibility when a patient experiences a negative health outcome. Further, qualifying an expert witness is a significant issue in malpractice litigation. It is apparent that Dr. Tanner is an expert in the field of speech-language pathology and has expertly and succinctly presented issues of importance to both plaintiff and defense attorneys. Everyone who is involved in the resolution of criminal cases where identity of the perpetrator is at issue or with medical malpractice litigation where responsibility for a patient's negative quality of life is in dispute will welcome this carefully documented, comprehensive, and authoritative book.

Ernest L. Cotton, JD
Attorney-at-Law

About the Author

Dennis C. Tanner received the Doctor of Philosophy degree in Audiology and Speech Sciences from Michigan State University where he was involved in voice print and speech pattern recognition research. Dr. Tanner's national and international scientific papers, diagnostic tests, and clinical programs address a wide range of topics in communication sciences and disorders. Books by Dennis Tanner include *The Family Guide to Surviving Stroke and Communication Disorders, The Forensic Aspects of Communication Sciences and Disorders, The Psychology of Neurogenic Communication Disorders: A Primer for Health Care Professionals, Exploring Communication Disorders: A 21st Century Introduction Through Literature and Media, The Forensic Aspects of Speech Patterns: Voice Prints, Speaker Profiling, Lie and Intoxication Detection* (with M. Tanner), *Anatomy and Physiology Study Guide for Speech and Hearing* (with W. Culbertson and S. Cotton), *Case Studies in Communication Sciences and Disorders,* and *An Advanced Course in Communication Sciences and Disorders.* Dr. Tanner has been named "Outstanding Educator" by the Association of Schools of Allied Health Professions and the College of Health Profession's "Teacher of the Year." He is the owner of Tanner Rehabilitation Services, Inc., and serves as an expert witness in legal cases involving Communication Sciences and Disorders. Dennis C. Tanner is currently Professor of Health Sciences at Northern Arizona University in Flagstaff, Arizona.

Acknowledgments

I am grateful to several people who helped me write this book. My colleagues, Dr. William Culbertson, Stephanie Cotton, M.A., CCC-SLP, and Dr. John Sciacca, gave me valuable advice and suggestions during the research phase for this book. I am also grateful to Krista Arendsen, J.D. and Eric Salo for their fine editorial assistance. As has been the case with all of my books, my wife Jody Tanner, M.A., CCC-SLP, served as a critical sounding board for many controversial issues, provided important and necessary clinical information, and continued to help me mature as a writer.

Part I
The Discipline of Communication Sciences and Disorders

Chapter 1

The Scope of *The Medical-Legal and Forensic Aspects of Communication Disorders, Voice Prints, and Speaker Profiling*

1.1 Chapter Preview

This chapter provides an overview of the subject matter covered in this book. *The Medical-Legal and Forensic Aspects of Communication Disorders, Voice Prints, and Speaker Profiling* provides lawyers, judges, and law enforcement personnel with a comprehensive resource addressing the major medical-legal and forensic aspects of communication sciences and disorders. This text addresses the important medical-legal aspects of speech-language pathology and audiology, and the forensic issues involved in voice prints and speaker profiling. The chapters in this book address several independent medical-legal and forensic topics in an interconnected general treatise on human communication and its disorders.

1.2 Communication in the 21st Century

Communication is any means of sending or receiving information; it is the act of sharing or exchanging thoughts, emotions, and information. The word "communicate" is Latin in origin and derived from *communis* "common" and *communicare* "to share." Communication is involved in every cooperative human endeavor. The world of the 21st Century would be dramatically different if it were not for the highly evolved human ability to communicate. Communication continues to be important in business, industry, medicine, and law, and rapidly becoming more so.

Ruben (2000) notes that at the beginning of the 1900s, about 80 percent of the American labor force was involved in manual labor jobs not requiring elaborate or sophisti-

cated communication skills, and today, 62 percent of workers have jobs where communication is all or a major part of their activities. Without communication, the practice of medicine would be dramatically different and there would be no law libraries, police-training academies, and universities as we know them. Without communication, FBI, CIA, ATF, Homeland Security, and police departments could not effectively function, lawyers could not litigate, or juries deliberate. All cooperative civilized activities rely on communication, and without it, the professions of law and medicine as practiced today would be dramatically different.

In the mid 1900s, communication theorist Marshall McLuhan published *The Medium is the Massage* and *Understanding Media,* postulating that communication will dramatically change the fundamental nature of human interaction. Indeed, mass communication with television, radio, newspapers, and the Internet has transformed the world into a "global village." Group communication is the foundation to teamwork in government, business, and industry; committees now do many tasks that individuals once did. In the business world, the higher a person goes up the corporate ladder, the more exclusive the job becomes "communication." Effective communication is the foundation to interpersonal relationships; the main cause of so many marital failures is a lack of it. It has been said that one "cannot not communicate" and even silence is a form of communication. Remarkably, every normal baby born into this world is neurologically wired for the ability to communicate. It does not matter the country, race, ethnicity, or society; all normal children learn the language to which they are exposed and they spend a lifetime engaging in communication. Communication is the highest mental, physical, and neurological ability of which humans are capable and there are thousands of defects, diseases, disorders, deficits, and disabilities that can lay waste to it. Communication is an integral part of human existence in the 21st Century. Advances in communication have also transformed medical malpractice litigation and the forensic sciences.

3

The practice of law, including medical malpractice litigation, has changed dramatically in recent years primarily due to the communication revolution. Televised trials of public figures, reporting of jury verdicts on twenty-four hour news channels, and the Internet give the public instant and in-depth access to legal cases that before were only available in newspapers or specialized legal books. Vast stores of Internet information provided by legal search engines such as Westlaw supplement law libraries and provide additional legal resources. Popular crime investigation television programs and movies reflect the public's appetite for the forensic sciences, and even jury deliberations have been affected by the media. Television programs and movies have raised jury expectations about the forensic sciences and what should be made available to it.. The Internet carries terrorists' messages to the world and the forensic sciences are called upon to examine and evaluate them. Communication lies at the heart of the practice of medicine, law, and the forensic sciences.

1.3 Overview of *The Medical-Legal and Forensic Aspects of Communication Disorders, Voice Prints, and Speaker Profiling*

There are three areas where lawyers, judges, and law enforcement personnel are involved in the discipline of communication sciences and disorders: (1) medical malpractice, (2) voice prints, and (3) speaker profiling. Part I of this book provides or overview of the discipline of communication sciences and disorders, defines and describes the diagnostic categories of communication disorders, and profiles the American Speech-Language-Hearing Association (ASHA) including its Code of Ethics. There is also a historical overview of the discipline including a review of the scientific method as the primary source of knowledge.

Part II addresses medical malpractice and particularly issues involving speech-language pathologists and audiologists. An increasingly frequent area of litigation for speech-language pathologists concerns the diagnosis and treatment of patients with swallowing disorders (Tanner, 2006; Tanner and Guzzino, 2002). Although not a communication disorder per se, the diagnosis and treatment of sucking, chewing, and swallowing disorder (dysphagia) are now primary clinical responsibilities for speech-language pathologists working in medical settings. Part II addresses the primary areas of medical malpractice litigation involving speech-language pathology and audiology, and also education-legal aspects of the Individuals With Disabilities Education Act (IDEA) and the Americans with Disabilities Act (ADA).

Part III of this book covers the forensic aspects of voice prints. Lawyers, judges, and law enforcement personnel may be involved in cases addressing speaker recognition based on voice prints and speech perceptual analyses. Voice prints and the perceptual analyses of speakers are conducted in several forensic and legal contexts including evaluating terrorists' messages to determine their authenticity.

Part IV of this book addresses an evolving forensic procedure: speaker profiling. Speaker profiling using accent, dialect, and other speech patterns can be used as a forensic tool to prevent crime and to apprehend and convict suspects. A suspect's speech pattern can provide important information about his or her psychological and emotional states, intoxication, socioeconomic background, and homeland. Speech, voice, and language patterns can also provide cues about a person's criminal intent, knowledge of a crime, and psychological status during forensic interviews and interrogations. Also reviewed in this section is voice stress analysis because many law enforcement agencies use these instruments for lie detection.

1.4 Organization of *The Medical-Legal and Forensic Aspects of Communication Disorders, Voice Prints, and Speaker Profiling*

Each chapter in this book contains a synopsis, chapter preview, summary, suggested readings and resources, and references. Synopses numerically list the chapters' subheadings, which are used liberally throughout the text, to give the reader quick access to pertinent topics. Synopses are useful to readers who do not read the chapters in their entirety, and only seek specific information regarding a medical-legal or forensic issue. Chapter previews and summaries are brief descriptions and reviews of the content of each chapter providing a context and closure for the material discussed therein. Suggested readings and resources list and describe supplemental books, films, Internet resources, journal articles, and documents considered important to each chapter.

Rather than one reference section at the end of the book, bibliographical information is provided at the conclusion of each chapter. Because the Internet is constantly changing, it is inevitable that some Internet addresses will close or change. If Internet information is to be relied upon as the basis of a legal opinion, the printed versions should supersede any downloaded version (Levin, 1999). The citations and references are in standard American Psychological Association (APA) style, which is the suggested and typical format for scholarly works in communication sciences and disorders. In several chapters, and particularly those in Part IV: Speaker Profiling, there is conjecture about the forensic value of information that can be gleaned from a speaker's speech and language. Every attempt has been made to clearly identify sections addressing theories, hypotheses, and conjecture from parts of this book where information is scientifically based.

A comprehensive glossary is provided at the end of the book. It contains relevant words and their definitions used in each chapter and also additional terms that may arise during investigations, depositions, and trials. Although several dictionaries and glossaries were consulted in the construction of the glossary, the definitions are those of the author and reflect the scientific and professional usage of the words. Some relevant terms were also selected from specialized books because they have entered the mainstream of professional usage.

This book supersedes *The Forensic Aspects of Communication Sciences and Disorders* (Tanner, 2003) and *The Forensic Aspects of Speech Patterns: Voice Prints, Speaker Profiling, Lie and Intoxication Detection* (Tanner and Tanner, 2004). Rather than create second editions of the above books, it was decided to incorporate the information into *The Medical-Legal and Forensic Aspects of Communication Disorders, Voice Prints, and Speaker Profiling* to give the reader an expanded, comprehensive resource for the medical-legal and forensic aspects of communication and its disorders.

1.5 Chapter Summary

The recent communication revolution has dramatically affected forensic sciences and the professions of law and medicine. There are three primary areas where lawyers, judges, and law enforcement personnel are involved in the discipline of communication sciences and disorders: medical malpractice, voice prints, and speaker profiling. This book addresses the major facets of medical malpractice litigation involving speech-language pathologists and audiologists including the diagnosis and treatment of swallowing disorders. Scientific advances in voice prints and their forensic and legal applications are also addressed. Included in this text is a treatise on speaker profiling and using accent, dialect, and other speech features as forensic tools.

Suggested Readings and Resources

Tanner, D. (2003). *The Forensic Aspects of Communication Sciences and Disorders*. Tucson: Lawyers and Judges Publishing Company. This book address communication disorders, medical malpractice, and many legal issues involved in the provision of special education services.

Tanner, D. and Tanner, M. (2004). *The Forensic Aspects of Speech Patterns: Voice Prints, Speaker Profiling, Lie and Intoxication Detection*. Tucson: Lawyers and Judges Publishing Company. This book provides a general overview of the forensic applications of speech patterns.

References

Levin, S. M. (1999). Screening the nursing home case. In P. Iyer (Ed), *Nursing home litigation: investigation and case preparation*. Tucson: Lawyers and Judges Publishing Company.

Ruben, R.J. (2000). Redefining the survival of the fittest: Communication disorders in the 21st century. *Laryngoscope, 110*: 241-245.

Tanner, D. and Guzzino, A. (2002, April). Westlaw search of litigation areas in communication sciences and disorders. A paper presented at the 2001-2002 Honors Day Program. Northern Arizona University, Flagstaff, Arizona.

Tanner, D. (2006, February). The forensic aspects of dysphagia: Investigating medical malpractice. *The ASHA Leader, 11(2), 16-17, 45*.

Chapter 2

A Brief History of the Study of Human Communication and Its Disorders

2.1 Chapter Preview

This chapter provides a condensed overview of the study of human communication and its disorders from ancient times to the present day. Included in this discussion is an overview of important past and current issues in communication sciences and disorders including the brain-mind leap, brain localization controversy, and the role of language in thought. There is also a discussion of the social status of people with communication disorders and advances in technology and recent legislation that have improved their lives.

2.2 Historical Overview of Communication and Its Disorders

Philosophers, scientists, and clinicians have studied communication for centuries, and communication disorders have existed presumably since people began to talk. The first recorded reference to communication disorders occurred in an ancient Egyptian surgical text. The text contained descriptions of medical disorders of about fifty cases, and Case Twenty-Two described a patient with a communication disorder (O'Neill, 1980). This account of speechlessness secondary to a neurological insult, a "smash in his temple," was written approximately four millennia ago. In this treatise, and in a subsequent "gloss" about the surgical text completed 800 years later, Ancient Egyptian scholars speculated about the role of the brain in the ability to speak and brain damage on speechlessness. It would be nearly 4,000 years later that Pierre Paul Broca, the pioneering French neurologist, would utter this famous statement: "We speak with the left hemisphere."

A persistent problem occurring throughout the centuries of philosophizing, theorizing, and researching human speech, voice, language, and hearing was vague or nonexistent definitions of terms. Too often, important terms central to theories about communication and clinical entities were inconsistently defined, ill-defined, or there was no attempt to define them. For example, Homer coined the word "aphasia" to refer to speechlessness caused by emotional reactions and associated with crying (O'Neill, 1980). Today, aphasia is considered a neurologically-based language disorder often seen in stroke patients, and not psychological in origin. Although more common early on, terminology controversies and definitional ambiguities have persisted into the 21st Century. Fortunately, with the increased emphasis on the scientific method, and its requirement that important research terms be clearly defined as part of the methodology section, terminology ambiguity has been reduced. Nevertheless, vague and indescript definitions of terms cloud the understanding of early scholarly contributions to the study of communication and its disorders.

In a trend that continues today, the Ancient Egyptians' curiosity about a speech pathology precipitated their theorizing about the nature of normal communication. Early speculation about the psychological, neurological, and physical bases to communication involved several contentious subjects that have yet to be resolved, and even today, they are controversial and spark debate. Today, as in ancient times, philosophers, scientists, and clinicians ponder the brain-mind leap, specific areas of the brain responsible for communication functions, and the role of language in thought.

2.3 The Brain-Mind Leap

Beginning with the Ancient Egyptians and continuing today, a primary and overriding theoretical issue about communication and its disorders is the so-called "brain-mind leap." The brain-mind leap is projecting the goings-on in a person's brain to what occurs in his or her mind. More generally, it is how the human brain creates consciousness—the awareness of self and the environment. After centuries of study, scientists, philosophers, and theologians have only scratched the surface in understanding how the brain functions to produce sensations, perceptions, thoughts, emotions, and the remarkable ability to communicate. According to Davis (2007), Leonardo da Vinci believed that the mind or soul inhabits little spaces inside the brain.

The brain functions by the complex interaction of neurons and changes in brain chemistry. Electrochemical impulses shoot from one neuron or tract of neurons to others, from white matter to cortex, from lobe to lobe, and from hemisphere to hemisphere. These impulses carry sound, the meanings of words, grammatical structures of utterances, speech sound production and execution plans, and the inner speech statements we use to plan, monitor, and adjust our actions in dealings with the world. At the heart of the brain-mind leap is how these neurological impulses – electrochemical changes in the brain – become thoughts, communication acts, and, on the most fundamental level, human consciousness. Communication is but one facet of individual and collective human consciousness.

Although the brain-mind leap has been pondered since the beginning of recorded history, arguments about it continue to permeate the discipline of communication sciences and disorders. At the heart of the arguments about the function of the brain, and the operation of the human mind, are the scientific and religious explanations of the origin of communication, and by extension, the fundamental nature of communication disorders. Today, creation and evolutionary views of the origin of communication and its disorders are contentious topics, and often, the subject of heated debate.

Currently, there are about 10,000 languages and dialects in use, and according to the creation argument, they exist because of divine imposition. In this belief system, the various languages and dialects of the world are a result of God confounding the "tongues" of the builders of the Tower of Babel. From this biblical parable, we get the term "babbling" to indicate confused and hard-to-grasp speech. By extension, communication disorders are also divinely created. In Exodus 4:10, there is a reference to communication and its disorders: "And Moses said unto the Lord, O my Lord, I am not eloquent, neither heretofore, nor since thou hast spoken unto thy servant; but I am slow of speech and slow of tongue. And the Lord said unto him, Who hath made man's mouth? or who maketh the dumb, or deaf, or the seeing, or the blind? have not I the lord?" Strict creationists believe in exorcism, laying on hands, faith healing, and other religious rituals to eliminate or minimize communication disorders.

The evolutionary or scientific explanation for human communication and the multiple languages of the world involves the isolation of prehistoric tribes and their arbitrary attachment of speech sounds to meanings. The meanings of words are based on the symbol-referent relationship. Over thousands of years of evolution, a language society agreed that a sound or series of sounds (symbol) refers to an aspect of reality (referent). The world's languages grew from this evolution of word meanings. This evolutionary theory of language ontogeny also played a role in the survival of the species. The ability to communicate was, and continues to be, a powerful survival tool enabling humans to be dominant over other creatures of the world. In the evolutionary view of language, the human ability to communicate is simply a more evolved animalistic function, and not unique to humans or divinely inspired. In the scientific treatment model, communication disorders are eliminated or minimized through surgeries, medications, instruction, counseling, and therapies.

2.4 Communication and the Brain Localization Controversy

The brain localization movement, the attempt to pinpoint areas of the brain responsible for specific functions, has also been around since the beginning of the study of human communication and its disorders. The Ancient Egyptians' linking the brain to the ability to speak was the first localization observation. Benson and Ardila (1996) and Sies (1974) provide detailed histories of the speech and language localization movement. In communication sciences and disorders, the brain localization movement continues to be central to the study of aphasia. Aphasia is a language disorder typically occurring in patients with brain tumors, traumatic brain injuries, and strokes.

The first localizationist with a large public following was Franz Joseph Gall. In the early 1800s, he popularized the Theory of Phrenology which postulated that a person's personality and intellect could be described by palpitations of the bones of the skull. Every human propensity from instincts to verbal skills could be discovered by feeling the bones of the skull. During that time, many affluent people in Europe and America had Phrenology readings to help plan their education, careers, and even marriage. Of course, the

Theory of Phrenology was fraught with error and based on unfounded assumptions. However, it clearly linked brain structures to the mind.

In the mid-1800s, Pierre Paul Broca did postmortem examinations of two aphasic patients, and in 1865, localized the expressive speech and language center to the left hemisphere, particularly the frontal lobe. He called this disorder "aphemia" noting that although the patient can understand speech, he or she can only utter a few words. (Pierre Marie, in 1906, reexamined the brains of Broca's patients and questioned attributing the disorder to a specific brain lesion). Sigmund Freud also questioned the strict localization view of communication functions.

Also in the mid-1800s, a German neurologist, Karl Wernicke, identified the sensory or receptive area of communication which is also found in the left hemisphere, particularly the temporal lobe. He noted that a patient with sensory aphasia has impaired understanding of speech not attributable to hearing loss or deafness.

Broca and Wernicke's research set the foundation for the localization movement which has continued unabated. At about the time of Broca and Wernicke's pioneering work on aphasia localization, John Hughlings Jackson, a neurologist, noted that the brain should be viewed as a functional unit where thought, language, and a person's psyche work together. Jackson developed the notion of "inner speech" as a form of verbal thought.

During the early 1900s, a British neurologist, Henry Head, became an outspoken critic of the aphasia localizationist movement. In his book, *Aphasia and Kindred Disorders of Speech*, he sarcastically labeled the localizationist as the "Diagram Maker." According to Benson and Ardila (1996) and Sies (1974), Head recognized that the brain operates holistically and that it was unproductive to create diagrams showing the areas of the brain responsible for all speech and language functions.

Today, researchers use sophisticated brain-scanning devices to identify areas of the brain responsible for everything from the perception of vowels to interpreting proverbs. The goal is to discover "modules," the functional speech and language areas of the brain (Owens, Metz, and Haas, 2000). While there are general module localizations that can be made about certain communication functions, especially motor and sensory representations, a strict localization philosophy is hard to justify because the brain operates holistically.

A strict localizationist philosophy of brain functioning is difficult to support. No single part of the brain functions completely independent from the others. For example, although there may be certain identifiable areas of the brain important in perceiving vowels and consonants, pointing a mass of brain cells completely responsible, in every person, for interpreting a proverb or understanding the implications of a Robert Frost poem is absurd. And, of course, there is the monumental task of identifying the neurochemical activities in the cells of the brain and projecting what happens in a particular person's mind (Tanner, 2003, p. 5).

As Figure 2.1 shows, given the complexities of brain localization and communication functions, five principles should be considered when discussing sites of lesions and aphasic disorders. Principle One addresses handedness as an indicator of hemisphere dominance. Handedness suggests hemispheric dominance, but so do dichotic listening tests, the presenting of auditory stimuli to the ears to decide ear-advantage. Additionally, eye preference is an indicator of hemispheric dominance. The statistics for handedness and language organization in Principle Two are obtained by noting that approximately 90 percent of right-handed people have language in the left-hemisphere, and approximately 60 percent of the left-handed people (11 percent of the population) and true ambidextrous individuals also have left-hemisphere dominance. Roughly 7 percent of the population is left-handed and left-hemisphere dominant. Principle Three addresses the anterior-posterior dichotomy in aphasia (relative to the Fissure of Rolando) and the importance of placing aphasic subjects in the two categories. The necessity of separating language-based neurogenic communication disorders (aphasia) from motor speech disorders (apraxia of speech) is addressed in Principle Four. Multiple etiologies of aphasia are addressed in Principle Five.

2.5 The Language-Thought Controversy

Throughout history, great thinkers have pondered the nature of thought, and more precisely, the role of language in thought. It is no wonder that when language is broadly defined, its role in cognition becomes essential to the human ability to understand the world. Language competence is broadly defined as the multimodality ability to encode, decode, and manipulate symbols for the purposes of verbal thought and communication (Tanner, 2006). Language per se is broadly defined as a symbolic code that is rule governed, uses several modalities and forms for expression, and serves as a communication code for social and societal interaction (Wiig, 2004).

Does language simply express thought, or is language itself a fundamental aspect of thinking? This notion was addressed early in the study of cognition as scholars realized that we think in words. Plato and Socrates believed that thought was a conversation with the soul and that speech is the outward expression of it. (Plato also thought that hearing was the exact reverse of speech and that the bloodstream conducted sound to the brain.) Socrates knew language was not only a means to self-exploration, to "know thyself," but also an end unto itself.

As reported previously, John Hughlings Jackson tied the totality of a person to language. As a result of studying patients with communication disorders, he considered it artificial to separate thought, language, and the patient's psyche. He also addressed propositional and nonpropositional speech acts and noted that single words are meaningless when communicating thoughts; the unit of speech is the proposition. According to Jackson (1878, p. 311):

> To speak is not simply to utter words, it is to propositionise. A proposition is such a relation of words that it makes one new meaning; not by a mere addition of what we call the separate meanings of the several words; the terms of the proposition are modified by each other. Single words are meaningless, and so is any unrelated succession of words. The unit of speech is the proposition. A single word is, or is in effect, a proposition, if other words in relation are implied.

In the early 1900s, Kurt Goldstein postulated the abstract-concrete imbalance in patients who are deprived of language. He suggested that because of the loss of language, aphasic patients are on a concrete level and have lost the "abstract attitude." This loss of an abstract attitude is present not only for verbal tasks, as would be expected, but also nonverbal tasks such as sorting according to categories such as color or shape.

Over the years, the two academic schools have surfaced about the role of language in thought and vice versa: the Associationists and the Cognitivists. The Association School of Thought believes that language simply expresses thought. Associationists regard intelligence as located outside the region bounded by the language centers (Benton, 1981). The Cognitive School of Thought takes a more holistic approach and believes that thought and language are functionally inseparable. The role language plays in thought continues to be an important and controversial issue in communication sciences and disorders. Today most neuroscientists recognize that language is a fundamental aspect of thought in adults. In young children, language probably only expresses thought.

Principle One: Handedness is an indicator of primary hemispheric language organization in most patients but not an absolute indicator of hemisphere dominance.

Principle Two: Based on handedness, language is localized primarily to the left brain hemisphere in approximately 87 percent of the total population.

Principle Three: In left hemisphere dominant aphasic patients, lesions anterior to the Fissure of Rolando usually cause predominantly expressive disorders and those posterior to the Fissure of Rolando usually cause predominantly receptive communication disorders.

Principle Four: Aphasia is a language disorder and inclusive of expressive and receptive grammar, syntax, phonology, and semantic impairments. Apraxia of speech and the dysarthrias are motor speech disorders.

Principle Five: Aphasia etiology is categorized as follows:
1. Aphasia resulting from unilateral strokes
2. Aphasia resulting from space occupying tumors
3. Aphasia resulting from focalized traumatic brain injury to the left-hemisphere
4. Aphasia resulting from multiple sites traumatic brain injury.
5. Miscellaneous aphasias resulting from infections, metabolic disorders, and degenerative disease process including multi infarct dementia and Alzheimer's disease.

Figure 2.1 Aphasia and brain localization.

2.6 Social Status of People with Communication Disorders

What are the consequences of communication disorders on the people who suffer them? Historically, how have disabled people, particularly those with communication disorders, been treated by society? What are the recent political and technological events that have occurred to bring communication disabled people into mainstream society?

People with communication disorders are a diverse group with varying degrees of disabilities. Some persons have communication disorders that are only nuisances such as lisping and mild stuttering. Others have more severe communication disorders that affect their day-to-day lives such as aphasia, severe stuttering, and articulation disorders that compromise speech intelligibility. Many people have severe communication disorders that substantially affect their social interaction and quality of life such as global aphasia, cleft lip and palate, traumatic brain injury, communication disorders related to severe mental retardation, and laryngectomy (surgical removal of the voice box). No matter the severity of their communication disorders, most people feel embarrassment and shame about their communication disorders, and strive to be more like the mainstream society concerning the ability to communicate. In school, children with communication disorders are in special education programs to help them "catch up" with their peers.

Historically, being communication disabled has been a significant deterrence to having even a modicum of a meaningful quality of life, and being born with a major communication disorder, or suffering one later in life, could be a death knell. It is likely that the word "handicapped" came from practice of disabled persons begging on street corners for food or money with caps in hand. For many communication-disabled people, their very lives depended on the kindness of strangers. At the core of the mistreatment and sometimes outright disdain for the communication disabled is their perceived inability to contribute to the survival of the tribe, community, and in a larger sense, the species. There is also an unfounded primal fear that reproduction among some individuals with communication disorders may propagate the worst of the gene pool.

In primitive societies, the value of an individual was based on his or her ability to contribute to the safety and survival of the tribe or community, and the communication disabled often had physical and mental disabilities that negated their value and resulted in brutal treatment. The inhabitants of ancient India cast the disabled into the Ganges; the Aztecs sacrificed them to the gods; the Melanesians buried them alive; and the Spartans hurled them from precipices (Van Riper and Erickson, 1996). More recently, during the 1930s and 1940s, the Nazis euthanized thousands of disabled individuals as part of their misguided attempts at racial cleansing and to purify the gene pool. Even recently in the United States, people with mental retardation were required to undergo mandatory birth control.

Van Riper and Erickson (1996) note that throughout history, societies have considered disabled people as nuisances, objects of mirth, pitiful beggars, challenging problems, and individuals who are challenged. Today, communication disabled people, as a group, continue to be economically and vocationally challenged. "In the United Kingdom men with a hearing or a speech handicap were found more frequently in the lowest classes. They were also more likely to be out of the labor force---three times more likely for the hearing impaired and eight times more likely for the speech impaired than non-disabled persons" (Ruben, 2000, p. 243). These class and employment patterns for disabled persons tend to be true for other industrialized countries as well. The plight of the communication disabled in non-industrialized countries is much more severe, rendering many of them beggars and social outcasts.

Several factors have played a role in the social status of people with communication disorders and continue to influence their progress toward social inclusion and equality. First, although the number of communication disabled is high—more than 40 million Americans—they are relatively politically effective. Communications disabled people, as a group, are not as politically powerful or socially effective as similarly large, politically active groups. Except for people with hearing loss, most individuals with significant communication disorders are young or old, economically and socially dependent on others, sometimes institutionalized, and often stricken by co-occurring physical and mental disorders that limit their political activism. Most importantly, their communication disorders per se obstruct or limit their political effectiveness. Acts of political activism are essentially acts of communication, and most communication disabled individuals are unable to fully engage in them.

The second factor that interferes with the communication disabled's progress toward social inclusion is the visibility of their disabilities. People with speech, voice, language, and hearing disorders, with few exceptions, only show their disabilities when engaging in acts of communication. Unlike many other disabled persons, such as amputees, the blind, and paraplegics who consistently show their disabilities, people with communication disorders only make their disabilities apparent when they attempt to communicate. Consequently, group cohesiveness for the communication disabled is less than what occurs with other groups of disabled persons because of the lack of continuity of identification. A particular person's identification with the larger group of communication disabled is irregular and dependent on communication. For many people with communication disorders, their disability is only partially a factor in their self-concept and this negatively affects the cohesiveness of their groups. Additionally, as noted above, there is a wide range of severity of communication disorders including those who are unable to communicate functionally, and others who only experience minor and barely noticeable speech and hearing impediments.

2.7 Social Inclusion through Accommodation

In the United States, two recent events have significantly improved the lives of many people with communication disorders: technological advances and the Americans with Disabilities Act. Both technological advances and legislation have increased the quality of life of people with communication disorders and improved their ability to contribute to society.

Most technological advances that benefit people with communication disorders are based on the silicon chip and the computer revolution it spawned. Speech synthesizers now produce speech for patients who have lost motor abilities due to degenerative diseases such as amyotrophic lateral sclerosis, multiple sclerosis, and Parkinsonism. No better example exists of the power of this technology to free the human mind from the confines of paralysis than that of Stephen William Hawking. Dr. Hawking, one of the premier mathematicians and theoretical physicists of our time, uses a speech synthesizer known as "The Equalizer." Although he cannot motorically produce speech, Dr. Hawking has written books and presented dozens of scientific papers using this advanced technology. Voice recognition devices that allow computers to follow speech commands permit people with communication disorders to use computers with the ease of non-disabled persons. Algorithms are available enabling computers to follow speech commands that are distorted and telegraphic. Suck and puff devices and specially adapted personal computers permit people with communication disorders mobility and unobstructed access to the World Wide Web and its vast stores of information. Digital hearing aids have improved the amplification of sound for millions of hard-of-hearing adults, and cochlear implants have opened the world of hearing for thousands of children previously isolated by their deafness.

The Americans with Disabilities Act was enacted in 1990. The purpose of this legislation is to improve educational, economic, and vocational status of people with disabilities. It was created to prevent discrimination against individuals with disabilities in communication, public accommodation, education, transportation, recreation, and access to public services. Other federal and state legislation complement the Americans with Disabilities Act such as the Individuals with Disabilities Education Act which guarantees disabled students access to free and appropriate public education. These political initiatives have broken down barriers many communication-disabled individuals previously endured.

The above technological advances and legislation have improved the lives, brightened the future, and increased the productivity of millions of individuals with communication disorders. Although there is no current data on the improved socioeconomic gains for people with communication disorders resulting from the above technological advances and legislation, they have clearly opened many doors previously closed.

2.8 Summary

The Ancient Egyptians wrote about communication and its disorders approximately 4,000 years ago. In these age-old records, they pondered many of the same issues about communication and its disorders that have transcended the centuries, and even today, spark heated debates among philosophers, clinicians, and scientists. In the 21st Century, the fundamental nature of communication and its disorders, the brain-mind leap, the brain localization movement, and the role of language in thought are issues yet to be resolved. Although controversy still exists over certain aspects of communication sciences and disorders, today, the social status of people with disabilities is improved. Recent advances in technology and legislation have significantly improved the quality of lives for many communication-disordered persons. Importantly, unlike in the past, the disabled in general, and communication-disordered in particular, have been brought into mainstream society making it possible for them to contribute to science, business, medicine, and industry.

Suggested Readings and Resources

Benton, A. and Joynt, R. (1960). Early descriptions of aphasia. *Archives of Neurology*, 3: 205-221. This journal article reviews early research and theories about aphasia.

Jackson, J. (1878). On affections of speech from diseases of the brain. *Brain*. 1: 301-330. This classic article written in the late 1800s addresses aphasia and related neurogenic communication disorders.

O'Neill, Y.V. (1980). *Speech and Speech Disorders in Western Thought Before 1600*. Westport, Connecticut: Greenwood Press. This text provides an historical overview of several communication disorders.

Tanner, D. (2006). *An Advanced Course in Communication Sciences and Disorders*. San Diego: Plural Publishing. Chapter three reviews the acquisition of knowledge in communication sciences and disorders from the Ancient Egyptians to the 21st Century.

References

Benson, D. and Ardila, A. (1996). *Aphasia.* New York: Oxford University Press.

Benton, A. (1981). Aphasia: Historical perspectives. In *Acquired aphasia*, M. Sarno (Ed.). New York: Academic Press.

Davis, G.A. (2007). *Aphasiology: Disorders and clinical practice* (2nd ed.) Boston: Pearson Allyn & Bacon.

Jackson, J. (1878). On affections of speech from diseases of the brain. *Brain.* 1: 301-330.

O'Neill, Y.V. (1980). *Speech and speech disorders in western thought before 1600.* Westport, Connecticut: Greenwood Press.

Owens, R., Metz, D., and Haas, A. (2000). *Introduction to communication disorders.* Boston: Allyn & Bacon.

Sies, L. (1974). *Aphasia: Theory and Therapy.* Baltimore: University Park Press.

Tanner, D. (2003). *The psychology of neurogenic communication disorders: A primer for health care professionals.* Boston: Allyn & Bacon.

Tanner, D. (2006). *Case studies in communication sciences and disorders.* Upper Saddle River, N.J.: Pearson, Merrill, Prentice Hall.

Van Riper, C., & Erickson, R. (1996). *Speech correction* (9th ed). Boston: Allyn & Bacon.

Wiig, E. (2004). Professional Correspondence: Manuscript review for *Case studies in communication sciences and disorders.* Upper Saddle River, N.J.: Pearson, Merrill, Prentice Hall.

Chapter 3

The Communication Sciences

3.1 Chapter Preview

This chapter examines the scientific disciplines involved in the study of human communication. There is a review of the academic specialties, disciplines, and professions related to communication sciences and disorders including physics, human anatomy and physiology, psychology, linguistics, and medicine. Several specialities in the speech and hearing sciences are also addressed.

3.2 Communication Sciences and Speech-Language Pathology and Audiology

Communication sciences and disorders is a broad discipline, and there are two related but academically divergent disciplines: communication sciences and speech-language pathology and audiology. Speech, language, and hearing scientists, usually employed by colleges and universities, primarily study normal human communication although communication disorders also may be studied. These doctoral-level scientists and professors are usually assigned to Departments of Communication Sciences and Disorders, Speech-Language Pathology and Audiology, Speech and Hearing Sciences, Special Education, Health Sciences, and Communication Disorders.

The study, evaluation, and treatment of speech-language pathologies and hearing disorders are primarily the responsibility of speech-language pathologists and audiologists (See Chapter 4). Speech-language pathologists and audiologists may be doctoral trained professionals, although the terminal degree for speech-language pathologists is the master's degree. In 2012, the clinical doctorate in audiology (Au.D.) will be required for individuals seeking certifica-

tion by the American Speech-Language-Hearing Association (ASHA). Although there is overlap, generally speech, language, and hearing scientists study normal human communication, and speech-language pathologists and audiologists study, evaluate, and treat communication disorders. In colleges and universities, both disciplines are typically administratively housed in Colleges of Medicine, Health Sciences, Education, Health Professions, Social Sciences, and Arts and Sciences.

3.3 The Speech, Language, and Hearing Sciences

Speech, language, and hearing scientists study the range of acoustic, muscular, neurological, and cognitive processes involved in human communication. According to Sphar and Malone (2002), scientists are employed in colleges and universities, governmental agencies, and private laboratories such as Bell Labs. The scientific study of speech, language, and hearing overlaps several related disciplines, and speech, language, and hearing scientists come from a variety of backgrounds. Powers (2000, pp. 6-7) notes that these diverse scientists engage in basic research to provide a better understanding of human communication processes:

> Some individuals are primarily speech scientists, others are hearing scientists, and others are language scientists. Because of this diversity, it is difficult, if not impossible, to define the limits of CSD [communication sciences and disorders] scientists. Suffice it to say, however, that the majority have strong backgrounds in the sciences and hold advanced degrees, most often a Ph.D. (Doctor of Philosophy). The degrees may be awarded in areas such as acoustics, anatomy and physiology, biological sciences, communication sciences and disorders, education, linguistics, physics, psychology, or speech communication.

Communication scientists engage in research to further our understanding of speech, voice, language, and hearing abilities. Sphar and Malone (2002, pp. 13-14) observe:

Researchers in human communication sciences and disorders (a) investigate the biological, physical, and physiological processes underlying normal communication; (b) conduct experimentation concerning fundamental processes and mechanisms in communication; (c) explore the import of psychological, social, and psychophysiological factors on communication disorders; (d) apply newly discovered basic knowledge and emerging technology to issues of clinical practice; and (e) collaborate with engineers, physicians, educators, dentists, and scientists from other disciplines to develop a comprehensive approach to individuals with speech, voice, language, hearing, and balance problems.

Funding for speech, voice, language, and hearing research comes from colleges and universities, federal, state, and local agencies, and private foundations.

The communication sciences draw from the related disciplines of human anatomy, physiology, acoustics, cognition, child development, and other fields as they pertain to all facets of communication. As Table 3.1 shows, speech and hearing anatomy concentration areas address gross or microscopic developmental, structural, and muscular facets of the physical aspects of speech production and hearing. Whereas anatomy addresses structure, physiology addresses function. Table 3.2 shows speech and hearing physiology concentration areas. According to Zemlin (1998), the application of physiological knowledge to medicine and industry is applied physiology. Cellular physiology concerns vital process and functional activities of cells and special physiology addresses the functional activity of some organ.

The discipline of acoustics, a branch of physics, addresses speech sound waves, resonance aspects of speech

Table 3.1
Speech and Hearing Anatomy Concentration Areas

Cytology and Histology	Study of cells and tissues
Practical Anatomy	Application of anatomy to several clinical disciplines (speech and hearing)
Embryonic and Fetal Anatomy	Development of the human organism from conception to birth
Gross Anatomy	Study of anatomy using the naked eye
Microanatomy	Study of anatomy using magnification

Table 3.2
Speech and Hearing Physiology Concentration Areas

Applied Physiology	Application of physiological knowledge to medicine or industry
Cellular Physiology	Cellular functional activities and vital processes
Special Physiology	Functional activity of some organ, e.g., organs of speech and hearing

Table 3.3
Communication Sciences and Focus Areas of Acoustics

Acoustic Phonetics	Physical properties of speech sounds
Physiological Acoustics	Functions of auditory systems in response to stimuli
Psychoacoustics	Perceptual features of a speech sound or environmental sounds

production, and voice prints (sound spectrography). Table 3.3 shows the acoustic focus areas of communication sciences. Acoustic phonetics concern physical properties of speech sounds such as wave forms and resonance. Physiological phonetics addresses the functions of auditory systems in response to stimuli. Psychoacoustics overlaps physiological phonetics, but it primarily is concerned with the perception of speech and other sounds.

In addition to drawing from the so-called "hard sciences" of anatomy, physiology, and acoustics, the discipline of communication sciences also draws from the social sciences of psychology and linguistics, and education. Cognitive psychology, a branch of psychology, and psycholinguistics, the union of psychology and linguistics, address the way humans think, and particularly the role of language in the thought process. Developmental psychology is concerned with the acquisition of speech and language in children. In the profession of education, communication sciences draws from childhood development and special education specialities involving children with special needs. Communication sciences also draws from pediatrics, a branch of medicine, with regard to physical, mental, and psychological development milestones.

In addition to drawing from related disciplines that also examine human communication, there are several communication sciences specialties. As Figure 3.1 shows, speech and hearing scientists develop expertise and become specialists in several communication sciences specialties. Currently, there are no official specialty designations in the profession of communication sciences and disorders. Nevertheless, some speech and hearing scientists focus their professional attention on the normal aspects of anatomy and physiology of the speech and hearing mechanism, articulation and phonology development in children, hearing sciences, motor speech production, phonetics, speech perception, acoustics, and voice production. Other scientists also address disorders such as aphasia, cleft lip and palate, motor speech disorders, hearing loss and deafness, and swallowing disorders to name a few.

3.4 Summary

Communication sciences is a broad discipline drawing on several related scientific fields and professions. Virtually any discipline involved in the study and treatment of communication and its disorders is part of the large group of concentration areas and specialties in the communication sciences. Of particular significance in communication sciences are human anatomy and physiology, acoustics, psycholinguistics, psychology, and education.

Anatomy and physiology of the speech and hearing mechanism
Aphasiology
Articulation and phonology acquisition and disorders
Cleft lip and palate
Hearing sciences
Language development and disorders
Motor speech
Neurogenic communication disorders
Phonetics
Speech perception
Speech acoustics
Stuttering
Voice and its disorders
Other less common specialties involve brain mapping of speech and language centers, syndromes affecting communication, birth defects, sound spectrography, cochlear implants, and swallowing disorders

Figure 3.1 *Selected specialties in speech and hearing sciences*

Suggested Readings and Resources

Tanner, D. (2003). *Exploring Communication Disorders: A 21st Century Introduction Through Literature and Media*. Boston: Allyn & Bacon. Chapter 1 describes communication sciences and Chapter 11 addresses scientific research in a question and answer format.

Tanner, D. (2006). *An Advanced Course in Communication Sciences and Disorders*. San Diego: Plural Publishing. Several chapters address the communication sciences in the overall structure of the "communication chain."

References

Power, G. (2002). Communication sciences and disorders: The discipline. In R. Gillam, T. Marquardt, and F. Martin (Eds.), *Communication sciences and disorders: From science to clinical practice*, (pp. 3-24). San Diego: Singular.

Spahr, F. T. And Malone, R.L. (2002). Human Communication Disorders: An Introduction. In G.H. Shames and N.B. Anderson (Eds), *Human communication disorders: An introduction* (6th ed.) (pp. 1-27). Boston: Allyn & Bacon.

Zemlin, W. (1998). *Speech and hearing science* (4th ed). Boston: Allyn & Bacon.

Chapter 4

Speech-Language Pathology and Audiology

4.1 Chapter Preview

This chapter explores the professions of speech-language pathology and audiology. The scope of practice is provided for both professions as are the educational and clinical requirements to obtain certification by the American Speech-Language-Hearing Association. The educational and clinical requirements for speech-language pathology assistants and audiometrists are detailed as are their scopes of paraprofessional conduct. Several medical and educational specialities involved in speech-language pathology and audiology are presented.

4.2 Scope of Practice for Speech-Language Pathologists

The scope of practice for speech-language pathologists is defined by the American Speech-Language-Hearing Association (ASHA) although some states may impose restrictions or permit additional privileges by their state licensing laws. Most speech-language pathologists are members of ASHA and hold the Certificate of Clinical Competence in Speech-Language Pathology (CCC-SLP). Speech-language pathologists are autonomous professionals in that they do not require supervision to perform their professional responsibilities. In general, a speech-language pathologist (SLP) is an independent practitioner and the primary pro-

vider of professional services to people with speech, voice, language, swallowing, and hearing disorders. The scope of practice for speech-language pathologists includes the evaluation and treatment of the cognitive and social aspects of communication and its disorders, and also accent and dialect reduction in individuals wanting this speech production modification. It should be noted, however, that accent and dialect differences are not speech pathologies.

There are three primary responsibilities of speech-language pathologists concerning the evaluation and treatment of individuals with communication and swallowing disorders. First, speech-language pathologists screen for communication disorders to decide the need for further assessment. Screening is a procedure to identify, but not comprehensively evaluate, persons at risk for communication and swallowing disorders. Second, speech-language pathologists comprehensively assess (diagnose) communication and swallowing disorders. In comprehensive assessment, the SLP decides the likely etiology (cause) of the communication disorder and determines the general and specific communicative or swallowing deficiencies. Third, speech-language pathologists provide nonmedical treatment of communication and swallowing disorders. These treatments include therapies, instructions, counseling, and other procedures for patients, clients, and students with communication and swallowing disorders. Training and instruction for family members of individuals with communication disorders is also part of the scope of practice for speech-language pathologists. Although audiologists are primary providers of nonmedical hearing services, speech-language pathologist conduct a variety of hearing tests and treat hearing-related speech, voice, and language disorders. Figure 4.1 details the scope of practice for speech-language pathologists as provided by the American Speech-Language-Hearing Association.

Assess, diagnose, treat, and provide follow-up services for people with communication disorders

Consult with professionals in medicine, education, psychology and dentistry

Counsel patients and their families

Make referrals

Engage in activities to prevent speech, voice, and language disorders

Train family members to participate in therapeutic activities

Select, prescribe, and dispense prosthetic/adaptive devices for speaking and swallowing

Conduct pure-tone air conduction hearing screening and screening tympanometery

Accent reduction therapy

Collaborate with teachers of English as a second language

Improve singing voices

Train and supervise support personnel

Conduct, disseminate, and apply research in communication sciences and disorders

Figure 4.1 *Scope of practice for speech-language pathologists (Source: American Speech-Language-Hearing Association, 2001)*

Speech-language pathologists work in two primary employment settings: medical and schools. In the medical setting, speech language pathologists provide services in hospitals, rehabilitation facilities, physicians' offices, nursing homes, and through home health agencies. In the medical setting, they primarily work with adults suffering from strokes, traumatic brain injuries, and diseases affecting communication and swallowing. In public, private, charter, and parochial school employment settings, speech-language pathologists work primarily with children with developmental delay and disorders, mental retardation, and learning disabilities. Speech-language pathologists working in medical settings also work with children with pediatric diseases, disorders, and traumas, and those working in the school setting may work with adolescents and adults with communication and swallowing disorders. Other types of employment for speech-language pathologists include schools for the deaf and hard-of-hearing, public health clinics, special schools and institutions, mental retardation facilities, and private and group practices.

4.3 Scope of Practice for Audiologists

Audiologists recognize two professional organizations. Most audiologists are members of the American Speech-

Language-Hearing Association (ASHA) and hold the Certificate of Clinical Competence in Audiology (CCC-A). In addition to ASHA, audiologists are also represented by the American Academy of Audiology (AAA), the world's largest professional organization of audiologists. It has an active membership of more than 10,000 members (American Academy of Audiology, 2005). Founded in 1988, AAA's mission includes enhancing the ability of audiologists to achieve their career objectives and to provide the highest quality of hearing healthcare service to children and adults.

As Figure 4.2 shows, the scope of practice for audiologists as determined and defined by the American Speech-Language-Hearing Association includes assessing and managing all aspects of hearing disorders including balance disorders. Balance disorders may occur with some diseases and traumas affecting the hearing mechanism. Audiologists fit and dispense hearing aids, and engage in auditory habilitation and rehabilitation. Newborn screening conducted by audiologists provides early detection of hearing loss and deafness in children. Audiologists train and supervise assistants, participate in interdisciplinary teams about hearing loss, deafness, rehabilitation, and habilitation, and engage in hearing loss prevention (hearing conservation) programs. Recently, audiologists have become more active in improving language development, teaching speechreading (lip reading), and maximizing existing auditory abilities in persons with hearing loss and deafness. Like the scope of practice for speech-language pathologists, some states may impose restrictions or permit additional privileges for audiologists in their state licensing laws. Audiologists are employed in hospitals, rehabilitation centers, clinics, schools, institutions, physician offices, and private and group practices.

4.4 Educational and Clinical Requirements for Speech-Language Pathologists and Audiologists

State licensing of speech-language pathologists and audiologists is a relatively recent event; before the mid-1900s, there were no states with licencing laws. Now all states set licensing standards for practicing speech-language pathologists and audiologists. States also may require background checks and fingerprinting for identification and verification. The educational and clinical requirements for speech-language pathologists and audiologists are set by the American Speech-Language-Hearing Association and most states accept the clinical and educational requirements. States grant licenses to individuals holding ASHA's Certificate of Clinical Competence in Speech-Language Pathology (CCC-SLP) or Audiology (CCC-A).

Assess and manage hearing disorders

Select, fit, and dispense hearing aides and related devices

Engage in activities to prevent hearing loss

Educate people to the effects of noise on hearing

Engage in audiological rehabilitation

Teach speechreading

Improve language development and auditory skills

Counsel persons with hearing loss and their families

Screen speech-language and use of sign language

Engage in research on the prevention, identification, and treatment of hearing loss and balance system dysfunctions

Train and supervise support personnel

Consult with individuals, public and private agencies, industry, governmental bodies, and attorneys about the effects of noise and hearing loss

Participate in interdisciplinary education and medical teams about habilitation and rehabilitation

Engage newborn screening procedures

Figure 4.2 *Scope of practice for audiologists (Source: American Speech-Language-Hearing Association, 2001)*

According to the American Speech-Language-Hearing Association (2005), to receive the Certificate of Clinical Competence, the applicant must have a Bachelor's Degree, either a Bachelor of Science or Bachelor of Arts in Communication Sciences and Disorders or related disciplines. The Bachelor Degree must include twenty-seven credit hours in the basic sciences including at least six semester credit hours in the biological/physical sciences and mathematics, six semester credit hours in the behavioral and/or social sciences, and at least fifteen semester credit hours in the basic human communication processes including course work in each of the following three areas of speech, language and hearing: the anatomic and physiologic bases, the physical and psychophysical bases and the linguistic and psycholinguistic aspects.

Following completion of the Bachelor's Degree, the applicant must obtain a Master's Degree in Communication Sciences and Disorders, or similarly titled degree, from an American Speech-Language-Hearing Association accredited program. The Master's Degree can be a Master of Science (M.S.), Master of Arts (M.A.), or Master of Education (M.Ed.). At the Master Degree level, a minimum of thirty-six semester credit hours in professional course work must be completed, and at least thirty of the thirty-six semester

credit hours of professional course work must be in the major area of concentration (speech-language pathology or audiology). At least six of the thirty-six semester credit hours of professional course work must be in the minor area of concentration (speech-language pathology or audiology). At least thirty semester hours of professional course work must be completed at the graduate level and a minimum of twenty-one of the thirty hours must be in the major area of concentration. Clinically, ASHA requires the applicant to complete 375 clock hours of supervised clinical observation/practice of which twenty-five hours are supervised observations and 350 hours are supervised clinical practicum. Of the total practicum hours, 250 must be completed at the graduate level. After completion of academic course work and clinical practicum, the applicant must successfully complete a thirty-six-week Clinical Fellowship under the supervision of an individual who holds the Certificate of Clinical Competence. Part-time, longer Clinical Fellowships are available for those not working full-time. Within two years from the date course work and practicum are approved by the ASHA Clinical Certification Board, the applicant for the Certificate of Clinical Competence in Speech-Language Pathology and/or Audiology must pass a comprehensive national examination administered by the Educational Testing Service (ETS).

4.5 Educational and Clinical Requirements for Assistants and Support Personnel

The American Speech-Language-Hearing Association recently set guidelines for speech-language pathology assistants (SLPAs). According to the American Speech-Language-Hearing Association (2004), the responsibilities for speech-language pathology assistant training and paraprofessional conduct are those of the supervising speech-language pathologists. Several principles and rules in the American Speech-Language-Hearing Association's Code of Ethics have been changed to encompass the supervising speech-language pathologists' ethical obligations concerning their assistants' education, training, and paraprofessional responsibilities. The responsibilities of a speech-language pathology assistant include helping with hearing screening (without interpretation), following treatment plans and protocols established by a certified speech-language pathologist, documenting patient/client performance, and helping in assessment, clerical duties, collecting data, and the maintenance of equipment. Speech-language pathology assistants are specifically prohibited from testing, screening, or diagnosing patients with feeding/swallowing disorders. Speech-language pathology assistants can collect data for monitoring patient/client improvement and must exhibit compliance with governing bodies' regulations and reimbursement requirements. Speech-language pathology assistants cannot write treatment plans, sign formal documentation, select patients for services or discharge, or counsel patients about their status or services. Speech-language pathology assistants must not represent themselves as speech-language pathologists. There are a variety of levels of training and educational requirements for audiology assistants who are also called audiometrists. They are audiology technicians working under the supervision of an audiologist or otologist. Audiologists and audiometrists must generally conform to the above with regard to provision of audiological services.

4.6 Medical and Educational Specialties Involved in Speech-Language Pathology and Audiology

As Figure 4.3 shows, several medical specialists are directly involved in the diagnosis and treatment of communication disorders. Otologists are physicians concerned with the diagnosis and treatment of diseases and disorders of the ear. Laryngologists and otolaryngologists diagnose and treat diseases and disorders of the larynx, and of the ear and larynx, respectively. Otorhinolaryngology, often called "ENT," is concerned with the medical management of disease and disorders of the ear, nose, and throat. Physicians who specialize in physiatry and physical medicine and rehabilitation evaluate and treat patients in need of rehabilitation. These patients often suffer from a variety of communication disorders related to their diseases, disorders, and injuries. Pediatricians and gerontologists are medical specialists concerned with diseases and disorders in children and the aged. Pediatricians diagnose and treat a variety of communication disorders because there is a high occurrence of communication disorders in children. Adults in the later decades of life have age-related disorders and disease that affect speech, voice, language, and hearing. Radiologists participate in video swallowing studies (VSS) for patients with sucking, chewing, and swallowing (dysphagia) disorders. A video swallow study is a comprehensive evaluation using barium to learn the structure and function of the three stages of the swallow. Many other branches of medicine are indirectly concerned with communication disorders because speech, voice, language, and hearing are frequently impaired in diseases, traumas, and disorders.

Clinical Psychology
Dentistry
Gerontology
Laryngology
Neurology
Neuropsychology
Orthodontics
Otolaryngology
Otology
Otorhinolaryngology
Pediatrics
Physiatry
Psychiatry
Radiology
Special Education

Figure 4.3 Medical and educational specialties involved in speech-language pathology and audiology

In education, several specialties address special education needs of children with communication disorders. Autism spectrum specialists address children with varying degrees of pervasive developmental disorders, the most extreme of which is severe autism. Teachers of the deaf-visually impaired help these children with their special education needs. The learning disability specialist, who also functions as a resource teacher in some schools, addresses dyslexia and other learning disabilities. The teacher of multihandicapped children works with children with multiple disabilities that often include severe communication disorders.

4.7 Summary

Speech-language pathology and audiology are autonomous professions and the primary providers of nonmedical services to individuals with speech, voice, language, and hearing disorders. Speech-language pathologists screen, evaluate, and provide therapies, instruction, counseling, and training to persons with swallowing and communication disorders. Audiologists assess and manage all aspects of hearing and balance disorder including fitting and dispensing hearing aids and engaging in aural rehabilitation. Certified speech-language pathologists and audiologists are licensed by the states and maintain certification by the American Speech-Language-Hearing Association.

Suggested Readings and Resources

American Speech-Language-Hearing Association (2005). Certification Requirements. Retrieved from the World Wide Web on December 16, 2005: http://www.asha.org/public/cert/. This website provides the general and specific certification requirements for speech-language pathology and audiology.

Justice, L. (2006). *Communication Sciences and Disorders: An Introduction*. Upper Saddle River, N.J.: Pearson Prentice Hall. Part I of this introductory textbook provides an overview of the professions of speech-language pathology and audiology.

Tanner, D. (2003). *Exploring Communication Disorders: A 21st Century Introduction Through Literature and Media*. Boston: Pearson Allyn & Bacon. Chapter 1 provides an overview of communication sciences and disorders. In Appendix B, three short stories show typical employment activities for practitioners in a public school, a hospital and nursing home, and what the practice of speech-language pathology and audiology may be in not-so-distant future due to the computer revolution.

References

American Academy of Audiology (2005). *About the Academy*. Retrieved from the World Wide Web on December 15, 2005: http://www.audiology.org/about/ (Author)

American Speech-Language-Hearing Association (2005). *Certification Requirements*. Retrieved from the World Wide Web on December 16, 2005: http://www.asha.org/public/cert/ (Author)

American Speech-Language-Hearing Association (2005). *Frequently Asked Questions About Speech-Language Pathology Assistants* (Updated 10/1/04). Retrieved from the World Wide Web on December 17, 2005: http://www.asha.org/about/membership-certification/faq_slpasst.htm#b1

Chapter 5

Economics, Prevalence, Incidence, and Diagnostic Categories of Communication Disorders

5.1 Chapter Preview

This chapter examines the costs of communication disorders and provides prevalence and incidence figures for industrialized countries. There are statistics for the incidence and prevalence of hearing loss, childhood speech impairments, neurogenic communication, and swallowing disorders. Seven categories of communication disorders are listed, defined, and discussed.

5.2 Economics of Communication Disorders

According to Ruben (2000), communication disorders are a significant economic loss to the United States, costing between $154 and $186 billion annually. Two factors are considered when examining the economic costs of communication disorders: loss of productivity and direct costs of medical and educational services.

When a communication disorder prevents a person from contributing to the goods and services of an economy, there is a loss to the nation's gross national product. Although technological advances and legislation have improved the opportunities for communication-disabled persons to enter the economic and social mainstream of society, many are still unable to participate fully because of

their disabilities (See Chapter 2). Consequently, many communication-disabled persons have unrealized potentials to contribute to law, business, medicine, industry, education, science, the arts, and other endeavors.

Besides the unrealized potential of communication-disordered persons, there are often high costs involved in evaluating and treating communication disorders. The costs of evaluating and treating communication disorders are borne by tax dollars and private funds. These expensive services can be major burdens for the communication-disabled person, his or her family, health insurance and maintenance organizations, and social welfare programs. For example, according to Northern and Downs (2002), a child with a severe hearing loss, over his or her lifetime, may have a staggering economic cost: $2 million. "Communication disorders will be a major public health concern for the 21st century because, untreated they adversely affect the economic well-being of a communication-age society" (Ruben, 2000, pg. 245).

5.3 Prevalence and Incidence of Communication Disorders

The incidence of a communication disorder is how many people have had it at some point in their lives and the prevalence shows how many people currently have it (Guitar, 1998). Accurate statistics on the total number of people with communication disorders (prevalence) and the number of new cases (incidence) are difficult to obtain for three reasons. First, communication skills and abilities are not mastered at precisely identifiable times; it takes months and even years for children to acquire them. Consequently, many children outgrow their apparent communication disorders. For example, stuttering and lisping occur in some children, but because of maturation, when they grow older, their communication disorders gradually become less apparent and eventually disappear. Additionally, some children acquire language slowly early on only to learn it rapidly later. Second, pinpointing exactly when a person gets a communication disorder is inexact because many speech, voice, language, and hearing pathologies develop slowly. In childhood stuttering for example, a child's self-report when he or she started to stutter, and when his or her parents noted its presence, can differ greatly. Often parents put the onset of the disorder earlier than what a child retrospectively reports. Some parents misdiagnose normal nonfluencies as stuttering and thus believe the child is stuttering before the child knows that he or she is a stutterer. A gradual onset of communication disorders is also seen in progressive neuromuscular disorders, hearing loss, and dementia.

The third reason for highly variable incidence and prevalence figures in communication disorders concerns the definitions and categorization of communication disorders. Researchers who study communication disorders come from a variety of backgrounds (see Chapter 3). Because of their professional backgrounds and perspectives, they may have different standards for what constitutes a communication disorder. Because definitions and categorizations may differ from one researcher to another, the incidence and prevalence figures may also vary.

In industrialized countries, the prevalence rate of all communication disorders ranges between 5 percent and 10 percent (Ruben, 2000). Overall, the United States has good reporting, identification, and treatment records for communication disorders, although individual states vary greatly in their record keeping of people with communication disorders. There are also degrees of communication disorders; not all speech, voice, language, and hearing impairments significantly affect the functional ability to communicate. For example, complex communication disorders, those individuals unable to meet their daily communication needs, occur in about eight to twelve of every 1,000 Americans or about 2 million persons (Beukelman and Ansel, 1995; ASHA, 1987).

In the United States, hearing loss and deafness are the most common communication disorders (Public Health Service, 1994). According to Justice (2006), approximately 10 percent of the population has a hearing loss, and the incidence of hearing loss increases with age. For example, in the age range sixty-five to seventy-four years, approximately 35 percent of that age group has a hearing loss, and in persons older than seventy-five years, 45 percent experience difficulty with hearing. The above prevalence statistics for hearing loss in the elderly is probably higher for mild hearing impairments due to the psychological defenses of denial and projection. Some people with mild hearing losses initially deny the disorder and engage in projection; they attribute the problem in communication to others'

mumbling. The prevalence of hearing loss in older persons is likely to increase in the near future as the population ages.

The incidence and prevalence of speech and language communication disorders are skewed to the younger and older age groups. The National Institute of Neurological and Communicative Disorders and Stroke (1988) reports that childhood speech and language disorders affect about 10 percent to 15 percent of school-aged children. About 4% of children have speech sound maturation and production problems, with boys and African-American children having slightly higher rates of these disorders than girls and European-American children (Justice, 2006). In older Americans, strokes are a leading cause of neuromuscular communication disorders. According to Justice (2006), approximately 750,000 Americans suffer a stroke each year and there are about 4 million stroke survivors in the United States, many of whom have communication disorders. According to Spahr and Malone (1998), approximately 15 million Americans have a swallowing disorder, which also often occurs with neurogenic disorders. Logemann (1995), and others, note that in nursing homes, as many as 50 percent of the residents have sucking, chewing, and/or swallowing disorders.

As can be seen by the above statistics, communication disorders occur in all age segments of society, but the numbers are higher for children and the elderly. Of course, people in the middle years also get communication disorders because of traumas, diseases, and acquired disorders. Roughly one in six Americans has a communication disorder (Bello, 1995). Spahr and Malone (1998) observe that rarely does a family not have at least one close relative with a communication disorder. In the future, the incidence and prevalence of communication disorders will increase overall due to better screening and identification methods, the aging of Americans and consequent age-related diseases and disorders, and the fact that more at-risk babies and individuals in catastrophic accidents survive—often with communication disorders.

5.4 Categories of Communication Disorders

Communication disorders may be classified by the communicative processes or functions affected by the disorders, diseases, or defects, by the site of neurological, structural, or muscular damage, and by the diseases and disorders that can cause them. In this book, a combination of classification systems is used to reflect the types of medical-legal issues addressed by in medical malpractice cases and other legal issues (see Table 5.1).

Table 5.1
Classification of Communication Disorders by Process

Process/Function	Disorder	Examples
Articulation and Phonology	Impaired or disrupted speech sound production	Lisping, w/r substitution, fronting
Fluency	Pathological disruption in the normal rhythm and flow of speech	stuttering, cluttering
Language (Children)	Delay or disorder in the acquisition of the structure and/or function of language	Delayed language, dyslexia, communication disorders related to mental impairment-mental retardation
Language (Adults)	Loss or impairment of previously learned aspects of language	Broca's aphasia, Wernicke's aphasia
Hearing	Hearing loss and deafness	Otosclerosis, otitis media
Motor Speech	Neuromuscular disorders of communication	Apraxia of speech, ataxic dysarthria
Intelligence/Cognition	Dementia and traumatic brain injury	Amnesia, disorientation, loss of mental executive functions, communication disorders related to Alzheimer's disease

5.5 Neurogenic Communication Disorders

Neurogenic communication disorders—aphasia and motor speech disorders—are caused by strokes, traumatic injuries, diseases, and disorders affecting the brain, nervous system, and muscles of speech. Aphasia is a multimodality language disorder and the motor speech disorders are neuromuscular speech impairments.

Aphasia occurs primarily in adults and is caused by damage to the speech and language centers of the brain. It is a multimodality disorder usually affecting all avenues of communication: speaking, writing, gestures, reading, and the ability to understand the speech of others. The ability to use mathematical symbols are also often impaired because mathematics is a language. In mild cases, the patient may only have minor word retrieval problems, and in severe cases, he or she may be completely unable to communicate functionally.

Motor speech refers to the motor, as opposed to sensory, aspects of the brain and nervous system that cause physical movements and drive the speech act. There are two categories of motor speech disorders: apraxia of speech and the dysarthrias. Mild cases of these disorders may only be a nuisance; in severe cases, they may render the patient mute.

Apraxia of speech is difficulty programming the speech mechanism. Although the patient knows the words he or she wants to say, there is difficulty getting the breathing apparatus, larynx, tongue, and lips to make the sounds. The person with apraxia of speech struggles to communicate verbally; programming the speech act is impaired, or in severe cases, nonfunctional. The dysarthrias are a group of neuromuscular disorders classified by the site of damage to the brain and nervous system. Here, speech disorders are a result of movement dysfunctions or flaccid, spastic, and ataxic muscles.

5.6 Communication Disorders Resulting from Head and Neck Injuries

The communication disorders occurring from traumatic brain injuries include aphasia, apraxia of speech, and the dysarthrias discussed above. This classification of communication disorders can also include global or specific memory loss, disorientation, behavioral disturbances, and loss of mental executive functioning occurring without damage to the primary speech and language areas of the brain. When traumatic brain injury occurs to the primary speech and language centers of the brain, and the patient has global or specific memory loss, disorientation, behavioral disturbances, and loss of mental executive functioning, patients often produce unusual and sometimes bizarre speech and language. Neck injuries result in communication disorders because the patient may be impaired in using and controlling his or her speech mechanism due to paralysis.

5.7 Voice and Resonance Disorders

Voice refers to sounds produced by the vibration of the vocal cords and the resonance characteristics of the speaker's neck and head. The frequency and force of vocal cord vibration are primary factors causing pitch and loudness characteristics. The quality of a speaker's voice is determined by the relationship between vocal cord vibration and the resulting resonance characteristics of his or her neck and head. Diseases, paralysis, tumors, vocal abuse, and psychogenic factors can cause voice disorders. Head trauma, surgery, paralysis, and the birth defect, cleft palate, can affect resonance and voice quality.

5.8 Childhood Communication Disorders

In this book, the primary childhood communication disorders are addressed as one category. The primary childhood communication disorders are language, articulation, and fluency disorders. Although there are other childhood communication disorders, such as dysarthria related to muscular dystrophy and cerebral palsy, they are addressed in appropriate categories involving the processes and functions of communication affected by pediatric disorders.

Children with language disorders may have difficulty with all or part of language, including understanding words, following directions, making sentences, socializing, reading, and writing. These language disorders may be part of larger cognitive problems such as occurs with mental retardation, autism, and Down syndrome, or they may occur independently of other disabilities.

Articulation disorders are impairments with the production of speech sounds. The child may substitute, omit, or distort speech sounds. Phonology is one aspect of language and includes the rules by which speech sounds are combined and articulated. Children with phonological disorders have problems combining and structuring speech sounds. Causes of language and articulation disorders include birth defects, mental retardation, head trauma, fetal alcohol syndrome, isolation from others during the speech and language development period, and improper or impaired learning.

Although there are many communication disorders affecting the rhythm, cadence, and flow of speech, there are two primary fluency disorders: stuttering and cluttering. The person who stutters repeats, prolongs, and blocks during speech and shows visible signs of speech struggle such as eye-squints, facial grimaces, and speech muscle tremors. The repetitions, prolongations, and gaps in the speech of stutterers are different in frequency and severity from the normal disfluencies seen in all speakers. Additionally, people who stutter often feel anxiety and other negative emotions during speech and may have reduced self-esteem related to aspects of social interaction.

Cluttering is a verbal thought-organization disorder. The person has trouble organizing his or her thoughts and typically, a short attention span. People who clutter revise, restate, stop, and start over during speech. Whereas people who stutter are aware of their stuttering, in cluttering there is often a complete lack of awareness of the disorder.

5.9 Communication Disorders and Dementia

In this book, dementia-related communication disorders are divided into Alzheimer's and non-Alzheimer's dementia. Several disorders and diseases can cause dementia. Alzheimer's disease is a common cause of dementia, and it frequently occurs in the later decades of life. Alzheimer's disease is the fourth-leading cause of death in the United States. Multiple brain infarcts primarily cause non-Alzheimer's dementia. The communication disorders seen in dementia include problems with reading, writing, producing speech sounds, constructing sentences, understanding the speech of others, and appreciating social-communicative contexts. These communication disorders are a result of generalized intellectual deterioration and are associated with memory, judgment, and orientation problems. Often these communication disorders gradually appear, but a rapid onset is also possible.

5.10 Hearing Loss and Deafness

Clinically, hearing losses range from slight to profound and the deaf person is functionally unable to hear with or without amplification. (Most deaf persons can sense vibration, however.) When hearing loss and deafness occurs at birth or during the major communication development period (approximately before the age of eight or nine), they can have major impacts on speech and language development. Additionally, the causes, severity, and frequency of the hearing loss affects speech and language development. Hearing loss that occurs in the later years of life often has a gradual onset, reaching a point where amplification may be necessary.

5.11 Dysphagia

As reported in Chapter 4, dysphagia is a sucking, chewing, and swallowing disorder, and although it is not a communication impairment, speech-language pathologists have accepted it as part of their clinical responsibilities. Dysphagia and the medical complications arising from it are increasingly frequent sources of medical malpractice litigation (Tanner, 2006). Dysphagia often occurs with motor speech disorders, but it can also be present without a communication disorder.

5.12 Summary

Communication disorders cost billions of dollars to treat them and in lost goods and services to the economy. Although statistics are inexact, there are approximately 40 million Americans with communication disorders ranging from mild hearing loss to complex communication disorders affecting about 2 million persons. Communication disorders occur in all age-segments of society, but they are particularly prevalent in the young and old. The categories of communication and related disorders in this book are (1) neurogenic, (2) communication disorders related to head and neck injuries, (3) voice and resonance, (4) childhood, (5) dementia-related, (6) hearing loss and deafness, and (7) dysphagia .

Suggested Readings and Resources

Justice, L. (2006). *Communication Sciences and Disorders: An Introduction.* Upper Saddle River, N.J.: Pearson Merrill Prentice Hall. This book reviews the incidence and prevalence statistics and examines each category of communication disorders.

Tanner, D. (2003). *Exploring Communication Disorders: A 21st Century Introduction Through Literature and Media.* Boston: Allyn & Bacon. Chapter 1 provides incidence and prevalence statistics and defines and describes each category of communication disorders.

References

American Speech-Language-Hearing Association (1987). Augmentative communication for consumers. Developed under contract for the U.S. Department of Education (Author).

Bello, J. (1995). Hearing loss and hearing aid use in the United States. *Communication facts.* Rockville, MD: American Speech-Language-Hearing Association.

Beukelman, D. and Ansel, B. (1995). Research priorities in augmentative and alternative communication. *Augmentative and Alternative Communication*: 11, 131-134.

Guitar, B. (1998). *Stuttering: An integrated approach to its nature and treatment.* Philadelphia: Lippincott Williams & Wilkins.

Justice, L. (2006). *Communication sciences and disorders: An introduction.* Upper Saddle River, N.J.: Pearson Merrill Prentice Hall.

Logemann, J. (1995). Dysphagia: Evaluation and treatment. *Folia Phoniatrica et Logopedica*: 47, 140-164.

National Institute of Neurological and Communicative Disorders and Stroke. (1988). *Developmental speech and language disorders: Hope through research.* Bethesda, MD: National Institutes of Health.

Northern, J. L. and Downs, M.P. (2002). *Hearing in children* (5th ed). Baltimore: Lippincott Williams and Wilkins

Public Health Service. (1994). Vital and health statistics: Prevalence and characteristics of persons with hearing trouble: United States 1990-91. Series 10: Data from the National Health Survey No. 188. DHHS Publication No. 94:1516.

Ruben, R.J. (2000). Redefining the survival of the fittest: Communication disorders in the 21st century. *Laryngoscope* 110:241-245.

Spahr, F. and Malone, R. (1998). The profession of speech-language pathology and audiology. In Shames, G., E. Wiig, and W. Secord (Eds.), *Human communication disorders: An introduction,* (5th Ed). Boston: Allyn and Bacon.

Tanner, D. (2006, February). The forensic aspects of dysphagia: Investigating medical malpractice. *The ASHA Leader, 11(2), 16-17, 45.* .

Chapter 6

Research Methodology in Communication Sciences and Disorders

6.1 Chapter Preview

This chapter examines the scientific method as it relates to the discipline of communication sciences and disorders and the dearth of evidence-based clinical research. There is a discussion of pure and applied research with an emphasis on experimental research design. The review of literature, definition of terms, ways of asking research questions, subjects and methodology, results and conclusions, and suggestions for future research are examined. There is also a section on evaluating empirical research in communication sciences and disorders.

6.2 Evidence-Based Clinical Practices in Speech-Language Pathology and Audiology

Recently, the American Speech-Language-Hearing Association (ASHA) emphasized that diagnostic and treatment practices in speech-language pathology and audiology should be evidence-based. In addition, the Code of Ethics of the American Speech-Language-Hearing Association requires that the effectiveness of clinical services be properly evaluated: "Individuals shall evaluate the effectiveness of services rendered and of products dispensed and shall provide services or dispense products only when benefit can reasonably be expected" (ASHA, 2006).

Although it is important that all clinical services in speech-language pathology and audiology be evidence-based, the reality is that there is a dearth of empirical research to support diagnostic and clinical practices. During the past three decades, the percentage of scientists in communication sciences and disorders has declined dramatically. At the same time, there are more practitioners than ever before, and they are performing a wider range of services. This has created a situation where the scientific base of applied clinical research has declined while practitioners need it now more than ever. This void of research is particularly apparent for speech-language pathologists practicing in medical settings. This shortage of clinically relevant, applied research is not new. Tanner and Gerstenberger (1996, p. 328) comment on the void of clinically relevant aphasia research in *Aphasiology*, an international, interdisciplinary journal:

> This unfortunate void of research extends to all aspects of clinician-patient interaction including the utilization of workbooks, apraxia and dysarthria drills, word recall assist strategies, techniques for reducing perseveration and bouts of emotional lability, reading and writing rehabilitation, orientation and stimulation and reinforcement techniques. Much of what a practising clinician must do has not been tested empirically. By necessity, therapy is a combination of borrowed teaching strategies from education, psychology, logical inductive and inductive reasoning, common sense direction and guidance. The limited body of applied research is certainly not desirable, but the practising clinician must perform; he/she does not have the academic luxury to close the lecture with the statement that "all the data are not in."

31

Ideally, speech-language pathologists and audiologists would provide only scientifically proven diagnostic and therapeutic methods and procedures for every category and subcategory of communication disorders. Further, they would have a body of research to support their application to individual patients, and have scientific studies addressing variables such as gender, age, ethnicity, race, and other case-by-case variables.

To provide optimal evidence-based clinical services, speech-language pathologists and audiologists need a large body of scientifically proven clinical methods and procedures from which they can select the appropriate evaluation procedures, instruction, and therapies. These scientifically based methods and procedures would have been studied in several clinical trials, and their indications and contraindications well-documented. Unfortunately, the applied research base for clinical services in speech-language pathology and audiology is far from optimal.

6.3 Pure and Applied Research in Communication Sciences and Disorders

As noted above, the dearth of clinical evidence-based research is caused by a shortage of communication scientists, and increasingly larger numbers of speech-language pathologists and audiologists performing wider ranges of services. The amount of pure research being conducted to the exclusion of applied research also exacerbates this problem.

Pure research is done to quench the thirst for knowledge and does not have a clinical objective in the research design. Pure research in communication sciences and disorders asks questions about the general nature of speech, voice, language, and hearing; it is conducted to help better understand how humans communicate. Examples of pure research in communication sciences and disorders include studies about respiratory physiology, how the larynx functions to change pitch and loudness, and the specific tongue muscles involved in the production of vowels and consonants. Other areas of pure research involve resonance characteristics of the speech production mechanism, and acoustic factors associated with auditory perception. Exciting areas of pure research, and arguably the most expensive, are brain localization studies that attempt to pinpoint areas of the brain responsible for this, that, or the other speech and hearing function (see Chapter 2). While pure research can provide a foundation for applied research, it does little to advance the clinical body of evidence-based information about the evaluation and treatment of persons with communication disorders.

Applied research, on the other hand, attempts to answer research questions or to prove or disprove hypotheses about

areas of evaluation and treatment. Applied research in communication sciences and disorders addresses a wide clinically based area of study, and the research is specifically designed to prove or disprove the value and merits of a specific evaluation procedure or treatment. Examples of applied research in communication sciences and disorders include investigating the value of voice rest on treating vocal nodules, polyps, and contact ulcers, the use of relaxation training to reduce stuttering, behavior modification in the treatment of aphasia, using mirrors to facilitate motor speech programming in stroke patients, and auditory bombardment of speech sounds to help children learn phonological rules.

6.4 Types of Research in Communication Sciences and Disorders

The type of research done in communication sciences and disorders is similar to all social and basic science research. In general, scientific research requires a statement of the study's purpose, e.g., the problem, concept, or issue to be examined, and the procedures followed to answer the research question or questions. These procedures are strictly detailed so that readers can understand the studies and criticize them. Equally important, this format gives scientists the methodological details of the studies so that they can replicate them with different subjects to learn whether the results were accurate, consistent, valid, and reliable. Catalog-epidemiologic, descriptive, and experimental research are three separate but related types of empirical research within the discipline of communication sciences and disorders.

As Table 6.1 shows, catalog-epidemiologic research is used to study the occurrences or factors associated with an aspect of communication or its disorders. Scientists catalog or profile some function of normal communication, list the frequency of occurrence of disorders overall, or catalog some aspect of a subgroup of the population. Although related to catalog-epidemiologic research, descriptive studies involve observing and describing some facet of communication and its disorders. For example, catalog-epidemiologic research may provide the psychological characteristics of patients with vocal nodules, and a descriptive study describe the muscular functions of the larynx. Whereas the above types of research are objective, the experimental method discussed below uses inductive reasoning to make generalizations about communication and its disorders. By sampling a small segment of a population and making observations in the past, inductive logic is used to make generalizations and predict laws and theories that will operate in the future (Velasquez, 2002).

6.5 Experimental Research Design

Although there may be variation in the format of experimental research, the following topics are addressed:

1. review of literature,
2. definition of terms,
3. hypotheses and research questions,
4. subjects,
5. results,
6. conclusions, and
7. suggestions for future research.

Institutions, journals, and scientific organizations may require that the above be combined into methodology sections, procedures, or data analyses sections. Nevertheless, each is addressed to show the primary elements of the study that can be criticized and the veracity of the conclusions drawn from it evaluated.

6.6 Review of Literature

The primary purpose of the literature review is to require the scientist conducting the study to become familiar with past research on the topic. All published research on the subject is reviewed including classic studies. However, the review of the literature concentrates on the research during the past ten years. The secondary purpose of the review of the literature is to provide readers of the published study, or the audience during a scientific platform presentation, with an overview of the relevant research conducted on the topic with particular emphases on their design and conclusions. The review of the literature provides the background and rationale for the design of the current study.

6.7 Definition of Terms

In Chapter 2, it was reported that a persistent problem in communication sciences and disorders is vague or nonexistent definition of terms. Since the beginning of the study of human communication and its disorders, the discipline has been plagued by researchers, theorists, and scholars who often only vaguely defined important terms or failed to define them at all. However today, in the experimental design, it is required that important terms be clearly defined either in a separate section of the study or when they are used in the text.

Clear and precise definitions of important terms are required for all communication sciences and disorders research, but particularly those conducted in the neurosciences. This is because the neurosciences include many disciplines with researchers from a variety of scientific backgrounds. For example, when describing the cortical and subcortical areas important to auditory understanding, the word "understand" must clearly be defined. The definition of the word must clearly describe, limit, and delimit the parameters of its meaning. Does the word "understand," as used in the study, encompass only the semantics of the smallest units of meaning (morphemes), individual words, or does it include decoding the much broader category of discourse semantics?

Table 6.1
Types of Research in Communication Sciences and Disorders

Type	Description	Example
Catalog-epidemiologic	A study to learn the number of entities and factors associated with a particular aspect of communication or its disorders.	How many kindergarten children stutter in the United States?
Descriptive	Systematic and methodical recording of observable events in communication sciences and disorders.	What is the cortical brain activity level of a patient with jargon aphasia?
Experimental	A study in which variables are manipulated to reach conclusions that can be generalized to larger populations.	Do intensive individual and group therapies benefit patients with global aphasia?

6.8 Research Questions and Hypotheses Testing

There are two ways of asking questions in communication sciences and disorders research: research questions and hypotheses testing. Research questions, more frequently used in catalog-epidemiologic and descriptive research, tend to be general and used when there is little information in the literature from which to form a hypothesis. A research question is a straightforward query such as, "Is there a difference between male and female stroke patients in their aphasic wordfinding strategies?" In this type of neutral research question, the scientist does not have evidence or a belief that either males or females differ in retrieving words from memory following a stroke. On the other hand, the hypothesis is more typically used in formal experimental research, and is a definite statement with a prediction of the outcome.

The hypothesis is written in the null form, i.e., that there is no statistically significant difference in the relationship being studied. The purpose of the study is to reject the null hypothesis. According to Maxwell and Satake (1997), the acceptance or rejection of the null hypothesis reflects the skepticism of scientists; nothing exists until proven to exist. In the above example of differences in aphasic word retrieval behaviors between the sexes, the hypothesis would be as such: "Female patients with stroke-related communication disorders are more successful in their word retrieval behaviors than male patients." The scientist would write the null hypothesis: "There is no statistically significant difference between the means and variances of male and female stroke patients on word retrieval tests." The result of the study either rejects or accepts the null hypothesis based on a level of statistical confidence.

6.9 Subjects

There are two general categories of subject selection in communication sciences and disorders research: random and convenience (nonrandom). A random selection of subjects (the sample) is representative of the larger group of persons (the population) from which conclusions can be drawn. The sample is selected by assigning potential subjects a number and using a computer program randomizer or a table of random numbers to get the participants in the study. Although many factors go into the power of a study to answer a research question and to prove or disprove a hypothesis, the larger the sample the greater power of the study. A sample of convenience is nonrandom and thus not representative of a larger population. Consequently, the scientist cannot make generalizations to a larger group of people. In a sample of convenience, the conclusions obtained from the study are limited to the subjects used in the

study. However, general inferences can be made, but not with statistical probability.

6.10 Control and Experimental Groups

The subjects in the control group are not subjected to the treatment; however, the experimental group is subjected to the independent variable. The scientist manipulates the independent variable to determine the effect on the dependent variable; the independent variable relates to the cause and the dependent variable relates to the effect. McReynolds and Kearns (1983) note that the purpose of a study is to isolate the effect of the independent variable from all other variables. For example, in a study to determine the benefit of a particular speech drill on stroke patients' abilities to speak clearly, the subjects in the control group would not be given the speech drill. The subjects in the experimental group would be given the speech drill, at the same frequency and duration, and by the same therapist or group of therapists trained to provide it in the same way. By minimizing as many variables as possible between the control and experimental group of subjects, except the experimental speech drill, the researcher can determine its effect on the subjects. Because the experimental group of subjects is randomly selected from the larger population, the scientist can generalize the results to all similar stroke patients.

6.11 Results and Conclusion

The results section of experimental research consists of objective numerical data tied to the research question or hypothesis. The results section consists of tables, figures, charts, and raw data (often located in the appendix), including the statistics used in the study. In the discussion section, the researcher describes the significance of the results, discusses their implications, and makes generalizations and inferences. In this section, it is important that the scientist logically base his or her conclusions on the obtained data. The conclusions reached from the study must be firmly based on the data and results. The conclusions should also summarize how the study is important to some aspect of communication sciences and disorders. This is most important in applied research; the discussion section should give clinicians a working understanding of the clinical implications of the experiment.

6.12 Suggestions for Future Research

The suggestions for future research is an often unheeded but very important aspect of the scientific method. Too often, the scientist only lists a few sentences at the end of the paper explaining how the study could be improved, its strengths and limitations, and the general course of future research on the subject. However, after a scientist has completed an experimental study, he or she is an authority on the subject and arguably the most qualified person to suggest areas and foci for future study. Science is cumulative and builds on itself, making the suggestions for future research an important aspect in the total creation of a body of empirical information about a subject. Ideally, every scientist would design her or his studies on previous suggestions for future research on the particular topic. The value of previous scientific contributions and guidance of earlier researchers is captured in Newton's refrain: "If I have seen farther it is by standing on the shoulders of giants."

6.13 Evaluating Empirical Research in Communication Sciences and Disorders

Not all statistically significant research is important research. Statistics are used to collect and evaluate large amounts of information and to decide whether the results are significant. A study that produces statistically significant results suggests that the findings are not due to chance. A statistically significant finding answers a particular research question and rejects the null hypothesis with a high level of confidence. In social science research, the usual required statistical level of confidence is 0.95 (0.05 level of significance). This confidence range suggests the margin of error; if the study were replicated with different subjects, ninety-five times out of 100 times, the results would be the same. Although there are many types of statistical analyses, most research in communication sciences and disorders either compares groups of subjects on some parameter of performance or looks at a correlation.

In group comparisons, a researcher examines whether the experimental group differs from the control group concerning the results of a particular treatment. For example, the researcher may look at children seen in pullout therapy, where they are removed from the classroom and given individual instruction, and compare their growth in vocabulary with children seen in inclusion therapy, where the therapist works with them in the classroom (Tanner, Weems, and Kendall, 1989). If the difference in the group is statistically significant, then therapists would have important information about providing speech pathology services to language-delayed children.

A correlation study may look at how two (or more) variable "co-relate." For example, the researcher may examine how the frequency of therapy for stroke patients with slurred speech correlates with a score on a test of speech intelligibility. A positive, statistically significant correlation would show that the more therapy given to the patients, the better the scores on the intelligibility test. If the results were statistically significant and negative, then speech intelligibility actually suffers with increased frequency of therapy. Research that is important and statistically significant answers critical research questions and provides high levels of confidence about the results.

6.14 Peer Review of Scientific Research

Published research is peer reviewed. Peer-reviewed research has been examined by several professionals in the field and either accepted or rejected for publication or presentation. Generally, published research is as influential as the journal in which it is published. In more prestigious journals, the research is examined in great detail concerning the methodology and conclusions. Often the researcher is provided with reviewers' comments and encouraged to make changes and additions based on them. Once the changes are made, the editor of the journal either accepts or rejects the revised paper. The publication process can take months and even years. Nevertheless, the product is often a carefully examined, reviewed, and edited research article. After publication, most journals accept letters criticizing the article. In some journals, a clinical forum is provided where they publish reviewers' comments and the researcher's responses to them together in the same edition. Many journals also have theory, essay, and tutorial sections allowing for these types of theoretical articles to be submitted to the scientific community. Although published research in respected journals is usually accurate and contributes meaningfully to the body of scientific information, sometimes studies are published with poor design or false data. However, this is rare and usually brought to the attention of the scientific world and corrected.

Scientific presentations, research papers given at scientific conferences, are also peer-reviewed. However, scientific papers at conferences are considered less rigorously reviewed and edited than those published in journals. The prestige of the research paper is dependent on the status of the scientific conference and the whether the paper is a poster or platform presentation; and as a rule, international conferences are more prestigious than national, state, or regional ones. Poster sessions are groups of papers provided at the same time and the audience walks through a hall and reviews them, and are considered less prestigious than platform presentations. A platform presentation is where several scientists present their studies sequentially to a seated audience who has the opportunity to question the researchers and their results. The veracity of scientific articles presented via the World Wide Web is generally considered suspect due to the lack of reliability, poor quality control, and the sheer vast amount of information available on the

Internet. However, this is not to say that articles are of high quality and major contributors to science; it is simply that today, Internet articles do not have the acceptance of those published in respected journals or presented at legitimate scientific conferences.

Sometimes, the popular media will report summaries of published scientific articles and papers. Media reporting of scientific advances in communication sciences and disorder gives the public important information about the process of communication and the prevention, diagnosis, and treatment of its disorders. However, newspapers and television programs often only superficially report the study's methodology and gloss over its implications and significance. Additionally, sometimes the media misconstrues the results or gives too much or little value to them. As a rule, reports of research in the popular media provide general information about scientific advances, but they should not be considered accurate reviews of the studies.

6.15 Summary

Although speech-language pathologists and audiologists attempt to provide evidence-based diagnostic and therapeutic services, the quantity and quality of empirical research in communication sciences and disorders are far from optimal. Experimental research provides the most credible diagnostic and therapeutic clinical evidence and involves a design format that gives clinicians a clear understanding of the methods used and conclusions reached. It also gives other scientists opportunities to replicate the study and further support or reject its conclusions.

Suggested Readings and Resources

Kent, R. D. (1997). *The Speech Sciences.* San Diego: Singular. This textbook reviews several important issues in the speech sciences including a chapter on applied speech sciences.

Tanner, D. (2007). *An Advanced Course in Communication Sciences and Disorders.* San Diego: Plural Publishing. Chapter 4 is a review of the scientific process in communication sciences and disorders.

References

American Speech-Language-Hearing Association (2006). Code of Ethics (Revised, 2003). Retrieved from the World Wide Web September 17, 2006: http://www.asha.org/NR/rdonlyres/F51E46C5-3D87-44AF-BFDA-346D32F85C60/0/v1CodeOfEthics.pdf.

Maxwell, D. and Satake, E. (1997). *Research and statistical methods in communication disorders.* Baltimore: Williams & Wilkins.

McReynolds, L. and Kearns, K. (1983). *Single-subject experimental designs in communicative disorders.* Baltimore: University Park Press.

Tanner, D. and Gerstenberger, D. (1996). Response to grief? Responses to commentaries. In C. Code and D. Muller (Eds), *Forums in clinical aphasiology* (pp. 328-331). Whurr Publishers Ltd.: London, UK.

Tanner, D., Weems, L, and Kendall, D. (1989). Pull-out versus classroom language intervention. A paper presented at the annual convention of the American Speech-Language-Hearing Association, St. Louis.

Velasquez, M. (2002). *Philosophy* (8th ed). Belmont, CA: Wadsworth/Thomson Learning.

Chapter 7

Professional Speech and Hearing Associations

7.1 Chapter Preview

This chapter examines professional speech and hearing associations including the International Association of Logopedics and Phoniatrics, the American Academy of Audiology, and the American Academy of Private Practice in Speech Pathology and Audiology. The American Speech-Language-Hearing Association, the largest speech and hearing professional association, is discussed including its mission, journals, and Code of Ethics.

7.2 International Speech and Hearing Professional Associations

Several international professional organizations represent communication scientists, speech-language pathologists, audiologists, and others professionals. Many third-world and nonindustrialized countries do not have strong, organized professional associations. In these countries, speech and hearing services are provided by physicians, teachers, nurses, therapists, and others who have a wide range of academic and clinical credentials. As a rule, the services provided to communication-disabled persons in third-world and nonindustrialized countries are of poor quality and inadequately funded by public schools and social welfare programs. However, wealthy persons may have the financial resources to obtain adequate speech and hearing services from professionals residing outside their countries. Some philanthropic and welfare organizations from industrialized countries send communication specialists to underserved areas of the world to provide speech and hearing services. The adequacy of a country's services to communication-disabled persons is often reflected by whether they have organized and active speech and hearing professional organizations. Table 7.1 provides a partial list of speech and hearing professional associations in industrialized countries. The major international speech and hearing professional association is the International Association of Logopedics and Phoniatrics (IALP).

The International Association of Logopedics and Phoniatrics was founded in 1924 and has approximately 400 individual members and affiliations with fifty national societies in more than fifty-five countries (IALP, 2006). Phoniatrics is the medical study and management of speech disorders, and logopedics is derived from the Greek for "word or discourse." The IALP professional organization represents persons involved in the scientific study and treatment of a broad range of communication disorders. The International Association of Logopedics and Phoniatrics publishes *Folia Phoniatrica et Logopaedica,* an international journal addressing communication, speech, and voice pathologies. The IALP provides a worldwide venue for sharing information, knowledge, and understanding about communication and its disorders (IALP, 2006).

7.3 The American Academy of Audiology

As reported in Chapter 4, currently about 10,000 audiologists are members of the American Academy of Audiology (AAA). The mission of AAA is to promote quality hearing and balance by advancing the profession of audiology. This is accomplished through leadership, advocacy, support of research, public education, and awareness of balance and hearing loss issues. Its slogan exemplifies the mission of the American Academy of Audiology: "Caring for America's Hearing."

Table 7.1
International Speech and Hearing Associations

Argentina	Associacion Argentina de Logopedia Foniatria y Audiologia
Australia	Speech Pathology Australia
Austria	Oesterreichische Gesellschaft für Sprachheilpädagogik
Belgium	Union Professionnelle des Logopèdes Francophones
Brazil	Sociedade Brasileira de Laringologia e Voz
Canada	Canadian Association of Speech-Language Pathologists and Audiologists
Czech Republic	Czech Phoniatric and Paedaudiologic Society Phoniatric Clinic
Denmark	Dansk Selskab for Logopaedi og Foniatri
Egypt	Egyptian Society for Phoniatrics and Logopedics
Finland	Finnish Association of Speech and Language Research
France	Societe Francaise de Phoniatrie et Pathologies de la Communication
Germany	Deutsche Gesellschaft für Sprachheilpädagogik
Greece	Panhellenic Association of Logopedics
Peoples Republic of China	The Hong Kong Association of Speech Therapists
Hungary	Ungarise Gesellschaft fur Phonetik, Phoniatrie und Logopadie
Iceland	The Icelandic Association of Speech Therapists
Ireland	The Irish Association of Speech and Language Therapists
Israel	The Israeli Speech, Hearing and Language Association
Italy	Societa Italiana di Foniatria e Logopedia
Japan	Japan Society of Logopedics and Phoniatrics
Malta	The Association of Speech - Language Pathologists
The Netherlands	Nederlandse Vereniging voor Logopedie en Foniatrie
New Zealand	New Zealand Speech Language Therapists Association
Norway	Norwegian Association of Logopedists
Poland	Polish Logopaedic Society
Portugal	Associacao Portuguessa de Terapeutas da Fala
Russia	Association of Phoniatricians and Speech Therapists
Singapore	The Singapore Speech-Language Hearing Association
South Africa	South African Speech-Language-Hearing Association
South Korea	The Korean Society of Logopedics and Phoniatrics
Spain	Association Espanola de Logopedia Foniatria y Audiologia
Sweden	Swedish Association of Phoniatrics and Logopedics
Taiwan	The Taiwan Speech-Language-Hearing Association
United Kingdom	The Royal College of Speech & Language Therapists
United States of America	American Speech-Language-Hearing Association

Source: The International Associacion of Logopedics and Phoniatrics (2006).

The American Academy of Audiology was founded in 1988 by Dr. James Jerger, a renowned hearing scientist and audiologist. According to the American Academy of Audiology (2005), the first national convention of the AAA was held in 1989 with approximately 600 attendees, and by the thirteenth conference, there were more than 7,300 attendees. This rapid growth showed the need for a professional association of audiologists, for audiologists, and by audiologists. The growth and success of AAA also demonstrated the dissatisfaction of audiologists with the American Speech-Language-Hearing Association in representing audiology and audiologists' professional interests (see below). Categories of membership in AAA include Fellows, Affiliates, International Members, Candidates, Retired, Disabled, Life, and Life Emeritus (AAA, 2005). The American Academy of Audiology's Code of Ethics is similar to those of other professions and defines the scope of ethical practices for audiologists. The AAA publishes the *Journal of the American Academy of Audiology* and *Audiology Today*.

7.4 American Academy of Private Practice in Speech Pathology and Audiology

The American Academy of Private Practice in Speech Pathology and Audiology (AAPPSPA) was founded in 1964 in San Francisco. It is a national nonprofit organization for speech-language pathologists and audiologists in private practice (AAPPSPA, 2006). The purpose of this professional association is to address the functions and concerns of those professionals in private practice which differ significantly from other areas of professional speech and hearing practice. Specifically, the American Academy of Private Practice in Speech Pathology and Audiology goals are to foster the highest ideals and principles of private practice in speech pathology and audiology, provide interaction and communication among members, create and elevate private practice professional standards, and provide ongoing interaction for the private practitioner (AAPPSPA, 2006). The American Academy of Private Practice in Speech Pathology and Audiology conducts conventions and workshops addressing clinical issues. The AAPPSPA provides Full, Affiliate, and Life memberships.

7.5 The American Speech-Language-Hearing Association

The American Speech-Language-Hearing Association (ASHA) is the largest scientific and professional association for speech-language pathologists and audiologists (ASHA, 2005). It has more than 120,000 members, certifi-

cate holders, and affiliates and maintains a permanent office in Washington, D.C. According to ASHA (2005), its mission is sevenfold:

1. Encourage basic scientific study of the processes of individual human communication, with special reference to speech, language, and hearing.

2. Promote appropriate academic and clinical preparation of individuals entering the discipline of human communication sciences and disorders and to promote the maintenance of current knowledge and skills of those within the discipline.

3. Promote investigation and prevention of disorders of human communication.

4. Foster improvement of clinical services and procedures addressing such disorders.

5. Stimulate exchange of information among persons and organizations thus engaged and to disseminate such information.

6. Advocate for the rights and interests of persons with communication disorders.

7. Promote the individual and collective professional interests of the members of the Association.

The American Speech-Language-Hearing Association sponsors national conventions, conferences, institutes, and workshops, and maintains a computerized database of federal and private funding sources for research into human communication and its disorders. It also accredits training programs in speech-language pathology and audiology. As reported in Chapter 4, ASHA provides two certificates: Certificate of Clinical Competence in Speech-Language Pathology and the Certificate of Clinical Competence in Audiology.

The American Speech-Language-Hearing Association publishes four journals:

American Journal of Audiology
American Journal of Speech-Language Pathology
Journal of Speech, Language, and Hearing Research
Language, Speech, and Hearing Services in the Schools

7.6 The Code of Ethics of the American Speech-Language-Hearing Association

The ASHA Code of Ethics lists and defines principles and rules of ethical conduct; however failure to specify particular responsibilities or practices in the code does not deny their existence. The ASHA Code of Ethics lists four principles of ethics with rules detailing individual conduct regarding them:

Principle of Ethics I: Individuals shall honor their responsibility to hold paramount the welfare of persons they serve professionally.

Principle of Ethics II: Individuals shall honor their responsibility to achieve and maintain the highest level of professional competence.

Principle of Ethics III: Individuals shall honor their responsibility to the public by promoting public understanding of the professions, by supporting the development of services designed to fulfill the unmet needs of the public, and by providing accurate information in all communications involving any aspect of the professions.

Principle of Ethics IV: Individuals shall honor their responsibilities to the professions and their relationships with colleagues, students, and members of allied professions. Individuals shall uphold the dignity and autonomy of the professions, maintain harmonious interprofessional and intraprofessional relationships, and accept the professions' self-imposed standards.

7.7 Student, State, and Local Professional Associations

Affiliated with the American Speech-Language-Hearing Association, the National Student Speech-Language-Hearing Association (NSSLHA) has chapters at most colleges and universities with programs in communication sciences and disorders. Two members of NSSLHA serve on the Legislative Council of ASHA. According to Spahr and Malone (2002), NSSLHA has about 20,000 members and was established in 1972. It is an outgrowth of Sigma Alpha Eta, the original student organization.

Most states have professional speech and hearing associations which may also sponsor annual conventions and publish journals. Spahr and Malone (2002) note that the District of Columbia, Puerto Rico, and Guam also have professional speech and hearing associations. Many larger cities in the United States also may have professional speech and hearing associations.

7.8 Summary

Local, state, national, and international professional speech and hearing associations represent speech-language pathologists and audiologists. The American Speech-Language-Hearing Association is the largest speech and hearing professional association and has approximately 120,000 members. The Code of Ethics of the American Speech-Language-Hearing Association details ethical conduct of its members through four Principles of Ethical Conduct and the rules pertaining to them.

Suggested Readings and Resources

American Academy of Audiology. *About the Academy*. http://www.audiology.org/about/ This is the Academy's home page and describes its mission.

American Speech-Language-Hearing Association. *About the Association*. http://www.asha.org/about/membership-certification. This is the Association's home page and describes its mission.

Tanner, D. (2006). *An Advanced Course in Communication Sciences and Disorders*. San Diego: Plural Publishing. Chapter 2 has a detailed discussion of the American Speech-Language-Hearing Association including a review of the Code of Ethics.

References

American Academy of Audiology (2005). *About the Academy*. Retrieved from the World Wide Web on December 15, 2005: http://www.audiology.org/about/ (Author)

American Academy of Private Practice in Speech Pathology and Audiology (2006). *About the Academy*. Retrieved from the World Wide Web on January 4, 2006: http://www.aappspa.org (Author).

American Speech-Language-Hearing Association (2005). Retrieved from the World Wide Web on January 5, 2006: http://www.asha.org/about/membership-certification/member-counts.htm (Author).

The International Association of Logopedics and Phoniatrics (2006). About the IALP. Retrieved from the World Wide Web on January 3, 2006: http://www.ialp.info/Frames/frames.html (Author).

Spahr, F. T. and Malone, R.L. (2002). Human Communication Disorders: An Introduction. In G.H. Shames and N.B. Anderson (Eds), *Human communication disorders: An introduction* (6th ed.) (pp. 1-27). Boston: Allyn & Bacon.

Part II
Medical-Legal and Forensic Aspects of Speech-Language Pathology and Audiology

Chapter 8

The Medical-Legal and Forensic Aspects of Dysphagia (Swallowing Disorders)

8.1 Chapter Preview

This chapter provides an overview of dysphagia litigation including incidence and prevalence statistics and a definition of the disorder. The neurology and musculature of the swallow are detailed as is the comprehensive swallowing evaluation. The role of the dysphagia expert witness is examined including the creation of a clinical timeline. The importance of the video swallow study in the diagnosis and treatment of dysphagia is also detailed. Several litigation issues are addressed including clinical documentation, communication among and between healthcare professionals, and clinical indications for radiographic and instrumental dysphagia assessments. There are also three case studies of litigation involving dysphagia management.

8.2 Overview of Dysphagia Medical Malpractice Litigation

Dysphagia is a sucking, chewing, and swallowing disorder. It can be an issue in medical malpractice litigation because it can cause aspiration pneumonia and lead to serious medical complications, including the death of the patient. Speech-language pathologists have assumed a pivotal role in the diagnosis and treatment of dysphagia: "It is the position of the American Speech-Language-Hearing Association (ASHA), that speech-language pathologists play a primary role in the evaluation and treatment of infants, children, and adults with swallowing and feeding disorders" (ASHA, 2001, p. III-1). Dysphagia medical malpractice litigation is increasingly common especially in nursing home patients (Tanner, 2006; Wright, 2004; Tanner and Guzzino, 2002).

Diet, eating, and swallowing abilities have always been important aspects of patient management, especially for the old and feeble and severely cognitively, neurologically, and physically compromised. Until the early 1980s, the role dysphagia played in medical management of these patients was not well understood, and little research had been done on its diagnosis and treatment. Most patients with significant dysphagia were simply given feeding tubes. Physicians and nurses usually addressed the neurological, anatomical, and physiological aspects of swallowing primarily in cases of oral cancer and progressive diseases such as amyotrophic lateral sclerosis and multiple sclerosis. Diagnosis of dysphagia and subsequent aspiration was limited to listening for coughing and gurgling sounds in the lungs. Occasionally, a radiologist did an upper gastrointestinal x-ray or general video swallow study to note gross deviations in the swallow. To complicate matters, no one specialist on the medical team was primarily responsible for this important aspect of patient management.

In the past twenty years, the management of dysphagia has evolved to a medical team approach. Research on swallowing and its disorders has increased significantly, and today, several books and one journal are exclusively devoted to dysphagia. Most communication sciences and disorders introductory books and professional textbooks addressing neurogenic communication disorders have sections or chapters devoted to the diagnosis and treatment of patients with swallowing disorders. In 1985, 35 percent of speech-language pathologists were involved in the delivery of dysphagia treatment (ASHA, 1987), and in 1995, 52 percent engaged in dysphagia diagnosis and treatment (ASHA, 1997). Today, dysphagia is the most common disorder seen by speech-language pathologists in medical settings. It is rare for a speech-language pathologist working in a medical setting not to spend a major part of his or her clinical time involved directly or indirectly in dysphagia management.

The advances in research, diagnosis, and treatment of dysphagia have also come with increased litigation. Dysphagia management is directly or indirectly an issue in many medical malpractice cases because of patient choking and aspiration pneumonia. A patient with dysphagia can choke to death if foods are not prepared properly and if he or she is not monitored carefully while eating. Pneumonia is a dangerous and life-threatening medical condition with a mortality rate of 43 percent in hospitalized elderly patients who develop it (Gonzalez and Calia, 1975). The occurrence of pneumonia is seven and one-half times greater in stroke patients who aspirate than in those who do not (Schmidt, Holas, Halvorson, and Reding, 1994).

8.3 Incidence and Prevalence of Dysphagia

Incidence and prevalence statistics for dysphagia are highly variable. Several studies suggest that approximately one-third of hospitalized patients have dysphagia and approximately two-thirds of nursing home residents may be compromised concerning eating and swallowing (Logemann, 1995; Cherney, 1994; Groher and Bukatman, 1986; Siebens, Trupe, and Siebens, 1986; and others). Although dysphagia can occur in any age group, the incidence and prevalence of dysphagia are skewed to the very young and old. According to Spahr and Malone (1998), approximately

15 million Americans have a swallowing disorder. The number of patients with dysphagia is likely to increase in the future, and so too will litigation involving dysphagia medical malpractice.

Future dysphagia incidence and prevalence rates are likely to increase for four reasons. First, more people survive serious motor vehicle accidents, gunshot wounds, and falls, but they often do so with sucking, chewing, and swallowing disorders. Improved emergency rapid transportation and trauma care have increased survival rates. In addition, more at-risk babies survive because of advances in medical care. Second, the population of the United States is growing. Consequently, there will be greater numbers of people with dysphagia. Third, the country is also aging, and there will be a higher percentage of elderly people who are susceptible to age-related diseases and disorders that often occur with swallowing problems. Finally, healthcare professionals are diagnosing and treating more people for dysphagia due to increased awareness of the disorder and its medical complications and legal implications. Because of litigation and large settlements from dysphagia malpractice suits, healthcare practitioners and administrators are increasingly more vigilant in identifying dysphagia patients and managing their sucking, chewing, and swallowing disorders.

8.4 Defining Dysphagia

The definition of dysphagia can be an important issue in dysphagia medical malpractice. The definition of dysphagia can include or exclude healthcare professionals and the medical institutions for whom they act as agents. Dysphagia can be defined narrowly to include only the ability of the patient to move food and liquid from the mouth to the stomach. Dysphagia, when defined broadly, can include the perceptual and cognitive awareness of the eating situation, and the physiologic responses to the smell of food (Leopold and Kagel, 1996). A broad definition of dysphagia can also include the interruption of eating pleasure (Buchholz, 1996) and consequent reduction in the patient's quality of life. In the broad definition of dysphagia, the patient's psychological responses to the smell of food and liquid, his or her cognitive abilities to recognize and understand what to do with them, and the motor and sensory aspects of moving substances from the mouth to the stomach are considered. In the narrow definition of dysphagia, only the motor acts of sucking, chewing, and swallowing substances are considered.

There are degrees of limitations caused by dysphagia. For example, according to Reilly (2004), some persons are "impaired" in swallowing such as occurs with restricted tongue movement, some are "handicapped" by needing a restricted diet, and others are "disabled" by an inability to chew. In both narrow and broad definitions, the role dysphagia plays in choking, aspiration, and the patient's ability to maintain hydration and nutrition can be an important issue in medical malpractice litigation. The following is the broadest definition of the disorder:

Dysphagia: Impairment of the emotional, cognitive, sensory, and/or motor acts involved with transferring a substance from the mouth to stomach, resulting in failure to maintain hydration and nutrition, and posing a risk of choking and aspiration.

The above definition of the dysphagia involves all relevant healthcare professionals in its management.

8.5 The Dysphagia Management Team

The patient's primary care physician is ultimately responsible for the medical management of dysphagia. He or she reviews histories, makes referrals, studies reports, participates in team meetings, prescribes diagnostic tests and procedures, and engages in monitoring and follow-up activities. In a rehabilitation unit, the patient's primary care physician is usually a specialist in physical medicine and rehabilitation. The registered nurse (RN) evaluates and monitors the patient's dysphagia, hydration, and ability to meet nutritional needs orally. The licensed practical nurse (LPN) and certified nursing assistant (CNA) feed the patient, and monitor, chart, and report dysphagia symptoms to responsible personnel. The registered dietician (RD) and nutritionist are responsible for temperature and texture of the patient's meals and any special dietary concerns such as allergies to foods, diabetes, vitamin deficiencies, etc. The radiologist, together with the speech-language pathologist (SLP), conducts videofluoroscopic swallowing studies (VSS). The occupational therapist (OT) is responsible for the patient's hand-and-arm coordination, posture, and sensory abilities during eating. The pulmonologist and respiratory therapist may be called on to deal with respiratory disease and disorders. The gastroenterologist evaluates and manages gastrointestinal disease and nutritional issues. The neurologist is important in conducting special muscular and neurological diagnostic tests. The social worker is involved with coordinating meetings, counseling family, and arranging home health care for dysphagia patients.

According to Arvedson and Brodsky (2002), dysphagia team members for infants and children with feeding and swallowing problems also may include a developmental pediatrician who manages pediatric and neuro-developmental issues and an otolaryngologist who manages medical and surgical issues related to drooling, aspiration, and gastro-esophageal reflux. Special education teachers, aides, and volunteers may see school children with dysphagia (see Table 8.1).

The speech-language pathologist is typically the dysphagia team leader. The speech-language pathologist's knowledge of neurology, anatomy, physiology of the speech production mechanism, and the processes of normal and deviant swallowing, provide the essential requisites to assume a leadership role in dysphagia management. In addition, swallowing disorders often occur with speech pathologies, and there is concurrent treatment of both disorders. In some hospitals and nursing homes, one or several speech-language pathologists may be exclusively assigned to patients with dysphagia.

8.6 Chewing, Swallowing, and Speech

Chewing is "mastication" and of Greek origin for "grinding the teeth." The first stage of digestion occurs in the oral cavity and includes biting, tearing, sucking, chewing, and swallowing many different types of foodstuffs. Humans have evolved the ability to sustain life by using the lips, teeth, tongue, and other structures of the oral cavity for digestive purposes. Humans have also evolved the ability to make sounds using the lungs, larynx, lips, teeth, tongue, and palate. Speech is an overlaid function; the muscles and structures of respiration and digestion have evolved to enable the production of speech sounds.

"Deglutition" is of Latin origin for the act of swallowing. Both speech and deglutition involve coordinated actions of the respiratory, laryngeal, and articulatory musculature. They share many neurological pathways and anatomical structures. For speech purposes, these head and neck structures are respiratory, while in swallowing they are digestive. According to Zemlin (1998), deglutition becomes successively more reflexive and ultimately autonomic. Swallowing is seen as early as the tenth week fetal life, and adults do it more than 500 times each day (Zemlin, 1998). Speaking and swallowing often occur concurrently, and there are momentary interruptions of speech while the speaker clears his or her mouth of food and liquid. Speaking and swallowing also differ in their directionality and rhythm. Swallowing movements are always ingressive, as food and liquid move inward, while speech movements are egressive, with air flowing out of the body.

Table 8.1
Professionals Involved in Dysphagia Diagnosis and Treatment

Primary Care Physician	Ultimately responsible for medical management of dysphagia
Registered Nurse	Evaluates and monitors dysphagia, hydration, and the patient's ability to meet nutritional needs orally
Licensed Practical Nurse/Certified Nurse Assistant	Feeds the patient, monitors, charts and reports status of dysphagia
Registered Dietician/Nutritionist	Responsible for temperature and texture of patient's meals and special dietary concerns
Radiologist	Conducts video swallowing studies (VSS) in conjunction with the speech pathology service
Occupational Therapist	Responsible for hand/arm movement and posture during eating
Pulmonologist/Respiratory Therapist	Responsible for management of airway diseases and disorders
Gastroenterologist	Manages gastrointestinal disease and nutritional issues
Neurologist	Responsible for special diagnostic tests
Social Worker	Coordinates meetings, consults with family and home health agencies
Speech-Language Pathologist	Responsible for diagnosis and therapeutic management of dysphagia
Others: Physiatrist, Pediatrician, Otolaryngologist, Special Education Teacher, Aides, and Volunteers	May be involved in management of dysphagia depending on age of patient and the site of services

8.7 The Normal Swallow

According to Reilly (2004), little time has been devoted to the description and measurement of normal swallowing. However, most authorities believe there are three interconnected phases to a normal swallow. The first is the oral phase, sometimes called the buccal stage. It is voluntary even if it is done unconsciously (Zemlin, 1998). In the oral phase, the food or liquid must be prepared for swallowing. Some authorities separate oral preparation from transport aspects of swallowing. Oral preparatory behaviors include chewing and liquid containment, and transportation involve moving the food or liquid to the back (posterior) of the oral cavity. Mastication involves breaking the food items into small pieces and the creation of a bolus. A bolus is a ball of food that can easily be moved to the back of the throat. The lips close and create a seal, and the soft palate closes down

on the back of the tongue to help form the bolus (Zemlin, 1998). Saliva and liquids in the meal lubricate the bolus. At the oral stage the tongue propels the substance posteriorly, triggering the swallowing reflex.

The second stage of the normal swallow is the pharyngeal stage. "The pharyngeal phase is complex, with many important physiological occurrences happening simultaneously and quickly" (Justice, 2006, p. 326). At the pharyngeal stage, several neuromotor events are involved in moving the bolus or liquid to a position necessary for swallowing. The velum elevates, closing off the nasal air passages. The vocal cords close, and the epiglottis covers the opening of the larynx (glottis) as a protective action. The larynx elevates and moves forward (anterior). The tongue pistons the mass of food or liquid posteriorly, and the laryngeal-esophageal stage is initiated. The third stage is called the laryngeal-esophageal rather than simply "esophageal." This is to show the importance of laryngeal protective actions during the combined stages of the swallow, particularly during the pharyngeal activities. Perlman and Christensen (1997) suggest the term "pharyngealolaryngeal" to better describe the laryngeal actions. Timing and coordination are very important to a normal swallow. These stages follow in rapid succession, and occur as often as 300 times per hour when a person eats (Zemlin, 1998). Figure 8.1 shows the movement of the bolus through the oral and pharyngeal cavities.

8.8 Neurology of Chewing and Swallowing

Swallowing is conscious, unconscious, voluntary, and involuntary. "Normal swallowing includes an integrated interdependent group of complex feeding behaviors emerging from interacting cranial nerves of the brain stem and governed by neural regulatory mechanisms in the medulla, as well as in the sensorimotor and limbic cortical systems" (Bass, 1997, p. 7). The vagus nerve is important in swallowing and may be damaged in surgery. See *Anderson v. Rengachary*, 608 NW2d 843 (Minn 2000). Table 8.2 shows the neurology of the swallow by stage/function, nerve, and muscle/tissues involved.

There are many muscles involved in swallowing, and the following discussion addresses the major ones. The most active muscle involved in chewing and swallowing is the tongue. The tongue consists of two groups of muscles: extrinsic and intrinsic. An extrinsic muscle has its origin outside the tongue and insertion (attachment) within it. The extrinsic tongue muscles, genioglossus, palatoglossus, sty-

loglossus, and hyoglossus, are involved in protruding, elevating, and depressing the tongue (Zemlin, 1998). The points of origin and insertion can often be gleaned from the names of the muscles. For example, the hyoglossus runs from the hyoid bone (hyo) to the tongue (glossus).

The intrinsic tongue muscles have both origin and insertion within the tongue. These tongue muscles have no bony attachments, and they function to shape the tongue. The intrinsic tongue muscles are classified by the orientation of the muscle fibers: longitudinal, vertical, and transverse (Perlman and Christensen, 1997).

The lips, cheeks, and jaw muscles are important in mastication. The orbicularis oris is a sphincter type muscle that opens, closes, and protrudes the lips. The buccinator flattens the cheek and holds food close to the teeth for chewing. Other muscles involved in mastication are the masseter, temporalis, and the pterygoid (medial and lateral). The palatopharyngeus and the levator and tensor palatini muscles elevate the soft palate (velum) and close off the nasopharynx. Several muscles in the larynx close and move the larynx during swallowing: thyroarytenoid, transverse arytenoid, oblique arytenoid, lateral cricoarytenoid, posterior cricoarytenoid, and thyroepiglottic muscles (Perlman and Christensen, 1997). The esophagus itself is a collapsed muscular tube approximately 23 to 25 cm long with a sphincter at each end (Logemann, 1998). Peristalsis is an important muscular function in digestion. It is the involuntary progressive contraction or "squeezing" of food and liquid for nutritional extraction.

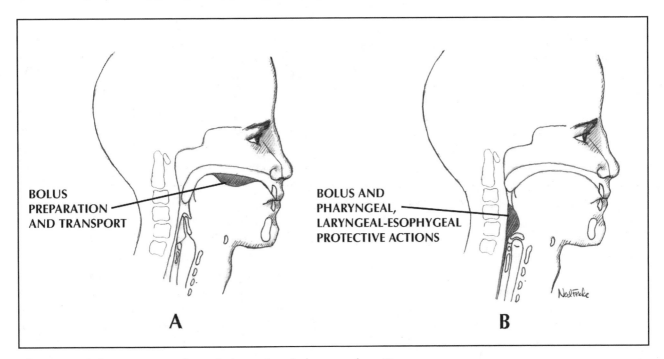

Figure 8.1 Bolus movement through the oral and pharyngeal cavities

Table 8.2
Neurology of the Swallow

Stage/Function	Nerve	Muscle/Tissue
Oral Stage (Mastication)	Trigeminal (V)	Temporalis, Masseter, Medial Pterygoid, Lateral Pterygoid
	Hypoglossal (XII) Ansa Cervicalis (C_1-C_2) Vagus (X)	Intrinsic Tongue Muscles Extrinsic Tongue Muscles Palatoglossus
Pharyngeal Stage	Glossopharyngeal (IX) Vagus (X) Trigeminal (V) $V_{(3)}$, VII, C_1-C_2	Stylopharyngeus Palate, Pharynx, and Larynx Tensor Veli Palatini Hyoid and Larynx
Laryngeal-Esophageal Stage (Completion of Swallow)	Facial (VII), Trigeminal (V), Vagus (X)	Opening of Cricopharyngeus Peristalsis
Sensation: Tongue	Lingual Nerve, Trigeminal Chorda Tympani, Facial (VII) Glossopharyngeal (IX)	General Sensation, Anterior Two-Thirds of the Tongue Taste, Anterior Two-Thirds of the Tongue Taste and General Sensation, Posterior One-Third of the Tongue
Oral Tract	Glossopharyngeal (IX), Vagus (X)	Pharynx, Larynx, Viscera

8.9 Geriatric and Pediatric Dysphagia

Although dysphagia can occur at any age, it is more frequently observed in the very old and young. Dysphagia is particularly common in elderly nursing home patients, and evaluation and treatment should be performed in a multidisciplinary/interdisciplinary team setting (Cefalu, 1999). In elderly patients, dysphagia is associated with aspiration pneumonia and death (Cowen, Simpson, and Vettese, 1997). Patients with dementia pose special problems concerning dysphagia. High-risk patients with dementia suspected of having dysphagia include those with significant weight loss or feeding difficulties, those requiring assistance with feeding, patients significantly below the ideal body weight, and those with concurrent depression or a history of cerebrovascular accidents (Cefalu, 1999). Significant weight loss is a 5 percent loss in six months or a 10 percent loss in twelve months.

Pediatric dysphagia is a rapidly evolving area of patient care. Pediatric swallowing and feeding problems are seen primarily in hospitals but also in schools. According to the American Speech-Language-Hearing Association (2006, p. 9), "Students with autism, developmental delay, mental retardation, multiple disabilities, orthopedic impairments, or traumatic brain injury may have accompanying or undiagnosed feeding and swallowing disorders." Sometimes, dysphagia in children involves nursing home services. See *Alexander v. State,* 727 So2d 1133 (Fla App 2 Dist 1999). There are important issues in pediatric patients requiring different diagnostic and treatment approaches than required in older children and adults. Pediatric dysphagia includes neurological and maturation assessment. Food tolerance and dysphagia in children have been considered in dysphagia litigation. Also, there are special dysphagia issues in children with craniofacial anomalies such as cleft lip and palate. The central difference between assessment and treatment of dysphagia in older children and adults revolves around anatomic differences. Arvedson and Brodsky (2002) list anatomic differences in the infant's and older child's upper aerodigestive tract. Important anatomical differences in the infant affecting the diagnosis and treatment of dysphagia include the following: mouth, tongue, mandible, larynx size, a narrow, vertical epiglottis, and no definite/distinct oropharynx. According to Logemann (1998), there are two important differences in the swallowing patterns of an infant and an adult. First, in the infant the laryngeal elevation is reduced since the larynx is elevated under the tongue base and does not need to move up during the pharyngeal swallow. Second, in infants the posterior pharyngeal wall moves farther anteriorly during swallowing. Figure 8.2 includes indications that an infant or young child should be referred for dysphagia evaluation.

Apnea during feeding

Dehydration

Diagnosis of neuromuscular disorders or diseases affecting swallowing

Excessive and persistent drooling

Failure to thrive

Frequent choking and/or aspiration

Frequent nasal reflux during feeding

Gastrointestinal disorders or diseases

Medications affecting alertness and/or swallowing mechanism

Presence of cleft lip and/or palate, other oral-facial anomalies affecting swallowing

Report from mother of child having sucking, swallowing and/or feeding difficulties

Significant loss of weight or failure to maintain weight

Figure 8.2 Indicators for pediatric dysphagia evaluation

8.10 Tracheotomies, Feeding Tubes, Intubation, Ventilation Devices

A tracheotomy tube is placed in a patient's neck below the vocal cords, usually between the third and fourth tracheal rings. A tracheotomy tube provides a direct route for air to enter the lungs and bypasses the larynx and upper air passageways, which may be obstructed. According to Logemann (1998), there are two important variations in tracheotomy tubes: cuffed or uncuffed and fenestrated and unfenestrated. A tracheotomy tube cuff is a balloon-like structure surrounding the lower part of the tube. When inflated the cuff presumably prevents food and liquid from entering the respiratory passageways. Obviously, an inflated tracheotomy cuff prevents a patient from producing voiced speech because no air can reach the larynx. A fenestrated tracheotomy tube, where a window is cut into the tube to allow for greater airflow, is used for patients having

difficulty producing voice with a normal tracheotomy tube (Logemann, 1998).

A common misconception is that patients with inflated tracheotomy tubes are unable to aspirate. Tracheotomy tubes may actually impede swallowing and provoke aspiration (McCulloch, Jaffe, and Hoffman, 1997). McCulloch, Jaffe, and Hoffman go on to note that the larynx is anchored by the tracheotomy tube, resulting in a decreased excursion during the swallow. Groher (1997, p. 101) reviewed several studies and concluded: "Tracheostoma tubes create a mechanical interference to swallowing by restricting normal laryngeal elevation. Loss of elevation compromises glottal protection and invites aspiration." In addition, even an inflated cuff creates a risk of aspiration because remnant food and liquid may enter the respiratory system when it is deflated. Fistulas, and improper inflation and placement of the cuffed tracheotomy tube, may also lead to aspiration. To test for adequacy of a cuff seal, a dye can be placed in the patient's mouth during the swallow. The dye should be a color not typically seen in body fluids. If it is present during tracheal suctioning or coughing (through the trach), then the cuff seal is insufficient. This is because the dye bypassed the seal into the patient's airway. Gastric tubes are used for patients who have a poor prognosis of dysphagia and are usually permanent. A gastric tube is placed directly into the patient's stomach and is sometimes called a PEG tube. The surgical procedure to create an opening in the stomach is called a gastrotomy (Dirckx, 1997).

Some patients require nasogastric feeding tubes. A nasogastric tube, sometimes called an "NG" tube, is placed through the patient's nose to his or her stomach. Liquid and nutritional supplements are supplied to the patient through the tube. Some authorities on dysphagia contend that nasogastric feeding tubes do not compromise swallowing, and others note a lack of research on the subject. Patients often report that nasogastric tubes are foreign and irritating. Lacking research on the effects of nasogastric feeding tubes and swallowing, it is prudent to assume they potentially disrupt and interfere with the swallow in some patients.

Intubation is the insertion of a tube into body structure to keep it open. The tube is placed through the mouth or nose or through the trachea to allow breathing. Schulze-Delrieu and Miller (1997) note: "Indwelling cannulas may interfere with swallowing, increase the risk of aspiration, and interfere with effective clearance of aspirated materials" (p. 140). According to Logemann (1998), prolonged tube placement can cause redness, edema, nodule or polyp formation, unilateral adductor paresis or paralysis, and consequently reduce laryngeal closure during the swallow.

A mechanical ventilator is a device for providing prolonged ventilation or breathing. Ventilators are used for patients who cannot breathe sufficiently on their own, and they disrupt swallowing. Most patients with chronic compromised breathing are mechanically ventilated through a tracheal tube. The tracheotomy tube interferes with swallowing in the manner described above. In addition, mechanical ventilators disrupt breathing-swallowing coordination and thus can contribute to dysphagia.

8.11 The Dysphagia Evaluation

The following describes a comprehensive dysphagia evaluation. It addresses the sensory and motor acts of transferring a substance from the mouth to stomach and the emotional and cognitive aspects associated with eating and meeting nutrition and hydration needs orally. The clinical/bedside assessment can be conducted by using a checklist format such as is used in the *Quick Assessment for Dysphagia* (Tanner and Culbertson, 1999). It is provided in Appendix B.

8.12 Review of Social and Medical History

Before the bedside assessment can be conducted, the patient's relevant medical history is reviewed. The patient's admitting diagnosis lists the reasons for admission to the facility. If the admitting diagnosis includes dysphagia, an automatic recommendation for a video swallow study (VSS) is warranted. The admitting diagnosis of dysphagia requires cinefluorographic examination of the swallow because the patient has sufficient medical history warranting comprehensive swallowing assessment. Biographical reports, social and medical history alluding to dysphagia, are also important. The admission diagnosis should be reviewed for indirect indications of dysphagia: terms such as "drooling," "eating difficulty," "dehydration" and the previous placement of a feeding tube.

Reviewing the chart for medical disorders that compromise the patient's respiratory function is also important. This is because aspiration pneumonia can exacerbate problems with respiration. Respiratory disorders, such as chronic obstructive pulmonary disease (COPD), suggest that the patient has compromised breathing. Chronic obstructive pulmonary disease is a general classification for diseases with permanent or temporary narrowing of the small bronchi in which forced expiratory flow is slowed and is used when more specific terms cannot be applied (Dirckx, 2001).

A history of speech and voice disorders also shows the need to provide comprehensive clinical/bedside assessment and instrumental diagnostic procedures. History or reports of changes in the patient's speech suggest neuromuscular

disorders associated with dysphagia. As noted previously, although dysphagia can occur independently of neuromuscular disorders, it is frequently a part of the symptoms presented with motor speech disorders. Strokes, head trauma, and progressive neuromuscular disorders such as multiple sclerosis and Parkinson's disease have a high occurrence of dysphagia, especially during late stages. Also, medical histories showing dementia should alert the team to the potential of dysphagia that can lead to malnutrition (Cefalu, 1999).

The medication regimen is reviewed to learn the effects on the patient's cognitive and physical abilities and salivation. Schulze-Delrieu and Miller (1997) describe product categories of medications and their potential effects on swallowing. Neuroleptics (psychotrophics) such as Elavil (tricyclic), Haldol, and Thorazine can cause drying of mucosa, drowsiness, altered mental status, muscle rigidity, and tardive dyskinesia (involuntary movements caused by long-term use of medications). Barbiturates and antihistamines can cause drowsiness. In addition, antihistamines and diuretics can dry the mucosa. Mucosal anesthetics, used to aid passage of fiberoptic nasopharyngoscopes, can suppress the gag and cough reflexes.

The nature of the patient's family and social support is reviewed. It is particularly important to note if family and friends of the patient feed him or her and whether this is done with medical supervision. Well-intentioned family members and friends can sometimes be unaware of the seriousness of dysphagia and secretly give the patient comfort foods and liquids. The patient's psychological adjustment to the disorder should also be noted. Is he or she depressed, angry, or anxious about the disorder? Functional dysphagia has been a litigation issue see *McDonald v. Bowen*, 818 F2d 559 (7th Cir1986).

Obtaining medical history includes more than chart review. Standards of practice require that nurses and aides be interviewed about the patient's swallowing status. Questions about the patient's abilities to meet his or her nutrition and hydration needs and issues related to tube feedings are asked before the clinical/bedside evaluation. Nurses can also report information about the patient's eating patterns, food likes and dislikes, and other information related to dysphagia. Nursing interviews provide the most current information about the patient's swallowing status and are essential to a comprehensive dysphagia assessment.

8.13 Appetite History

Obviously, a patient whose appetite is suppressed may refuse food and liquid. Reduced appetite can complicate feeding and attempts to meet the patient's nutrition and hydration needs orally. In the broad definition of dysphagia reported above, dysphagia can be inclusive of suppressed appetite and reduced eating pleasure.

Reduced eating pleasure may be associated with impairments or reductions in the sense of smell and taste. The patient is asked about his or her senses of smell and taste and possible effects they may have on appetite. Three cranial nerves are important to smell and taste. The olfactory nerve conveys odors to the central nervous system. This sense is closely associated with the sense of taste, which is the function of the several cranial nerves. Loss of taste and smell is associated with radiation therapy. Groher (1997) reviewed several studies and found that over half the patients undergoing irradiation experienced loss of appetite due to disruptions of the sense of taste, feelings of nausea, and a general dissatisfaction with diet. Taste typically returned within two to four months following radiotherapy. Aversion to foods such as meat and vegetables was noted. Sour and bitter tastes may be suppressed more than sweet and salty ones.

Psychological factors influencing appetite and eating pleasure can include anorexia nervosa. Anorexia nervosa is a psychological disorder involving fear of becoming obese and an aversion to eating. In some patients negative emotions may be conditioned to eating due to choking and aspiration. These patients may have anxiety and fear about eating because of classically conditioned (Pavlovian) negative emotions to certain food and eating stimuli. These negative emotions may also cause hypertense face and neck muscles and consequently impair the swallowing reflex.

8.14 Clinical/Bedside Assessment of Swallowing

The American Speech-Language-Hearing Association (2000) separates the clinical/bedside dysphagia evaluation from the instrumental one. They are two related but clinically separate activities. The clinical/bedside examination includes the above review of medical records, assessment protocols, and observations. According to the American Speech-Language-Hearing Association (2000), the clinical/bedside examination may include cervical auscultation and pulse oximetry to monitor clinical symptoms of dysphagia. Also included in the clinical/bedside examination are the structural and functional assessments of the muscles and structures discussed below.

After reviewing the chart and interviewing family, nurses, and aides, the clinical/beside evaluation is conducted. Sometimes a patient is designated "NPO," which means that he or she should not be given food or liquids orally. In most hospitals and nursing homes, it is understood

that the speech-language pathologist may provide food and liquid to the patient as part of the swallowing evaluation. However, prudent practice dictates that the clinician check with the attending physician for authorization to give the NPO patient food and liquid orally. If it is learned that the patient remains NPO, then an indirect clinical/bedside evaluation is conducted by observing speech production and oral motor and sensory functioning.

Bedside Assessment: Oral Stage

Accept food and create bolus
Lip seal
Mastication
Dentition
Salivation and drooling
Pocketing
Tongue mobility
Mandibular movements
Impulsivity

Figure 8.3 *Salient aspects of the oral stage of swallowing assessment (Source: Tanner and Culbertson, 1999)*

There are several ways clinicians quantify and qualify the patient's swallowing behaviors. Some clinicians operationally describe the swallow. Others simply use a yes/no system to identify those behaviors the patient is capable of performing and those he or she is incapable of doing. A modified Likert Scale is useful in recording the results of the clinical/bedside evaluation (Tanner and Culbertson, 1999). The scale ranges from "0," clearly abnormal or nonfunctional, to "5," indicating clearly normal or functional behaviors. This scale can be used for test-retest comparisons, and combining of the categorical scores.

8.15 Oral Stage

Some speech-language pathologists do not make clinical distinctions between oral preparation and transportation during the clinical/bedside evaluation. This is because both facets of the oral stage use essentially the same musculature and the therapies are not fundamentally different for problems arising at this level. Clinical/bedside assessment of the oral stage involves learning whether the patient can accept food and liquid, create a bolus, and successfully move it along the palatal vault to the back of the throat. Factors to assess include whether the patient can create a lip seal and chew successfully. The patient's teeth are examined to see whether they are adequate for chewing. A determination is made whether the patient has enough salivation to moisten the food, and whether tongue and mandibular mobility are adequate. Some patients are unable to swallow their oral secretions and thus drool. Drooling can be caused by inattention, excessive mucous buildup, sensory deficits, and deficient swallowing. Tongue mobility is usually assessed for protrusion, retraction, lateralization, elevation, and depression. Speed of the movements can be determined by assessing the oral diadochokinetic rate. Oral diadochokinetic rate is the speed of sequential oral movements, usually assessed by having the patient rapidly repeat: "puh," "duh," and "kuh." For young children, a word such as "buttercup" can be used for assessment. The adequacy of the patient to propel the bolus along the palatal vault is determined as is whether he or she pockets particles of food or liquid in his or her cheeks. In addition, there is assessment of the patient's cognitive and perceptual abilities to recognize food and liquids, and a determination is made about whether he or she is impulsive. Figure 8.3 lists the salient aspects of the oral stage of the clinical/bedside assessment.

8.16 Pharyngeal Stage

The pharyngeal stage of the swallow is initiated when the bolus or liquid reaches the pharynx. At this stage there is velopharyngeal closure, which is a valving action. Velopharyngeal closure is the closing of the nasal cavity from the oral cavity. The velum (soft palate) and the muscles at the back of the throat (posterior pharyngeal wall) meet, thus separating the oral and nasal cavities. Velopharyngeal incompetence is the lack of this closure due to muscular weakness or paralysis. Velopharyngeal insufficiency is usually a result of a cleft or other structural deficiency of the velum. If there is velopharyngeal incompetence or insufficiency at this stage of the swallow, the patient may have food or liquid penetrate the nasal cavity.

The gag reflex provides information about the patient's oral sensation, muscular strength, and control. According to Schulze-Delrieu and Miller (1997), the sensory and motor neurons of the IXth and Xth cranial nerves mediate the gag reflex. Although the gag reflex can provide valuable information about neuromotor control of the oral mechanism, several authors have noted that either diminished or hyperactive gag reflexes have little predictive value about the patient's swallowing safely.

Peristalsis is the rhythmic contraction of muscles in a tube to propel food. At the pharyngeal level, there is a peristalsis effect, an automatic contraction-relaxation. It is important that the oral stage be coordinated with the pharyngeal stage. According to Logemann (1998), delayed pharyngeal swallow occurs when the bolus enters the pharynx before the pharyngeal swallow has been triggered, causing problems with swallowing liquids. "If the pharyngeal swallow has not been initiated as the liquid passes the tongue base, there is increased risk that the liquid will enter the open airway before the pharyngeal swallow has been activated" (Logemann, 1998, p. 93).

8.17 Laryngeal-Esophageal Stage

"The cervical esophageal phase of deglutition involves the initial peristaltic wave in the esophageal musculature" (Logemann, 1998, p. 110). The esophagus is a muscular tube capable of peristalsis and connects the oral cavity with the stomach. The cervical esophagus begins at the level of the second and third thoracic vertebrae and ends at the thoracic inlet (Perlman and Christensen, 1997). Logemann (1998) notes that the esophageal stage of the swallow cannot be modified by therapy. According to Ravich (1997), esophageal dysphagia can be caused by structural abnormalities and motor dysfunctions. Structural abnormalities include luminal stenosis and deformity, and motor impairments include abnormalities of peristalsis and sphincter function. Diagnosis of a perforated esophagus and interpretation of a video swallow study have been forensic issues. An important aspect of the laryngeal-esophageal stage is the strength of throat-clearing, and a determination is made about the productivity of the patient's cough.

8.18 The Dynamic Swallow

The clinical practice of artificially separating swallowing into as many as four independent and distinct stages, i.e., oral preparation, transportation, pharyngeal, and laryngeal-esophageal, is misleading regarding the actual nature of chewing and swallowing. These are artificial clinical distinctions used to evaluate the swallow, show the need for radiologic evaluation, and for therapy purposes. The reality is that people put food in their mouths, chew, and then they swallow it. Artificially dividing swallowing into several independent movements is analogous to viewing running as many independent movements. For example, swallowing, as with running, cannot be completed by any of the acts occurring independently. Running and swallowing are dynamic acts. When evaluating swallowing, the beside examination can only determine "possible" structural, neurological, or muscular deficiencies that may interfere with the movement of the bolus or liquid. There can be no certainty that a patient will or will not choke or aspirate at any level or stage based on clinical/bedside swallowing examination. If there is sufficient reason to believe that a patient has compromised swallowing, regardless of the deficient stage, the prudent clinical course is to conduct one or more instrumental evaluations of the sequentially occurring swallow. Neglecting to conduct an instrumental evaluation of the swallow in cases of suspected dysphagia is analogous to refusing to X-ray a leg for suspected fractures.

Structural and functional assessment of the muscles and structures used in swallowing

Functional assessment of actual swallowing ability

Assessment of adequacy of airway protection and coordination of respiration and swallowing

Screening of esophageal motility and gastro-esophageal reflux

Assessment of the effect of changes in bolus delivery:

Textural alterations/bolus characteristics

Use of therapeutic postures

Use of maneuvers on the swallow

Figure 8.4 *Instrumental assessment of dysphagia [Source: American Speech-Language-Hearing Association (2000)]*

8.19 Clinical Indicators for Radiologic and Instrumental Assessment of Dysphagia

The American Speech-Language-Hearing Association (2000) executive summary on clinical indicators for instrumental assessment of dysphagia provides guidance but not official standards for the association. Instrumental examination involves fluoroscopy, ultrasound, and manometry. Instrumental assessment includes functional assessment of actual swallowing and assessment of adequacy of airway protection (see Figure 8.4). A video swallowing study, also called a videofluoroscopic swallowing study (VFSS), is the most common instrumental assessment. The speech-language pathologist is present during the test and may give the patient liquid barium and several barium soaked foods of differing consistencies. In addition, during the test, the speech-language pathologist tries several compensatory actions with the patient to see if there are ways to prevent choking and/or aspiration. Endoscopic assessment of the swallowing function is gaining acceptance among some speech-language pathologists. In this instrumental assessment, a fiberoptic endoscope is passed through the nose, permitting inspection of the swallowing mechanisms and functions, including the potential for aspiration (ASHA, 2002). According to the American Speech-Language-Hearing Association (2000), the signs and symptoms indicating instrumental dysphagia examination include complaints or sensations reported by the patient and/or caregivers and variables derived from the medical history. Daniels, McAdams, Brailey, and Foundas (1997) found several factors predicting the severity of dysphagia. Dysphonia, dysarthria, abnormal volitional cough, abnormal gag reflex, abnormal cough reflex, cough after swallow, and voice change

had predictive value in determining the severity of dysphagia and the need for instrumental examination.

Clinical/bedside and instrumental assessments of dysphagia have the potential for false positive and negative results. A false positive test result says a patient has dysphagia/aspiration when in reality he or she is free from the disorders. A false negative test result says a patient does not have dysphagia/aspiration when in reality he or she is dysphagic and/or aspirates. Repeated tests are necessary to check the reliability of an assessment. Reilly (2004, p. 176) notes: "In summary, although the worthiness of the instrumental and non-instrumental examinations would not be questioned by clinicians, the scientific validity and psychometric properties of procedures in common use are some way from being established."

8.20 The Treatment of Dysphagia

The ultimate objective of dysphagia treatment is to improve the patient's swallowing abilities to the extent that he or she can meet hydration and nutritional needs orally. This requires elimination of the risks of choking and aspiration pneumonia. It is hoped that the patient can attain oral neuromuscular levels of functioning that will allow his or her diet to be normal in taste and dietary consistency, thus improving the overall quality of life.

In the treatment of dysphagia the thickness of liquids and the texture of foods are adjusted and modified. Thin liquids tend to be more difficult to manage, and a thickener is added. The amount of thickener determines the consistency. There are liquids that are naturally thick, such as some soups, sauces, and gravies. As a rule, food textures are adjusted by the kitchen staff. Dry and hard-to-manage foods can be made more manageable by the addition of gravy or sauces. The temperature of the food and liquid is also an important part of dysphagia management. Foods and liquids that are either hot or cold can better be tracked in the mouth and throat. They help the patient, particularly those with compromised sensation, to monitor his or her swallow. Tepid foods and liquids are typically avoided.

Patient positioning is also important in dysphagia therapy. Patients swallow better when sitting up rather than lying down. The goal is to permit gravity to help the swallow. In addition, some patients do better when leaning a little forward or backward, with a chin-up or chin-down posture during different stages of the swallow, and in the case of laryngeal paralysis or paresis with their heads turned.

There are several non-swallowing exercises and activities used to improve the strength, range-of-motion, and coordination of the swallowing stages. Specific muscles and muscle groups are targeted. When possible, these exercises are combined with speech drills for patients with dysarthria.

In swallowing therapy, the clinician instructs the patient on how to improve muscle coordination during the swallow. In addition, there are demonstrations of how to swallow and clear food from the posterior cavity. There are also instructions, exercises, and demonstrations on how to remove pooled liquid and food particles from above the glottis. For example, in some patients, it is helpful to push air out of their lungs by producing a voiced sound such as "ah" at the end of each swallow. This prevents seepage of liquids and food particles into the lungs. Dry swallows are also encouraged where the patient swallows one or more times after the food and liquid have been swallowed. There is gradual step-by-step progression of drills designed to help the patient either compensate for the swallowing problem or eliminate it. Patient feedback is an important aspect of this therapy. Feedback about swallowing abilities is provided on a daily, weekly, and monthly basis. Sometimes redoing a video swallowing study, or other instrumental test, to assess the success of treatment is necessary. Most patients maintain high levels of motivation in dysphagia therapy because of the improvement they have in eating and the likelihood that they will again be able to meet hydration and nutrition needs orally.

8.21 Dysphagia Management Malpractice Litigation and the Expert Witness

When litigating dysphagia management malpractice, the primary expert witness is often a professor of speech-language pathology or a speech and hearing scientist who also has extensive clinical experience and whom the plaintiff's attorney has retained (Tanner, 2006). It is important that the dysphagia expert witness have extensive clinical experience because pure academic experts may be unfamiliar with practical dysphagia management issues in hospitals, nursing homes, and home health agencies. Although academics may be competent to testify about theoretical issues in dysphagia, choking, and aspiration, they have an incomplete understanding of the complexities of managing dysphagia in several medical settings and through a team approach. When an academic is used as a dysphagia expert witness, he or she may be unable to opine as to the pragmatic issues involved in the specific case, and his or her testimony may be impeached. Depending on the type of dysphagia management negative outcome being litigated, the dysphagia expert witness will testify as to the adequacy of clinical documentation, swallowing evaluation, competency and proficiency of the speech-language pathologist in dysphagia

management, professional communication, and dysphagia effects on the patient's quality of life. The structure for preparing an expert opinion is usually established through the creation of a clinical timeline.

The dysphagia expert witness will prepare a timeline of events to show what the healthcare professionals did concerning dysphagia diagnosis and treatment by examining extensive amounts of medical information, usually involving several medical facilities. The goal is to determine "who did what, when, and where, and the probable clinical outcome." All relevant medical records are reviewed, but especially dysphagia referrals and orders, bedside evaluation reports, progress notes, video swallow studies, and communications with the patient, the patient's family, and other healthcare professionals. The timeline of events shows whether members of the medical team engaged in commissions or omissions that may have resulted in or contributed to the negative outcome. It is likely that the alleged dysphagia malpractice occurred several years previously, so the medical records are critical in reconstructing the clinical events. Each page is stamped with a number for easy reference during conferences, depositions, and trials. Once the timeline is created, the expert witness and the attorney confer about the important legal issues and merits of the case.

To ensure maximum objectivity, the dysphagia expert witness and his or her staff should create and review the timeline independently. Each party to the eventual final expert opinion should reach independent decisions about the primary healthcare professionals involved, omissions and commissions concerning the management of dysphagia, what facility or facilities for whom they were acting as agents, and "probable" clinical outcomes of their actions or inactions. The distinction between "possible" and "probable" can be an important issue in dysphagia litigation especially concerning the clinical timeline.

A health care provider's action that "possibly" resulted in a negative dysphagia management outcome suggests that his or her actions were capable of causing the clinical effect. However, this opinion is essentially useless because virtually anything is possible. A statement that an action was "probably" the cause of a negative dysphagia management outcome shows that it likely caused the clinical effect. There can degrees of probability in assessing a healthcare provider's action in a dysphagia malpractice lawsuit and the expert witness can provide confidence levels of the opinion by providing percentages. For example, expert can state that he or she is 60 percent, 75 percent or 90 percent certain that the action resulted in or contributed to the negative dysphagia management outcome.

8.22 Dysphagia Management Malpractice Litigation and Clinical Documentation

As noted above, in dysphagia litigation, who did what, when, and where and the clinical outcomes may become an issue in patient management. "Clear and comprehensive records are necessary to justify the need for treatment, to document the effectiveness of that treatment, and to have a legal record of events" (ASHA, 1994, p. 355). Speech-language pathologists and audiologists have official guidelines from the American Speech-Language-Hearing Association about clinical record keeping (see Figures 8.5, 8.6, and 8.7). There are also indirect requirements for documentation in the Code of Ethics of the American Speech-Language-Hearing Association and other professional guidelines. In addition, medical care facilities, Medicare, Medicaid, private insurance carriers, and accrediting bodies have general and specific requirements for documentation. According to Swigert (2002), for Medicare claims there should be documentation that the speech pathology services are specific, effective, skilled, and the treatment goals must be likely to achieve improvement within a reasonable period. In addition, a speech-language pathologist must have a documented physician's order for an evaluation. For treatment, effective documentation must show the frequency and length of the sessions. Swigert notes that irregularities in documentation may include allegations that the therapy goals were too ambitious, the patient had met the goals but the services continued, and the patient was not meeting the goals but a reevaluation was not completed. "The therapy must require the knowledge, skills, and judgment that only the certified and licensed SLP can provide" (Swigert, 2002, p. 14). Daily progress notes must be kept for each session. Many clinicians use a modified "SOAP" format (subjective, objective, assessment, plan).

Treatment plans must contain short-term and long-term goals. A long-term goal might be independent oral eating ability, i.e., the patient can meet hydration and nutrition needs orally. Short-term goals are sequential objectives to meet the long-term ones. According to the American Speech-Language-Hearing Association (1994), clinical records should be stored in a secure place and accessed only by authorized personnel. Fifteen working days is the specified time frame for sending reports and information to other professionals. Historical clinical records should be transferred to microfilm, maintained through computer storage, and secure in a less accessible place but away from current files. The length of time records must be kept varies with facilities, state laws, and the age of the patient/client. According to ASHA (1994), seven years is usually the maximum length except for minors. It may be necessary to keep some records permanently, or for several years after the patient attains the age of majority. Hospitals and medical care facilities have medical records divisions that comply with these requirements.

The following are miscellaneous factors that may become issues in dysphagia litigation and are detailed in ASHA standards for clinical record keeping (ASHA, 1994):

- Writing should be accurate, concise, and informative.

- Writing should be neat and legible.

- Clinical records need to be organized with entries recorded chronologically.

- Blank spaces should not be left to be filled out at a later time.

- Current symbols or abbreviations from an approved facility list can be used.

- There should be proofreading of documentation to verify accuracy.

- There should be avoidance of personal or flippant remarks.

---

1. Date of initial assessment/reassessment
2. Initial functional status of client in present facility based upon:
   a. Baseline testing (using standardized and nonstandardized measures)
   b. Interpretation of test scores/results
   c. Other clinical finding (including those from other specialists)
3. Documentation that speech-language pathology evaluations considered a client's hearing status
4. Statement of prognosis
5. Recommendations based on the client's functional needs (including referrals as appropriate)
6. Signature and title of qualified professional responsible for the assessment (and that of the documentor, if different)

Figure 8.5 *Required clinical record keeping for speech-language pathology assessment (Source: ASHA, 1994)*

- All medical/clinical records are the property of the facility and confidential unless otherwise provided by law.

- Clinical records must be treated as legal documents, including typing and using ink for permanence, signing all record entries with name and professional title, and dating and initialing materials from other facilities before entering them into a permanent record.

8.23 Dysphagia Management Malpractice Litigation and Clinician Proficiency

In dysphagia litigation, the clinical competence of a speech-language pathologist may be called into question. Although speech-language pathologists are certified clinically competent by the American Speech-Language-Hearing Association and states have licensure laws, there are special knowledge and skills required of them in dysphagia management. The following dysphagia management competencies are based, in part, on a task force report prepared by the American Speech-Language-Hearing Association (1990). Below is a condensed summary of that official position statement that can be used to explore competence in dysphagia patient management.

Identification of Individuals at Risk for Dysphagia: Clinicians should be proficient in identifying individuals at risk for dysphagia. The knowledge base and skills necessary for this proficiency include, but are not limited to, recognizing signs and symptoms of dysphagia, review of the client/patient's medical status, assessment of cognitive, communication, behavioral, and social status, and oral intake situations. In addition, clinicians should be knowledgeable of medical diagnoses and the methods for communicating a client/patient's need for instrumental dysphagia assessment, and the interpretation of risk factors for dysphagia.

Clinical Oral-Pharyngeal and Respiratory Examination with a Detailed History: Clinicians should be proficient in conducting a swallowing mechanism examination. The knowledge base and skills necessary for this proficiency include, but are not limited to, identification of normal and abnormal structure, function, symptoms, medical conditions, and medications pertinent to dysphagia. Clinicians should possess knowledge of the limitations of the clinical/bedside examination, specifically regarding detecting aspiration. In addition, clinicians should possess a knowledge of tracheotomy tubes and ventilators affecting the swallowing mechanism.

---

1. Date plan of treatment established
2. Short-and long-term functional communication goals
3. Treatment objectives
4. Recommended type and expected amount, frequency and duration
5. Follow-up activities
6. Statement of prognosis
7. Date treatment plan was discussed with client and/or family
8. Date interdisciplinary conferences were held
9. Statement of the schedule for review of the plan
10. Signature and title of qualified professional responsible for treatment plan (and that of the documentor, if different)

Figure 8.6 *Required clinical record keeping for speech-language pathology treatment plan (Source: ASHA, 1994)*

---

1. Date client began treatment at present facility
2. Time period covered by the report
3. Summaries of assessment and treatment plan in treatment reports
4. Number of times to date that treatment was rendered in present facility and length of sessions
5. Current client status
6. Any changes in prognosis
7. Any changes in plan of treatment
8. Follow-up recommendations or description of need for continued intervention
9. Signature and title of professional responsible for treatment services (and that of the documentor, if different).

Figure 8.7 *Required clinical documentation of treatment for speech-language pathology (Source: ASHA, 1994)*

Instrumental/Structural Physiologic Examination with Related Professionals: Clinicians should be knowledgeable and proficient in identifying available and appropriate testing resources and be able to recommend such tests as videofluoroscopy, manometry, electromyography, and ultrasonography. Clinicians should be able to interpret information from those tests and make appropriate recommendation jointly with a physician. The knowledge base and skills necessary for this proficiency include, but are not limited to, knowing the advantages and limitations of instrumental tests with a particular patient or type of swallowing disorder, and being able to interpret the data resulting from instrumental assessments.

Patient/Client Management Decisions Regarding Methods of Oral Intake, Risk Precautions, Candidacy for Intervention, and Treatment Strategies with Related Professionals: Clinicians should be able to identify acceptable oral intake methods, educate support personnel, and document management decisions including long-term and short-term goals. Specifically, the clinician should be proficient in the identification of risk and appropriate precautions in dysphagia. The knowledge base and skills necessary for this proficiency include, but are not limited to, precautions to reduce medical risks associated with alternate and supplemental oral intake devices, existing treatment procedures, and use of support personnel. The clinician should be knowledgeable about the client/patient's medical status.

Treatment with Related Professionals as Appropriate: Clinicians should be able to identify the client/patient's need for modification of diet and oral intake in the provision of all types of direct and indirect dysphagia treatment. In addition, the clinician should interpret, quantify, and revise the client's responses to treatment and communicate them to appropriate professionals. The knowledge base and skills necessary for this proficiency include, but are not limited to, learning theory, behavior modification, anatomy and physiology of swallowing, and cognitive factors associated with dysphagia management. Clinicians should be knowledgeable of treatment strategies described in the literature.

Education, Counseling, and Training to Patient, Family, Significant Others, Dysphagia Team, and Health Professionals: Clinicians should be able to identify educational needs and provide programs of continuing education, counseling, and patient advocacy regarding swallowing. In addition, clinicians should be able to instruct other health care professionals in dysphagia management. The knowledge base and skills necessary for this proficiency include, but are not limited to, education, behavior modification, counseling principles, and patient monitoring.

Manage and/or Participate in Interdisciplinary Dysphagia Team: Clinicians should identify team members and supportive services and engage in appropriate communication and facilitation of the team's activities. The knowledge base and skills necessary for this proficiency include, but are not limited to, roles and responsibilities of team members in dysphagia management.

Archives of Physical Medicine and Rehabilitation
Dysphagia Journal
Gastroenterology
Journal of the American Geriatric Society
Journal of Head and Neck Cancer
Journal of Medical Speech Pathology
Journal of Pediatric Gastroenterology and Nutrition
Journal of Speech and Hearing Research/Journal of Speech, Language, and Hearing Research
Neurology

(Pediatric)

Developmental Medicine and Child Neurology
American Journal of Diseases of Children

Figure 8.8 *Journals addressing dysphagia in children and adults [Source: American Speech-Language-Hearing Association (1997)]*

Knowledge base and skills about dysphagia diagnosis and treatment can be documented in several ways. First, university programs in communication sciences and disorders provide a broad education in swallowing disorders. Most programs offer at least one course specifically on dysphagia, usually at the graduate level, and many other courses indirectly address it. University programs also provide basic practicum experiences in dysphagia where clinicians can develop requisite skills in its management. To obtain the Certificate of Clinical Competence in Speech-Language Pathology, the graduate must also pass the national examination. It addresses dysphagia. Second, the American Speech-Language-Hearing Association requires continuing education of members, and most states require it as part of their annual licensing of speech and hearing professionals. Dysphagia management courses are included in authorized areas of continuing education. Third, members of the American Speech-Language-Hearing Association (ASHA) also receive journals with articles on dysphagia. Those journals, and others, are also available in college libraries, and some are now retrievable on the World Wide Web. Journals give the clinician current scientific advances in the diagnosis and treatment of dysphagia. Figure 8.8 lists journals addressing dysphagia in children and adults. Fourth, ASHA sponsors an annual national convention. Papers, miniseminairs, short courses, and poster sessions are offered on dysphagia. Annual conventions are also offered by most state associations. Finally, clinicians can improve their knowledge base and skills in the diagnosis and treatment of dysphagia through inservice training programs. These programs are offered by universities, hospitals, schools, and some are now available on the World Wide Web. Many hospitals require their employees and consultants to attend them. In dysphagia litigation a clinician's proficiency in dysphagia diagnosis and treatment, at least partially, can be learned from his or her participation in the above educational and training opportunities and programs.

8.24 Dysphagia Management Malpractice Litigation and Adequacy of Professional Communication

Many professionals are directly or indirectly involved in dysphagia diagnosis and treatment (see Table 8.1), and clear and timely professional communication is vital to proper patient management. The patient's primary care physician is involved in all relevant communication regarding the patient's dysphagia for he or she is ultimately responsible for the medical management of the disorder. Both formal and informal modes of communication are provided to the primary care physician. Formal written clinical reports and histories are available to the physician in a timely manner in the medical chart, through consultation copies placed in his or her hospital mailbox, and through email and faxes. Informal verbal communication about the patient's dysphagia occurs in staff meetings, telephone conversations, and through personal contacts during rounds. The registered nurse is also kept in the communication loop through the formal and informal modes of communication available to the attending physician. The licensed practical nurse and certified nursing assistant note dysphagia issues formally through nursing notes and also with verbal reports to the registered nurse. The registered dietician and/or nutritionist attend regularly scheduled staff meetings and communicates issues related to the temperature and texture of the patient's meals and special dietary concerns. Changes in patient dysphagia status and diet are noted in the chart and verbally. The radiologist and speech-language pathologist conduct videofluoroscopic swallowing studies together, review swallowing status, and report the results to members of the dysphagia team. Formal and informal avenues of communication are open to occupational therapists, pulmonologists, respiratory therapists, gastroenterologists, neurologists, pediatricians, and otolaryngologists as needed by a particular patient. The social worker is responsible for seeing that communication is open and unimpeded and for soliciting family and patient input.

Timely communication is important in dysphagia management because of the health risks. Many hospitals require dysphagia evaluations to be conducted within twenty-four hours of referral. Designation of patients as NPO is communicated immediately to staff and others who may be involved in providing the patient with food or liquid orally. This is done by chart notation and verbally.

Because of the problems that can arise in medical communication, many hospitals and medical care facilities have developed critical pathways. A critical pathway is a set of required tests, consultations, and other procedures automatically ordered and prescribed for a particular injury or disease. A goal of a critical pathway is to insure that all necessary medical diagnostics and treatments for a particular injury or disease are provided to a patient and not omitted through a failure of communication. For example, under a critical pathway, a stroke patient admitted with a history of dysphagia requires an automatic referral to the speech pathology service for a swallowing evaluation. Critical pathways are created by medical committees and set minimum diagnostic and treatment guidelines for a particular type of admission.

There are several checks provided by hospitals and medical care facilities for review of dysphagia communication and management. Quality assurance and medical utilization review committees are used by hospitals and medical care facilities to oversee diagnostic and treatment practices. In addition, regulating and certifying agencies at the state and federal level do regular reviews, including site visits, of hospitals and medical care facilities. These committees and regulating and certifying bodies address the provision of dysphagia communication and services.

8.25 Dysphagia Management Malpractice Litigation and Patient Quality of Life

Dysphagia disability determination is not often an issue because most patients are severely disabled by the medical condition or conditions causing it. Pure dysphagia, swallowing problems occurring independently of other medical conditions, is rare. Return to gainful employment is not an option for the majority of patients with dysphagia because of other medical factors such as paralysis. For patients returning to employment, the disabilities resulting from dysphagia are usually temporary. Either the patient can return to gainful employment because the dysphagia is resolved, or a permanent gastric tube is placed and the patient can function relatively independently. The patient provides himself or herself with nutrition and hydration through the gastric tube four or five times per day. Patients with partial dysphagia usually can meet oral nutrition and hydration needs by liquid meals or special diets. Although there are certain inconveniences with chronic dysphagia, the limits to employment are minimal. Quality of life, however, may be significantly reduced by chronic dysphagia.

There are several factors to be considered in assessing a dysphagic person's quality of life. Lawton (1991) defines quality of life in a multidimensional framework inclusive of both subjective and objective criteria: objective environment, behavioral competence, perceived quality of life, and psychological well-being. In Lawton's model, these four critical domains interact among each other. The patient's objective environment and behavioral competence are generally unaffected by dysphagia. Even patients who must take food and liquids through gastric tubes or make accommodations for special diets are not environmentally deprived by the inconveniences associated with gastric tube feedings or special diets. The environment can still provide the requirements to meet basic needs and to thrive. The patient is not behaviorally incompetent. The patient with pure dysphagia can interact with and exercise basic control over his or her environment. The patient's mobility and abilities to interact with his or her environment are not necessarily affected by pure dysphagia. However, the patient's perceived quality of life and psychological well-being can be dramatically affected by loss of oral eating abilities. Oral eating is a satisfying human social ritual, and for some patients, one of the few pleasurable abilities remaining to them. It often provides time and opportunity for interaction with others. Chronic dysphagia can affect the patient's subjective judgment about his or her satisfaction with life in general. As a subjective judgment, the previous role oral eating played in the patient's satisfaction with life is weighed. For some patients oral eating may have been a minor contributor in their perceived quality of life, while with others it may have been substantial. For the latter, dysphagia may result in a sense of loss. Loss of function, one aspect of loss of self, may result in several adjustment stages, including depression (Tanner, 2003; Tanner and Gerstenberger, 1996).

8.26 Case Studies in Dysphagia Malpractice Litigation
A. Case Study Number One: Silent Aspiration; Failure to Place Patient on NPO Status

This case involved the death of a seventy-six-year-old male who had previously undergone coronary bypass surgery. During the surgery there was a possible allergic reaction to medication. Subsequently the patient experienced loss of appetite, and family members noted difficulty swallowing, which nursing staff confirmed. Also, there were several indications that the patient suffered a stroke during or after the heart surgery; his face sagged, and he became disoriented and lethargic, and experienced judgment impairments, disorientation, and short-term memory loss. He was weak and had difficulty breathing.

Depositions from family members said that the patient would have a "hard time" swallowing foods, would take very small bites, and complained of swallowing problems. There were chart notations that the patient had "occasional non-productive coughs." The patient's daughter noted that he would chew for a very long time and attempt to swallow but the food would not go down. The daughter gave him pureed food, cut solids into small bites, and spoon-fed him. Medical reports and nursing notes showed loss of weight, weak coughing, and bilateral rales in his lungs. (Rales are extraneous sounds usually heard with a stethoscope.) Portable chest X-rays revealed persistent diffuse infiltrates with pleural fluid in the left lung.

The reports by nurses and family members confirmed that the patient experienced dysphagia and they alluded to the seriousness of the dysphagia. Loss of appetite, while also a symptom of postsurgical depression, can be a manifestation of fear of eating and anxiety associated with choking. If a patient chokes, coughs, and aspirates food, there can be negative emotional learning. This classical, or Pavlovian, conditioning occurs when negative emotions associated with the choking, coughing and aspiration are paired with oral eating. After several occurrences of negative emotions paired with dysfunctional eating, the patient may develop classically conditioned negative emotional responses to food and eating stimuli. Therefore, the patient can become negatively conditioned and consequently refuse and avoid food and liquids. This negative learning can also interfere with the normal swallowing reflex by disrupting the finely coordinated reflex due to hypertense muscles. The patient's loss of appetite and weight loss may have been symptoms of the dysphagia.

Terms and statements used by nurses to indicate dysphagia included that the patient needed "full assist pureed diet," "patient only ate 10% by mouth at dinner," "... needed help with feeding and encouragement," "eats approximately 20% of meal," "dry cough and poor effort," "fine scattered rales, partially clears with cough," "lungs were auscultated with coarse rhonchi bilaterally . . ." and "occasional non-productive cough." X-ray reports of persistent diffuse infiltrates with pleural fluid in the left lung were strong indicators of dysphagia. One report said "diminished crackles in the bases bilaterally," and that his chest X-rays suggest "... vascular congestion and possibility of pending pneumonia." Silent aspiration was also probable given the severity of his obvious swallowing difficulties. The nutritionist noted that the patient was "not able to tolerate solids." The patient also had a constant low-grade fever.

Besides the psychogenic considerations discussed above, several other factors may have caused or contributed to the patient's dysphagia. There were reports and observations of the patient experiencing a stroke during the coronary bypass surgery. Strokes can destroy or damage motor and sensory nerves which can cause dysphagia. One indication of the possibility of a stroke affecting the swallowing mechanism was the patient's facial sag. X-rays and brain scans do not always show mild strokes early postonset. Intubation can also irritate the vocal cords and other oral and laryngeal structures. Intubation can also cause problems with coordination and timing of the stages of the swallow, and there can be vocal cord abrasions affecting the protective closure of the vocal cords. Given the neurological and psychological complexity of swallowing, a patient may have dysphagia that X-rays and brain scans do not confirm.

Standards of practice provide that, given the patient's indications of post-surgery dysphagia, the patient should have been placed on NPO status and a speech-language pathology referral made. Competent management of the dysphagia would have included a clinical/bedside swallowing evaluation and video swallow study (VSS). The patient was transferred to a nursing home soon after the surgery, and the comprehensive dysphagia evaluation report should have been forwarded with the discharge summary.

According to the daughter's deposition the patient continued to show signs of dysphagia. During this two-month period he also continued to lose weight. Reportedly, food would get caught in his throat, and there were episodes of gagging and coughing. Clear liquids caused more difficulty than other types of foods. The home health nurses were aware of the patient's eating and swallowing problems and created a calendar to record daily weights. The patient reported that he "feels like he has to cough," and a physician noted "probable left pleural effusion." The patient was so weak that he had to be taken to an emergency room and was admitted to the hospital. Given the patient's persistent symptoms of dysphagia, standards of practice required that the patient be seen for a comprehensive dysphagia evaluation during this period. Yet, the patient did not receive one, continued to eat orally, and likely aspirated food particles and liquids.

A specialist in cardiology consulted on the patient. The consultant noted that the patient was on oxygen therapy since his bypass surgery but not on it before the operation. The patient was disoriented and appeared to have sensations that time was passing extremely slowly or very fast. The patient was talking slowly and continued to have a poor appetite. He also continued to have a low-grade fever. The diagnosis was made of chronic obstructive pulmonary disease (COPD) with chronic hypoxia, dementia, and mild congestive heart failure. He was not helped with eating, nor was there a swallowing evaluation ordered during his stay at the hospital. Again, the patient was discharged to home with home health care, and he continued to show signs of dysphagia. The patient was subsequently admitted to a nursing home where records continued to document dysphagia. The nursing home admitting diagnosis was "swallowing difficulties unable to eat."

When a dysphagia evaluation was ordered, the speech-language pathologists conducted a limited clinical/bedside assessment. The speech-language pathologist observed the patient swallow water, but not food, and noted that he took three attempts to clear each drink of water. The patient reported to the speech-language pathologist that he did not have a swallowing problem, but this report was probably unreliable due to his dementia or confusion about the question; it was inconsistent with previous reports. Based on the limited and brief clinical/bedside evaluation, the speech-language pathologist reported that the patient's swallowing was "within normal limits."

The clinical/bedside evaluation was insufficient and below acceptable professional standards. Given the patient's history of dysphagia, the admitting diagnosis of "swallowing difficulties unable to eat" and likely confirming clinical/bedside symptoms, the speech-language pathologist's conclusions and conduct were improper and substandard. An ongoing clinical/bedside evaluation should have been conducted using several types of foods and during different times of the day. A video swallow study (VSS) should have been recommended, and the patient placed on NPO status until the results were obtained.

The proper test to have been ordered by the attending physician was a "video swallow study," sometimes in the past called a "barium esophagram." The physician ordered an "upper GI." With the video swallow study, the radiologist and the speech-language pathologist would use several types and textures of barium-soaked foods and liquids to assess the three stages of the swallow. Although an upper gastrointestinal examination indirectly addressed the barium movement above the larynx, it was not the appropriate test for assessing dysphagia.

The patient continued to lose weight, and the dysphagia symptoms persisted. He was dehydrated and incontinent to bowel and bladder. A shift nurse noted that the patient "lies in fetal position most of the time." An NG tube was ordered, and there were more attempts to feed him orally. The patient was sent by ambulance to a nearby hospital for observation. The chief complaint given to the ambulance attendant was the patient had "difficulty swallowing." A social worker at the hospital filed a "report of abuse, neglect or exploitation of an incapacitate or vulnerable adult." Later, the patient returned to the home care of his daughter and continued to receive oral feeding. The patient was found passed out at his daughter's house, taken to an emergency room in code arrest, and subsequently died. The cause of death was listed as "pneumonitis due to inhalation of food or vomit." It was also noted that he had anemia indicative of malnutrition that contributed to his death. The autopsy found vegetable material in the lungs and indications of chronic aspiration pneumonia.

The patient displayed classic symptoms of dysphagia from the time of his coronary bypass surgery. These were well documented. They included family and self-reports of swallowing problems, low-grade fever, wheezing and rales, choking, facial sag, voice changes, gagging, refusal to eat, weight loss, and anxiety associated with eating. It is likely that the severity of the dysphagia fluctuated over time. The medical and autopsy reports confirmed chronic aspiration pneumonia.

This illustrates the results of misdiagnosis and improper medical management of dysphagia. Proper standards of care would have resulted in early diagnosis of the dysphagia. The patient would have been tube fed and gradually provided with oral nutrition and hydration under the supervision of a speech-language pathologist. If the patient responded to dysphagia therapy, he would have been weaned from tube feeding and carefully monitored for aspiration. If the patient did not respond to dysphagia therapy, a permanent gastric tube would have provided him with hydration and nutrition and eliminated the potential for aspiration and choking. Had the above been provided, the patient would likely have survived the dysphagia. This case was settled out of court.

B. Case Study Number Two: Dysphagia Misdiagnosis; Delayed Video Swallow Study

This case involved an elderly male and dysphagia management at one hospital and two nursing homes over an approximately two-year period. The patient had a history of anorexia before the medical events leading to the alleged dysphagia management malpractice. He suffered a cerebrovascular accident (CVA) and presented with signs and symptoms of dysphagia at the first admission to the hospital. The major signs and symptoms of dysphagia were right-sided hemiplegia and dysarthria. Although there were medical, nursing, family, and therapist reports of swallowing problems, the patient did not receive an immediate video swallow study (VSS), nor was he placed on NPO (nothing orally) status before the VSS. The plaintiff alleged that all three facilities misdiagnosed and mismanaged the patient's treatable dysphagia. Other alleged medical malpractice included failure to adequately monitor and prevent patient elopement from a nursing home and improper management of decubitus ulcers (bedsores). Defendants asserted that patient did not present with clear signs and symptoms of dysphagia, and that facilities and staff met general and accepted standards of professional care concerning the patient.

Other factors addressed in this case included the presence of a severe bilateral hearing loss in the patient allegedly making nursing observations and the medial diagnoses of disorientation, aphasia, and dementia suspect. Throughout the course of the patient's illness, hearing aids were either unavailable or insufficient amplifiers. Especially during dysphagia, orientation, and aphasia testing, the speech-language pathologist relied on patient responses to verbal questions and did not adequately address the patient's hearing sensitivity in the veracity of the patient's responses. The patient was also diagnosed with clinical depression following the initial CVA and prescribed an antidepressant (Zoloft). The role dysphagia, anorexia, and depression played in his weight loss and compliance with treatment were also addressed.

At issue in this case were inconsistent reports about the patient's sucking, chewing, and swallowing functions at all three facilities. In several instances, medical and nursing reports concluded that the patient's speech was normal, yet identified deficits. There were remarks that patient was hard to test, yet documentation that swallowing was unimpaired or minimally affected. Other reports suggested significant dysphagia and communication impairments. According to the plaintiff, there was little continuum of care for the dysphagia.

The summary opinion rendered by the plaintiff's dysphagia expert witness in this case was that the communication disorders and dysphagia management of the patient were substandard, incompetent in several aspects of diagnosis and treatment, and plagued by miscommunication among and between facilities and healthcare professionals, and with disregard for the seriousness of his condition. Specifically, the healthcare professionals at one facility continued to give the patient food and liquid orally, and although indicating possible aspiration risks and recommending a modified barium swallow study, did not engage in proper precautions to prevent it. This case was settled out of court after mediation.

Table 8.3
Primary Dysphagia Litigation Issues

Dysphagia Issue	Plaintiff Position	Defendant Position
Clinician/healthcare professional proficiency in dysphagia management	Clinician/healthcare professional fell below current, general, and accepted standards of professional conduct in the dysphagia management.	Clinician/healthcare professional met or exceeded current, general, and accepted standards of professional conduct in the dysphagia management.
Professional Communication	Dysphagia diagnostic and treatment orders, referrals, and test results were not clearly and timely communicated among and between facilities, clinicians/healthcare professionals to the detriment of the patient.	Professional communication among and between facilities, clinicians/ healthcare professionals were standard and customary, and did not contribute to the negative dysphagia management outcome.
Accuracy, appropriateness, and timeliness of clinical bedside assessment	Dysphagia patient's signs and symptoms warranted additional swallowing diagnostics	Bedside dysphagia assessment was appropriate and yielded accurate results.
Video swallow study (VSS)	Patient displayed signs and symptoms of dysphagia, choking, and aspiration risks warranting a video swallow study.	Bedside assessment did not warrant additional dysphagia diagnostic testing.
Diet-NPO status-tube feeding	Patient's signs and symptoms of dysphagia warranted diet changes, NPO status, and/or tube feeding.	Patient's signs and symptoms of dysphagia did not warrant diet changes, NPO status, and/or tube feeding.

C. Case Study Number Three: Reflux and Silent Aspiration, Respiratory Failure Due to Recurrent Aspiration

This case involved the alleged improper management and misdiagnosis of dysphagia in an elderly female confined to a nursing home. Cause of death was listed as respiratory failure due to recurrent aspiration and right lower lobe infiltrates. (Having infiltrates in the right lung as opposed to the left lung is consistent with the direct passage of aspirated food and liquid to the right lung.) The patient suffered multiple cerebrovascular accidents which were confirmed by several CT and MRI scans. The plaintiff alleged that the speech-language pathologist at one medical facility observed that the patient was at risk for aspiration but did not recommend NPO status nor a video swallow study. The patient continued to receive thin puree-mechanical soft foods and liquids.

The patient's attending physician recommended NPO status for the patient but qualified the recommendation with the order that if the VSS study could not be completed in a timely manner, there should be a resumption of the oral diet. There was a significant delay in scheduling and conducting the video swallow study. The patient did receive an esophagogastroduodenoscopy to determine the patient's swallowing functions, but plaintiffs contend that this procedure is not accepted as a definitive test to determine the risk of aspiration during a dynamic swallow.

During admission to a regional hospital, a speech-language pathologist diagnosed dysphagia and silent aspiration, yet recommended thin liquids and a pureed diet. The patient had a PEG tube in place at the time. The plaintiff alleged that physicians and the speech-language pathologist at the regional hospital fell below current, general, and accepted standards of dysphagia management by failing to enforce the NPO status of the patient. In addition, upon return to the nursing home, the attending physician, on the patient's admission sheet, diagnosed severe dysphagia and aspiration as revealed by the video swallow study, yet ordered a puree diet.

The summary opinion rendered by the plaintiff's dysphagia expert witness in this case was as follows: "It is remarkable that the modified barium swallow ... using multiple barium tainted media from thin liquids to solids showed almost immediate aspiration of thin liquids, thicker liquids, and semi-solids. Standards of professional conduct concerning dysphagia management would warrant immediate rigid adherence to NPO status yet patient received various orders for puree, liquids, and ice chips. Either the results of the modified barium swallow were not available to medical staff or they were disregarded to the significant detriment of the patient."

Table 8.3 provides a summary of litigation issues in dysphagia management in the above case studies.

8.27 Chapter Summary

The diagnosis and treatment of dysphagia involve several medical professionals, and the speech-language pathologist is a pivotal member of the team. Because dysphagia is a potentially life-threatening condition, competent evaluation and treatment of the disorder may be an issue in medical malpractice litigation. It is important that patients at risk for choking and aspiration be properly evaluated at bedside and through instrumental procedures. Clinician competence, standards of care, and the efficiency of medical communication are important factors to consider in medical malpractice cases involving dysphagia.

Suggested Readings and Resources

Arvedson, J.C. and Brodsky, L. (2002). *Pediatric Swallowing and Feeding: Assessment and Management* (2nd ed.). San Diego: Singular. This book is a comprehensive treatise on the unique aspects of pediatric dysphagia and feeding problems.

Carrau, R. and Murry, T. (2006). *Comprehensive Management of Swallowing Disorders*. San Diego: Plural Publishing. This text, written by physicians, addresses the medical management of dysphagia.

Cefalu, C. (1999). Appropriate dysphagia evaluation and management of the nursing home patient with dementia. *Annals of Long-Term Care*, 7(12): 447-451. This article, written by a physician, addresses the diagnosis and treatment of swallowing in demented patients. It includes an overview of the swallowing evaluation with particular reference to patients with dementia.

Logemann, J.A. (1998). *Evaluation and Treatment of Swallowing Disorders*. Austin, Tx: Pro-Ed. Many consider this book to be the definitive treatise on dysphagia and is frequently the text used by university training programs.

Perlman, A.L. and Schulze-Delrieu, K. S. (Eds.) (1997). *Deglutition and its Disorders: Anatomy, Physiology, Clinical Diagnosis, and Management*. San Diego: Singular. This book is a comprehensive discussion of dysphagia. The chapters are written by several medical specialists.

Tanner, D. (2006, February). The forensic aspects of dysphagia: Investigating medical malpractice. *The ASHA Leader, 11(2), 16-17, 45.* This article addresses the investigative process in medical malpractice cases involving negative dysphagia management outcomes.

Zemlin, W. (1998). *Speech and Hearing Science* (4th ed). Boston: Allyn & Bacon. This text provides a comprehensive review of general anatomy and physiology of the speech and hearing mechanism.

References

American Speech-Language-Hearing Association. (1990). Knowledge and skills needed by speech-language pathologists providing services to dysphagic patients/clients. *ASHA, 32 (Supplement,* 2), 7-12. Rockville, MD. Author.

American Speech-Language-Hearing Association. (2000). Clinical indicators for instrumental assessment of dysphagia (guidelines). *ASHA Supplement,* 20, 18-19. Rockville, MD. Author.

American Speech-Language-Hearing Association. (2001). Roles of speech-language pathologists in swallowing and feeding disorders: Position statement. *ASHA Supplement.* Rockville, MD. Author.

American Speech-Language-Hearing Association. (2002). Knowledge and skills for speech-language pathologists performing endoscopic assessment of swallowing. *ASHA Supplement.* Rockville, MD. Author.

American Speech-Language-Hearing Association (2006, September). Managing dysphagia in the schools. *ASHA Leader,* Vol 11, No. 13.

Arvedson, J.C. and Brodsky, L. (2002). *Pediatric swallowing and feeding: Assessment and management* (2nd ed.). San Diego: Singular.

Asha, (1987, April). Dysphagia. Vol. 29, pp. 57-58. Rockville, MD. Author.

Asha, (1994, May). Clinical record keeping in audiology and speech-language pathology. Vol. 36, pp. 40-43. Rockville, MD. Author.

ASHA Special Interest Division 13: Swallowing and Swallowing Disorders (Dysphagia). (1997). Graduate curriculum on swallowing and swallowing disorders (adult and pediatric dysphagia). Asha Desk Reference, Vol 3, 248a-248n.

Bass, N.H. (1997). The neurology of swallowing. In M. E. Groher (Ed) *Dysphagia: Diagnosis and management* (3rd ed). Boston: Butterworth-Heinemann.

Buchholz, D.W. (1996). What is dysphagia? *Dysphagia,* 11:23.

Cefalu, C. (1999). Appropriate dysphagia evaluation and management of the nursing home patient with dementia. *Annals of Long-Term Care,* 7(12): 447-451.

Cherney, L.R. (1994). Dysphagia in adults with neurologic disorders: An overview. In L. R. Cherney (Ed) *Clinical management of dysphagia in adults and children.* Gaithersburg, M.D.: Aspen.

Cowen, M., Simpson, S., and Vettese, T. (1997). Survival estimates for patients with abnormal swallowing studies. *J. Gen. Intern. Med.,* 12:99-94.

Daniels, S., McAdams, C., Brailey, K., and Foundas, A. (1997). Clinical assessment of swallowing and prediction of dysphagia severity. *American Journal of Speech-Language Pathology,* 6, 17-24.

Dirckx, J. H. (2001). *Stedman's concise medical dictionary for the health professions* (4th ed). Philadelphia: Lippincott Williams & Wilkins.

Gonzalez, C. and Calia, F. (1975). Bacteriologic flora of aspiration-induced pulmonary infection. *Archives of Internal Medicine,* 135, 711-714.

Groher, M. and Bukatman, R. (1986). Prevalence of dysphagia in two teaching hospitals. *Dysphagia,* 1:3.

Groher, M.E. (1997). Mechanical disorders of swallowing. In M.E. Groher (Ed) *Dysphagia: Diagnosis and management* (3rd ed.). Boston: Butterworth-Heinemann.

Justice, L. M. (2006). *Communication sciences and disorders: An introduction.* Upper Saddle River, N.J.: Pearson, Merrill, Prentice Hall.

Lawton, M. (1991). A multidimensional view of quality of life in frail elders. In J. Birren (Ed) *The concept and measurement of quality of life in frail elders.* San Diego: Academic Press.

Leopold, N.A. and Kagel, M.A. (1996). Prepharyngeal dysphagia in Parkinson's disease. *Dysphagia,* 11, 14-11.

Logemann, J. (1995). Dysphagia: Evaluation and treatment. *Folia Phoniatrica et Logopedica:* 47, 140-164.

Logemann, J.A. (1998). *Evaluation and treatment of swallowing disorders*. Austin, Tx: Pro-Ed.

McCulloch, T.M., Jaffe, D.M., and Hoffman, H.T. (1997). Diseases and operation of head and neck structures affecting swallowing. In A. L. Perlman and K.S. Schulze-Delrieu (Eds) *Deglutition and its disorders: Anatomy, physiology, clinical diagnosis, and management* (pp. 343-381). San Diego: Singular.

Perlman, A.L. and Christensen, J. (1997). Topography and functional anatomy of the swallowing structures. In A. L. Perlman and Schulze-Delrieu, K. S. (Eds.) *Deglutition and its disorders: Anatomy, physiology, clinical diagnosis, and management* (pp. 15-42). San Diego: Singular.

Ravich, W. J. (1997). Esophageal dysphagia. In A. L. Perlman and K. S. Schulze-Delrieu (Eds) *Deglutition and its disorders: Anatomy, physiology, clinical diagnosis, and management* (pp. 107-130). San Diego: Singular.

Reilly, S. (2004). The Evidence Base for the Management of Dysphagia. In *Evidence based practice in speech pathology*, S. Reilly, J. Douglas, and J. Oates (Eds). London: Whurr Publishers.

Roberts, K. (2002, February). Documentation in long-term care. *ASHA Leader*, Vol. 7, No. 2., p. 15.

Schmidt, D., Holas, M., Halvorson, K. and Reding, M. (1994). Videofluoroscopic evidence of aspiration predicts pneumonia and death but not dehydration following stroke. *Dysphagia*. 9, 7-11.

Schulze-Delrieu, K.S. and Miller, R.M. (1997). Clinical assessment of dysphagia. In A. L. Perlman and Schulze-Delrieu, K. S. (Eds) *Deglutition and its disorders: Anatomy, physiology, clinical diagnosis, and management*. (pp. 125-152). San Diego: Singular.

Siebens, H., Trupe, E., Siebens, A.A. (1986). Correlates and consequences of eating dependency in institutionalized elderly. *Journal of the American Geriatric Society*, 34:192.

Skrine, R. B. (2002, February). Home care documentation. *ASHA Leader*, Vol. 7, No. 2., p. 16.

Spahr, F. and Malone, R. (1998). The profession of speech-language pathology and audiology. In G. Shames, E. Wiig, and W. Secord (Eds), *Human communication disorders: An introduction*, (5th ed.). Boston: Allyn and Bacon.

Swigert, N.B. (2002, February). Documenting what you do is as important as doing it. *ASHA Leader*, Vol. 7, No. 2, p. 1.

Tanner, D. and Guzzino, A. (2002, April). Westlaw search of litigation areas in communication sciences and disorders. A paper presented at the 2001-2002 Honors Day Program. Northern Arizona University, Flagstaff, Arizona.

Tanner, D. and Gerstenberger, D. (1996). Clinical forum 9: The grief model in aphasia. In *Forums in clinical aphasiology*, C. Code (Ed). London: Whurr Publishers

Tanner, D. and Culbertson, W. (1999). *Quick Assessment for Dysphagia*. Oceanside, CA: Academic Communication Associates.

Tanner, D. (2003). *The psychology of neurogenic communication disorders: A primer for health care professionals*. Boston: Allyn & Bacon.

Tanner, D. (2006, February). The forensic aspects of dysphagia: Investigating medical malpractice. *The ASHA Leader, 11(2), 16-17, 45*.

Wright, H. M. (2004). Personal correspondence. Mesa and Phoenix: Udall, Shumway, and Lyons, P.L.C.

Zemlin, W. (1998). *Speech and hearing science* (4th ed.). Boston: Allyn & Bacon.

Chapter 9

The Medical-Legal and Forensic Aspects of Neurogenic Communication Disorders

9.1 Chapter Preview

This chapter provides a comprehensive overview of neurogenic communication disorders and the medical-legal and forensic issues associated with them. Neurogenic communication disorders—aphasia, apraxia of speech, and the dysarthrias—result from damage to the central or peripheral nervous systems and the muscles they enervate. They are caused by strokes, traumatic brain injuries, and diseases. Addressed in this chapter are medical-legal and forensic issues related to efficacy of treatment, evaluation philosophy, malingering, standards of care, quality of life, disability de-

termination, and determining mental competence. There is also a case study involving medical-legal and forensic aspects of neurogenic communication disorders.

9.2 Overview of Neurogenic Communication Disorders Litigation Issues

There are two primary areas where attorneys are involved with neurogenic communication disorders: mental competence determination and compensation-damages issues. Both areas of litigation address a wide range of related issues including standards of institutional care, quality of patient management, postonset quality of life, malingering, and disability determination. In this chapter, the discussion is limited to adult neurogenic communication disorders such as occur in patients who have suffered strokes, traumatic brain injuries, and adult-onset diseases. Neurogenic communication disorders are complex language and motor speech disabilities and they are caused by hundreds of diseases, disorders, and defects. Litigation issues related to neurogenic communication disorders require that attorneys be well-versed in their etiology, diagnosis, and treatment.

9.3 Etiology of Neurogenic Communication Disorders

Strokes, traumatic brain injuries, diseases, and other types of injuries and defects cause neurogenic communication disorders. As a rule, the site and size of the brain damage determine the severity of the communication disorder. However, small areas of brain damage can cause severe communication disorders, and relatively large ones can result in patients having few symptoms. Strokes are the third leading cause of death in the United States (Owens et al., 2000). There are two categories of strokes: hemorrhagic and occlusive.

Hemorrhagic strokes occur where there is a rupture or bursting of a blood vessel in the brain. These hemorrhagic events are also called "cerebral bleeds." They are primarily caused by traumatic head injuries (see below) and high blood pressure. When hemorrhages deprive blood to the speech and language areas of the brain, neurogenic communication disorders result. Not only do hemorrhages result in an interruption of the flow of blood to parts of the brain, they also can cause blood to be spilled into the cranial cavity. This can cause increased intracranial pressure (IICP) which is sometimes called increased cranial pressure (ICP). Increased intracranial pressure can affect the patient's speech and language abilities, and be life-threatening.

Occlusive strokes occur when there is a blockage, restriction, or "plug" in an artery. The blockage can be a clot or other type of obstruction. When there is an occlusion of blood supply to the brain, it is called a cerebral thrombosis. When the blockage originates elsewhere in the body and eventually lodges in the brain, it is called a cerebral embolus. A shower of emboli occurs when several obstructions lodge in the brain. A transient ischemic attack (TIA) occurs when blood flow is interrupted to the brain for fewer than twenty-four hours and the symptoms are temporary. Transient ischemic attacks are sometimes called "ministrokes." The aphasia resulting from TIAs is sometimes called transient aphasia and can be involved in litigation. See *Lewis v. Seidman, 976 F2d 587 (9th Cir 1992)*.

Traumatic brain injuries and neurogenic communication disorders are discussed in Chapter 10. However, there are three factors to be considered when discussing the etiology of neurogenic communication disorders and traumatic brain injuries. First, traumatic brain injuries can cause focalized damage to the speech and language centers of the brain, similar to what occurs in a stroke. Second, some patients suffer traumatic brain damage not affecting the major speech and language centers. Although these patients may have problems communicating, the fabric of language and motor speech processes remain largely unaffected. Many of these patients have problems with arousal, orientation, behavior, judgment, and memory. Third, patients can have neurogenic communication disorders complicated and compounded by arousal, orientation, behavior, judgment, and memory problems.

There are many diseases of the brain and nervous system that can cause neurogenic communication disorders. Cancerous tumors, nonmalignant growths, infections, and progressive diseases can disrupt language and motor speech processes. Neuromuscular disorders such as multiple sclerosis, muscular dystrophy, amyotrophic lateral sclerosis, and Parkinson's disease are common causes of neurogenic communication disorders.

9.4 Aphasia and Motor Speech Disorders

Neurogenic communication disorders are typically divided into aphasia and motor speech disorders. Aphasia is a language disorder and the motor speech disorders are apraxia of speech and the dysarthrias. This approach of separating neurogenic communication disorders into those that eliminate or disrupt the fabric of language from those that are primarily motor speech impairments was based on research conducted by Darley, Aronson, and Brown (1975), the results of which were published in their landmark book: *Motor Speech Disorders*. Darley's (1982) equally influential book, *Aphasia,* further clarified the neurogenic language-motor speech disorder dichotomy with the first aphasia-motor speech disorder distinction: "Aphasia is not a speech disorder." Most, but not all, present-day speech and hearing scientists and clinicians view neurogenic communication disorders in the Darley tradition, and it is adhered to in this text because it clearly provides a logical basis for many litigation issues related to neurogenic communication disorders.

A. Aphasia

As reported previously, aphasia is the loss of language due to stroke, head trauma, disease, or other type of brain damage. Technically, "aphasia" means the complete loss of language, whereas "dysphasia" means partial loss or impaired language. However, most scientists and clinicians use the term "aphasia" also to refer to partial loss of language; a patient may be said to have partial aphasia. Although there are many varieties of aphasia and hundreds of clinical manifestations, this disorder is primarily a form of amnesia. At its core, aphasia is primarily the loss of memory for words.

Aphasia can be considered a syndrome where there is a combination or cluster of symptoms. Most types of aphasia can be classified as predominantly expressive or predominantly receptive communication disorders. The expressive disorders affect speaking, writing, and using expressive gestures. The receptive disorders affect reading and understanding the speech and gestures of others. These two categories of aphasia are called "predominantly" expressive and receptive disorders because usually aphasia affects all modalities of expression and reception. It may take detailed and sophisticated testing to discover the deficiencies, but aphasia usually cuts across all modalities of communication. Because mathematics is a language, a form of symbolic expression and reception, aphasia also disrupts the ability to do and understand simple arithmetic.

Scientists and clinicians use several terms to refer to expressive and receptive neurogenic communication disorders. Table 9.1 shows common expressive and receptive categories of aphasia. In Table 9.1, anterior and posterior refer to the major speech and language centers lying in front (anterior) or behind (posterior) the fissure of Rolando, also called the central sulcus, which separates the frontal and parietal lobes (see Figure 9.1). Motor and sensory refer to the neuromuscular process of making body structures move and obtaining sense information of the body and environment.

B. Predominantly Expressive Aphasia

When there is damage to the expressive language centers of the brain, the patient has difficulty recalling and producing sounds, syllables, words, and phrases. His or her speech is typically nonfluent. It is produced with hesitations, repetitions, fillers, and revisions. A common label for this type of disorder is Broca's aphasia. Broca's aphasia has both motor speech and language components to it. Patients with Broca's aphasia have trouble remembering words for expression; this is the language component. This type of amnesia for words is sometimes called wordfinding or naming deficits. For example, when an examiner asks a patient with Broca's aphasia to provide the name of an eating utensil, he or she might call a "knife" a "fork" or be unable to remember any word for the object.

Even when a name can be remembered, the patient may have trouble programming his or her speech mechanism to produce the word; this is the motor aspect of Broca's aphasia. He or she may struggle, overshoot, undershoot, and complicate the physical acts of speaking. Some Broca's aphasia patients will be so impaired with language and/or the motor acts of speaking that they will be mute.

One of the frustrating aspects of predominantly expressive aphasia is the tip-of-the-tongue phenomenon. As the label suggests, the patient senses that he or she is close to being able to say a word, but correct production of it is just beyond his or her reach. The word lacks a trigger to be recalled or produced. Patients displaying the tip-of-the-tongue phenomenon are aware of their word-finding errors; they know when they have made a mistake. However, they may only be partially able to self-correct, and the tip-of-the-tongue phenomenon is part of their self-correction behaviors.

When patients say words that rhyme with the correct ones, they produce literal paraphasias or approximations: "pork" for "fork." When patients say words related in meaning to the correct one, they produce verbal paraphasias or association errors: "knife" for "spoon." Random errors occur when there is no rhyme or reason to the naming mistakes. When speaking, patients with predominantly expressive aphasia often telegraph utterances. They use content words to the exclusion of grammatical and functional ones. The notion of telegraphing speech came from the time when people sent messages via the telegraph. Because they had to pay for the message by the word, they would only use ones essential to carry the meaning. A patient with telegraphic speech might say, "Eat here now" to express through telegraphic speech his or her desire to eat in the bedroom rather than to go to a dining room at lunch time.

Table 9.1
Expressive and Receptive Categories of Aphasia

Predominantly Expressive Aphasia	Predominantly Receptive Aphasia	Severe Aphasia Affecting Both Expressive and Receptive Modalities
Anterior aphasia	Posterior aphasia	Complete aphasia
Motor aphasia	Sensory aphasia	Global aphasia
Nonfluent aphasia	Fluent aphasia	Irreversible aphasia syndrome
Broca's aphasia	Wernicke's aphasia	Severe expressive-receptive aphasia
Telegraphic speech	Jargon aphasia	Profound aphasia

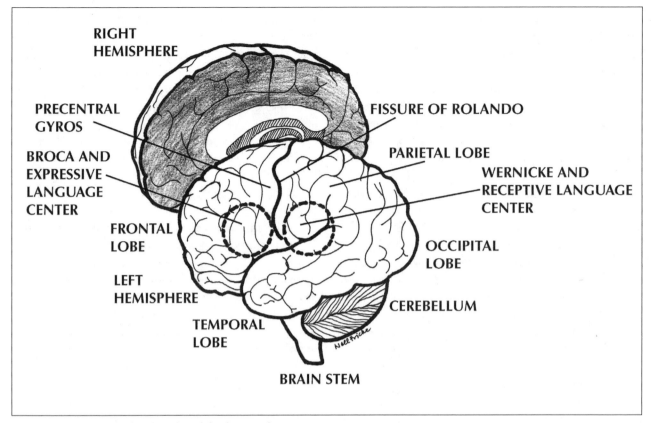

Figure 9.1 *Important landmarks of the human brain*

Another frequently occurring aspect of predominantly expressive aphasia is agrammatism, which is the impaired ability to use words in their proper sequence or according to their grammatical functions. The use of grammar and syntax is impaired. In addition, patients with predominantly expressive aphasia often have automatic speech. When speaking purposefully and thoughtfully, the patient with automatic speech will have difficultly with word retrieval, and complicate the speech act, only to be able to say sounds, words, and even phrases easily and correctly when little thought and attention are given to them. Although purposeful and volitional utterances are difficult or impossible to say, nonpurposeful and involuntary utterances can sometimes be spoken easily. This phenomenon is also called subcortical speech. Automatic speech often occurs with swear words and over-learned phrases. The following is an example of the impaired speech typical of a patient with moderately severe predominantly expressive aphasia:

> I, swant, uh, want, to say, play, choker; not choker, uh, (pause) choker. No. Poker. I want to say poker today, uh, tonight, with my daught . . . , strife, uh strife, uh, (pause) wife. I bet quarter. Straw choker, uh, uh, foker, uh, forker, forker, puh, orker is game. Damn it, draw poker is my game.

Strokes, tumors, head traumas, and diseases causing aphasia often, but not always, result in right hemiplegia. Hemiplegia is paralysis of one side of the body. Patients with expressive aphasia often have right hemiplegia because the left side of the brain controls the right side of the body and vice versa in most persons. Motor control of the right arm and hand is found in the precentral gyrus of the frontal lobe in the left hemisphere. The precentral gyrus is also known as the motor strip. Consequently, motor control for writing is adjacent to the expressive speech and language centers. Thus, in most patients, strokes, tumors, head traumas, and diseases affecting expressive speech and language are also likely to affect motor control of the right arm and hand.

Agraphia is the inability to write *not* attributable to arm or hand paralysis. Dysgraphia is a less severe writing problem where the patient maintains some ability to express himself or herself graphically. Agraphia and dysgraphia are disorders of the ability to use graphic symbols for expression. Although patients with Broca's aphasia often have weak or paralyzed right arms, their difficulty or inability to write is not because of motor deficits. Arm and hand weakness or paralysis can cause the patient to have difficulty grasping and holding a writing device. Nevertheless, the writing problem goes beyond legibility factors. Patients with agraphia or dysgraphia are unable, or impaired in the ability, to write even when they do so with their nondominant hands. Certainly, when a person tries to write with the nondominate hand, it is usually done less legibly, but thoughts can be expressed nonetheless. Even if these patients' arms and hands were not paralyzed or weak, they would be impaired with the ability to write. Agraphia and dysgraphia are part of the language disorder. In aphasia, reading and writing disorders tend to occur together, but there is a form of dysgraphia where the patient has significant problems writing, and reading is only slightly impaired. This rare disorder is called pure dysgraphia or pure agraphia.

Aphasic patients tend to write like they speak. Although there are exceptions, the patient with nonfluent aphasia writes haltingly, with poor penmanship. Writing often occurs with revisions and letter substitutions. The patient complicates the writing act. The nonfluency of speech is reflected in the patient's writing. In severe cases, the patient has difficulty copying letters, numbers, and geometric forms. Often, the last letter of a written word trails off to a straight line (see Figure 9.2). For many aphasic patients, writing to dictation is extremely difficult. Patients often appear perplexed at the task of writing.

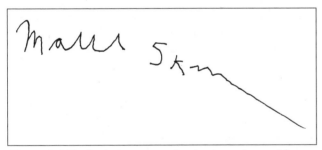

Figure 9.2 *Typical signature of aphasic patient with dysgraphia*

Patients with predominantly expressive aphasia usually have difficulty expressing themselves gesturally. This is particularly true of those with moderate to severe aphasia but usually only for complicated gestures. Most aphasics, even severely involved ones, can turn away to communicate avoidance and refusal. They can use gross gestures for expression. However, it is usually beyond their capabilities to use complicated serial gestures for expression. For example, it would be difficult or impossible for most patients with predominantly expressive aphasia sequentially to point to a bathrobe, slippers, toilet and gesturally to show the need to go to the bathroom. Similarly, teaching a patient to use sign language, even a modified version using one

hand, is futile because of the language deficits. Sign language is a language per se; teaching it would be like teaching the patient a foreign language. Although the basic ability to use gross gestures for expression is retained in most patients, complicated and sophisticated use of expressive gestures is beyond their reach. Even the accuracy of "eye-blinking" in response to questions can be an issue during litigation. See *Downs v. Hoyt,* 232 F. 3rd 1031 (9th Cir 2000).

> Predominantly expressive aphasia
>
> Impaired verbal expression
>   Broca's aphasia
>   Wordfinding and naming deficits
>   Motor speech programming deficits
>   Verbal (association) and literal (approximation)
>   paraphasias
>   Agrammatism
>   Automatic speech
> Agraphia and dysphasia
> Impaired gestural expression

Figure 9.3 *Primary aspects of predominantly expressive aphasia*

Figure 9.3 shows the primary symptoms of predominantly expressive aphasia.

C. Predominantly Receptive Aphasia

In most patients, the major site of brain damage in predominantly receptive aphasia is the temporal-parietal region of the left hemisphere (Zemlin, 1998). Some scientists and clinicians limit the area damaged to the temporal lobe, but they probably are referring to auditory comprehension deficits and excluding other impaired modalities such as reading. A common label for aphasic auditory comprehension deficits is Wernicke's aphasia. Patients with predominantly receptive aphasia are impaired, to various degrees, in comprehending the speech, writing, and gestures of others. In severe cases of receptive aphasia, patients are completely unable to understand the speech, writing, and gestures of others. They do not understand simple words and cannot follow even rudimentary instructions and commands.

For forensic purposes, it may be necessary to determine if a patient can (or could) follow commands and instructions and, if not, what reasons accounted for the impairment. When addressing the issue of why a patient cannot (or did not) follow verbal directions, there are several possibilities. First, the patient may have body weakness, paralysis, or limb apraxia. Walking, grasping an item, or wheeling a chair from one place to another may be impossible because of the weakness or paralysis. Body apraxia, sometimes called limb apraxia, also may prevent the patient from following verbal directions. Body apraxia is when the patient cannot program his or her body to perform voluntary movements. The patient overshoots, undershoots, or cannot grasp the idea of the body movements necessary to accomplish the motor act. Usually, there is a voluntary-involuntary dichotomy. Although the patient cannot perform purposeful, volitional body movements, he or she will be able to complete them normally when little or no conscious attention is given to them. For example, when an apraxic patient is asked: "Show me how you light and smoke a cigarette," he or she will be unable or impaired in following the instructions. However, after the diagnostic session, when the patient feels the urge to smoke, he or she will be able to light and smoke the cigarette when little conscious thought is given to the task.

The second reason the patient cannot follow verbal instructions may be that he or she has a hearing loss affecting the speech frequencies or deafness. Consequently, he or she cannot hear the verbal instructions. Obviously, a person who cannot hear instructions, cannot be expected to follow them. The third reason is that he or she may have attention and memory deficits and be unable to focus on instructions or remember them. There are two patterns of attention and memory problems that can contribute to difficulty following instructions. First, the patient may have slow rise time. Slow rise time is when the patient attends to the final aspects of a series of requests and does not attend to or forgets the initial ones. Auditory fade is the opposite of slow rise time and occurs when the patient attends to the initial aspects of a series of requests and does not attend to or forgets the final aspects. For example, if a patient is asked to touch his or her nose, then hold up two fingers, and then point to the window, slow rise time would result in the patient only pointing to the window. Because of auditory fade, the patient may only touch his or her nose. Fourth, the patient may have receptive aphasia and not be able to comprehend the grammar, phonology, and semantics of utterances. Fifth, the patient may be disoriented; he or she may be confused about who is giving instructions and/or why and how to follow them. Finally, the patient may be cognitively and intellectually impaired. He or she may be demented or retarded and thus be unable to cognitively process the situation. Figure 9.4 lists the common reasons some patients cannot follow verbal instructions. Of course, some patients do not follow instructions because they are not inclined and willing to do so.

Body weakness or paralysis
Limb apraxia
Hearing loss and/or deafness
Attention and memory deficits
   Slow rise time
   Auditory fade
Receptive language deficits
Disorientation
Cognitive and intellectual deficits

Figure 9.4 Reasons a patient with neurogenic communication disorders may not follow instructions

Whereas expressive aphasia is typically nonfluent, the speech of many patients with predominantly receptive aphasia is fluent. It is fluent but without meaning. The fluent, meaningless speech often occurring with damage to the left temporal-parietal lobes is called jargon aphasia.

There are two forms of jargon speech. First, the patient may produce sounds which have no meaning when they are combined to make words. For example, the patient may say, "tula, est dool, dool, dool." The words are not recognizable in the language being used. A made-up word is called a neologism. Second, the patient may say words that when combined do not make sense. For example, he or she may say, "The acrylic thus far is preponderance." Most patients with jargon aphasia combine the above types of errors and produce a mixture of meaningful and meaningless words and statements. Their writing usually reflects this fluent jargon output.

Attorneys, judges, and jurors may wonder why patients with damage to the receptive centers of the brain also have problems with expression. After all, there is little, if any, damage to the major expressive speech and language centers. There is no general agreement among scientists and clinicians why many patients with damage to the receptive language centers speak jargon. There are four possibilities. First, as stated previously, the brain operates as a whole, especially concerning language. No one area operates completely independently of another; the strict localization view of language is insufficient when explaining jargon aphasia (see Chapter 2 for a detailed discussion of the localization controversy). Second, jargon speech results from the patient being unable to monitor and understand his or her output. The patient cannot understand his or her own speech any better than he or she can understand the speech of others. Because the patient has trouble understanding, he or she does not know when nonsense is being uttered. The third possibility concerns the language-thought controversy. Jargon speech may simply be the expression of disordered or disrupted verbal-thought patterns. The patient's semantic processors are damaged for verbal expression, auditory association, and inner speech; the patient is expressing mixed-up ideas. Finally, a contributing factor to persistent jargon speech is the psychological defense of denial. Even though patients are clearly unable meaningfully to communicate to doctors, nurses, therapists, and family members, many continue to speak jargon. Some patients act as though their speech is perfectly normal, and if the listener would simply try harder, he or she would be able to understand them. Many patients with persistent jargon speech deny its existence and project the communication disorder onto the listeners (Tanner, 2003a; Tanner, 2003b). All of the above may combine to explain why some patients with damage to the receptive language centers of the brain speak jargon.

Technically, a patient with alexia is completely unable to read, while dyslexia refers to a less severe form of the disorder. Recently, some scientists and clinicians have referred to the reading problems found in neurogenic communication disorders as complete or partial alexia. The trend is to disregard the term dyslexia when referring to neurogenic patients because it is a commonly used label for the type of reading problem diagnosed and treated in school children. Dyslexia seen in educational settings is often different from the alexia seen in patients with neurogenic communication disorders. The learning disability of dyslexia is often a visual perceptual disorder where letters are juxtaposed, reversed, or inverted. Aphasia alexia can include the above but often is primarily a loss of written word meanings. In addition, using the label "word blindness" to refer to the reading problems seen in patients with neurogenic communication disorders is misleading because it suggests that the core of the problem lies in eye-blindness. A common visual field cut, a type of eye-blindness, seen in neurogenic communication disorders is homonymous hemianopsia. It is the loss of the same visual half-field of both eyes. Patients can have right or left homonymous hemianopsia where they are blind in either the right or left fields of both eyes. Although strokes, head traumas, and diseases causing aphasia can result in blindness, tunnel vision, and cuts in the visual fields, the reading disorder of alexia is not a result of the patient having problems seeing the printed or handwritten word.

The language disorder of alexia results from the patient's loss of the ability to remember the meaning of written words. Although there may be perceptual deficits, where the patient has problems recognizing and appreciating letters similar to what occurs in dyslexia, the primary problem in aphasia is amnesia for words. Other factors are also involved in alexia. The patient may have reduced attention and have difficulty grasping the entire idea of a text.

There is a rare reading disability in neurogenic communication disorders called alexia without agraphia. With this disorder, the patient has trouble reading, but writing is done relatively well. Some patients with alexia without agraphia cannot read what they have just written. Although reading is represented throughout the brain, damage to the parietal lobe of the left hemisphere is often associated with alexia.

Alexia is an important issue in determining whether a patient is competent to drive. Although many factors go into driving competency, including overall mental and physical status, the patient's ability to read traffic signs is important. Obviously, a patient who is compromised in reading can create a traffic hazard unless he or she can recognize traffic signs by their shapes. Additionally, a patient may be competent to drive, but his or her alexia can prohibit passing the written test.

Whereas patients with predominantly expressive aphasia have problems expressing themselves with gestures, predominantly receptive aphasia impairs the ability to understand gestures. Similar to the problems seen in predominantly expressive aphasia, the gestural problems in predominantly receptive aphasia are usually limited to understanding complicated, serial gestures. Basic gestures such as shaking the head "no" or using the finger to beckon the patient can be understood by most aphasic patients. However, patients with moderate to severe predominantly receptive aphasia are usually unable to comprehend and follow complicated gestures. Figure 9.5 shows the primary symptoms of predominantly receptive aphasia.

Predominantly receptive aphasia

Impaired auditory comprehension
    Wernicke's aphasia
        Jargon
        Neologisms
Alexia, dyslexia, and word blindness
Impaired gestural comprehension

Figure 9.5 *Primary aspects of predominantly receptive aphasia*

D. Mathematical Expression and Reception

Words are symbolic; they are symbols that refer to ideas, objects, emotions, actions, and so forth. They are also arbitrary in that a language society has agreed on the symbol or word to represent a particular referent. Mathematics has been called the universal language; there are semantic, syntactic, and grammatic bases to it. In addition, doing mathematical problems also involves speaking, reading, and writing. Consequently, in aphasia, patients often have difficulty with simple arithmetic and complex mathematics. This disorder is called acalculia (dyscalculia), and it is an important consideration in determining the competence of a patient for independent living, understanding and writing wills and trusts, and participating in business and corporate affairs.

Acalculia is the inability to perform and understand simple mathematics due to brain damage, and dyscalculia is a less severe form of the disorder. Patients with acalculia and dyscalculia have problems doing simple mathematics; it is not restricted to complex formulas and problems involving calculus, algebra, or statistics. Patients with acalculia cannot do even simple computations such as knowing how much change to receive from a dollar for a purchase costing $0.85.

The difficulties patients have with mathematics include appreciating the significance of money and financial decisions. The inability to do simple arithmetic can impair self-sufficiency. Basic activities such as shopping for groceries and clothes can be problematic for the patient because he or she is impaired in knowing how much to spend and on what items. Business persons may be compromised about decisions concerning corporate expenditures, budgets, and purchases. Not only do acalculia and dyscalculia affect the ability to perform even simple mathematical problems, they can eliminate or impair the ability of the patient to appreciate monetary values. Thus, the patient's financial competence is suspect, but not because of intellectual or cognitive deficiencies such as dementia and mental impairment-mental retardation. It is brought into question because the patient cannot compute numbers correctly and does not appreciate numerical values and processes.

E. Perceptual Disorders

The perceptual disorders are referred to as the agnosias. In the broadest definition of the word, agnosia means lack of recognition (Benson and Ardila, 1996). It is the impairment of the ability to recognize and appreciate the significance of a stimulus in one sense modality. It can occur in all of the five senses: vision, hearing, taste, touch, and smell. Agnosia is the breakdown in information processing occurring between the senses and associative functions of the cortex. Whereas aphasic disturbances are multimodality, affecting all avenues of communication, the agnosias are modality specific. In agnosia, the patient has difficulty recognizing stimuli in only one sense but can recognize them in other senses.

Visual, auditory-acoustic, and tactile agnosias are the most relevant perceptual problems in neurogenic communication disorders. Perceptual problems are an important aspect to dyslexia. Visual agnosia also impairs the patient's ability to read, recognize, and appreciate the significance of objects. For example, a patient with visual agnosia, during lunch, may try to suck milk from a glass using a knife or spoon rather than a straw. The patient has lost the ability to recognize and appreciate the significance of objects, in this case, eating utensils. Although patients who are retarded, demented, or delirious may also engage in the above types of behavior, the patient with visual agnosia does so because of perceptual, not global cognitive and intellectual, deficits. There is a rare type of agnosia, prosopagnosia, where the patient loses the ability to recognize familiar faces. Because the perceptual disorder is limited to the visual sense, the patient can often recognize the voices of the familiar people.

Auditory perception plays an important role in the comprehension of speech and environmental sounds. Auditory agnosia is the impaired perception of all auditory input and includes speech and nonspeech stimuli. A patient with auditory agnosia may have difficulty perceiving and appreciating the significance of the ringing of a telephone, a knock at a door, or the sound of a smoke alarm. The patient might answer the door when a fire alarm goes off, pick up a telephone when there is a knock at a door, or do nothing at all. Acoustic agnosia is a specific type of auditory perceptual disorder where the patient has difficulty distinguishing between speech sounds. He or she has lost the ability to appreciate the perceptual differences between speech sounds, particularly ones acoustically similar to each other. This disorder is sometimes called pure word deafness. This label is misleading because the patient does not have a hearing loss; the deficiency is perceptual. Tactile agnosia is an issue with regard to vision-impaired patients who use Braille. The patient loses the ability to recognize and appreciate the significance of raised dots used for reading. Tactile agnosia may also be an inconvenience to patients when they try to find objects in their purses or pockets by the sense of touch. Olfactory and gustatory agnosias affect the perception of stimuli from the sense of smell and taste. Table 9.2 shows the senses, agnosias, and higher level deficits.

Table 9.2
Senses, Agnosias, and Higher Level Cognitive Functions

Sense	Perception	Higher Cognitive Functions
Vision	Visual agnosia	Visual association deficits
Hearing	Auditory-acoustic agnosia	Verbal association deficits
Touch	Tactile agnosia	Tactile association deficits
Taste	Gustatory agnosia	Gustatory association deficits
Smell	Olfactory agnosia	Olfactory association deficits

F. Motor Speech Disorders

Motor speech production involves five basic processes: respiration, phonation, articulation, resonance, and prosody. Respiration is the compressing of air in the lungs so that speech sounds can be made. Phonation is voicing. It is the vibration of the vocal cords as air passes through the larynx. Articulation is the act of shaping the voiced and unvoiced air and sound into speech sounds. This shaping is done by several valving actions of the articulators. Resonance is amplification and damping of energy in the resonating chambers in the neck and head. The soft palate (velum) opens and closes the nasal passageway, permitting some sounds to have more or less nasal resonance. Too much and too little nasality are called hypernasality and hyponasality, respectively. Prosody is the rhythm and flow of speech. It includes emphasis, stress, and intonation of speech. Motor speech disorders disrupt, to various degrees, respiration, phonation, articulation, resonance, and prosody.

G. Apraxia of Speech and Oral Apraxia

Apraxia of speech, sometimes called verbal apraxia, is usually an aspect of Broca's aphasia, and rarely does it occur alone. Davis (2007), and others, also consider apraxia of speech to be related to certain fluent types of aphasia. When it does occur independently of aphasia, it is usually mild in severity. Apraxia of speech is the disruption of the motor plan of the speech act. In the majority of people, it results from damage to Broca's area of the frontal lobe in the left hemisphere of the brain. The articulatory plan may occur in other areas of the left hemisphere of the brain, specifically the anterior insula and lateral premotor cortex (Wise, Greene, Büchel, and Scott, 1999). Apraxia of speech in children is associated with poor auditory discrimination abilities, suggesting a relationship between auditory processing and motor speech programming (Groenen, Maassen, Crul, and Thoonen, 1996). The motor plan for speech, especially articulation, is tied to the ability to distinguish auditorially between sounds. Although apraxia of speech can affect all aspects of motor speech programming, usually articulation is the primary process that is impaired. Apraxia of speech usually presents with the voluntary-involuntary dichotomy. Utterances that are off-the-cuff can sometimes be said easily and normally.

The following is a classic example of mild to moderate apraxia of speech. It is called the "Tornado Man" passage and represents relatively pure apraxia of speech. The example below is a transcription of a taped recording of a patient describing a family fleeing from a tornado:

I am looking an a drawing or a-a pec-picture of what is apparently a tor-nuh-ner-nor-tornatiuhd blew-brewing in the c-country side. This is having an nuh-nuhmediate and frightening ef-f-ff-fuh-feck on a fairm famerly num-ber-ing---six uh humans and af-ff-sss-uh-sh-suh-sorted farm uh animals. There are quick-uh-ly going into a-a sss-sor-sormb uh cellar with fright in their ar-uh-eyes and in their every-movement " (Darley et al. 1975, p. 250).

In the above example, the patient has no intellectual deficits. He can appreciate and describe the actions in the picture. There is little, if any, language deficit. The patient has no apparent wordfinding deficits. He is also aware of errors and occasionally self-corrective.

In severe cases of apraxia of speech, the patient may be unable to plan and coordinate exhalation and speech. Some patients are unable to blow air from their lungs to move a tissue held close to their mouths when the attempt is purposeful and voluntary. Voluntary tongue movements may be impossible in severe cases of the disorder.

The hallmark of apraxia of speech is struggle. The patient complicates, confounds, and entangles the speech act. The patient with apraxia of speech overshoots and undershoots the articulatory targets during speech. Overshooting is also called an anticipatory error, and undershooting is a perseveratory one. The patient makes articulatory errors in anticipation of the next sound, or the previous one contaminates the program. For example, an anticipatory error is when the patient says "carp" for "car" in the question: "Where is the red car parked." A perseveratory error would result in "dar" for the word "car." The sounds preceding and following the target word disrupt the articulatory plan.

Oral apraxia, sometimes called bucco-facial apraxia (Katz, Bharadwaj, and Carstens, 1999), is similar to apraxia of speech, except it involves nonspeech oral behaviors like puckering or biting the lips and attempting to touch the tongue to the nose. Oral apraxia is difficulty performing oral nonspeech movements. This apraxia also has the voluntary-involuntary dichotomy. Oral nonspeech acts are impaired or impossible when the patient consciously and purposefully tries to perform them. However, usually they can be done when the patient gives little attention and thought to how they are done. Oral apraxia and apraxia of speech usually occur together. However, in rare instances, they can occur independently of each other.

H. The Dysarthrias

The dysarthrias are a compendium of neurogenic communication disorders classified by the site of the neuromuscular impairment and subsequent type of weakness, paralysis, or movement impairments that disrupt motor speech. Duffy (2007) considers dysarthria to result from damage to the motor cortex of the brain and below. Dysarthrias can also be functional, occurring without apparent organic causes, and a source of litigation. See *Cooper v. Nieman Marcus,* 125 F3d 786 (9th Cir 1997). They are sometimes called neuromuscular communication disorders. The dysarthrias affect, to various degrees, respiration, phonation, articulation, resonance, and prosody. When a patient is rendered mute because of dysarthria, he or she is labeled "anarthric." When pure dysarthria occurs, there are no language impairments. Pure dysarthria involves only motor speech. The types of dysarthria are spastic, flaccid, ataxic, hypokinetic, hyperkinetic, and mixed-multiple.

Spastic dysarthria results from bilateral upper motor neuron damage. Bilateral means both sides of the brain, and the upper motor neurons are the tracts of the motor strip and associated areas. Duffy (1995) has also identified unilateral upper motor neuron dysarthria. It results in weakness on the opposite side of the body and resulting speech characteristics. Because of the proximity of the motor strip to the expressive speech and language centers, spastic dysarthria commonly occurs with predominantly expressive aphasia. The speech of patients with spastic dysarthria often includes harsh or hoarse voice quality, hypernasality, and distorted speech sound production.

Flaccid dysarthria results from damage to lower motor neurons, and the motor unit is impaired. The motor unit is the muscle and the nerve which enervates it. The motor unit is sometimes called the final common pathway because all motor commands ultimately go through it. The speech of patients with flaccid dysarthria often includes hypernasality, distorted speech sound production, and breathy voice quality.

Ataxic dysarthria occurs when the cerebellum and the tracts leading to and from it are damaged. The cerebellum is called the great modulator of muscular movements. Ataxic dysarthria is primarily a coordination problem because damage to the cerebellum causes movements that are ill-timed and jerky. The speech of patients with ataxic dysarthria includes disruptions of pitch and loudness, distorted speech sound production, and prosodic disturbances.

When there is damage to the extrapyramidal system, hypokinetic dysarthria can result. The extrapyramidal system is a tract of nerve fibers involved in automatic aspects of motor coordination. It is sometimes called the indirect motor system and is important in regulating posture and walking. Parkinson's disease, caused by a deficiency of the neurotransmitter dopamine, is the usual cause of hypokinetic dysarthria. The speech of patients with hypokinetic dysarthria includes a slow rate of speech, voice tremor, and reduced volume. These speech patterns occur in most patients, including those who take antiparkinson medication.

Hyperkinetic dysarthria also results from damage to the extrapyramidal system. In this type of dysarthria, there is too much movement that occurs either quickly or slowly. Quick unwanted movements affect speech because ticks and jerks can disrupt respiration, phonation, and articulation muscles and structure. Tourette's syndrome causes quick hyperkinetic dysarthria and can include coprolalia. Coprolalia is the uncontrolled use of profanity. Slow unwanted movements can cause the patient to have writhing contractions affecting one muscle after another, such as in athetoid cerebral palsy.

Mixed and multiple dysarthria occurs when two or more of the above dysarthrias exist simultaneously or when the type of dysarthria changes over time. For example, progressive neurological disorders such as amyotrophic lateral sclerosis (Lou Gehrig's disease) often have more than one of the above dysarthrias. Additionally, in some patients, the type of dysarthria changes as the diseases progresses. Approximately 50 percent of all dysarthrias are of the mixed and multiple types.

9.5 Psychological Concomitants of Neurogenic Communication Disorders

There are five major psychological concomitants of aphasia and related disorders: catastrophic reaction, emotional lability, response to loss, perseveration, and organic depression (Tanner, 2006; Tanner, 2003a; Tanner, 2003b). While not all patients experience all of them, they are frequently occurring aspects of neurogenic communication disorders. Few patients are spared one or more of them.

A catastrophic reaction can be viewed as an anxiety attack. Eisenson (1984) considers it to be a psychobiological breakdown. When a patient is placed in a frustrating and anxiety-provoking situation, he or she can feel overwhelmed with communication impotence and the possibility of failure. For some patients, there is a sense of impending doom and loss of integrity of self. Physiologically, the patient experiences rapid respiratory rate, increased blood pressure, hypertense muscles, sweating, and dry mouth. The biological reactions are related to the fight or flight response. The patient feels the need to either fight or flee from the threatening situation. The stimuli setting off a catastrophic reaction need not be profound, and they are usually related to too many demands being placed on the patient. They can be as simple as trying to remember the name of a relative or getting the articulators to produce it. Two factors are primary triggers of a catastrophic reaction. First, temporal urgency can stimulate one. Temporal urgency is the need to do something in a hurry. The patient must deal with an imposed deadline. For example, a therapist can inadvertently stimulate a catastrophic reaction in a patient prone to one by trying to get him or her to say something in a hurry or to read a passage rapidly. The second factor prompting a catastrophic reaction is sensory bombardment. Too much noise in a hospital or nursing home room, loud overhead paging systems, vacuums, television noise, and other patients' chatter can precipitate a catastrophic reaction.

Review of the research on catastrophic reactions show that they are more common in patients with predominantly expressive aphasia. Some authorities believe that they are related to damaged brain cells in, around, and below Broca's area and the consequent neurochemical imbalances that create anxiety. A more compelling reason is that predominantly expressive aphasia tends to be frustrating. The more nonfluent the speech output, the more likely the occurrence of a catastrophic reaction. There may be a relationship between post stroke depression and catastrophic reactions (Craig and Cummings, 1995).

Observable catastrophic reactions can take many forms. Some patients cry, throw objects, upturn dinner trays, physically accost medical staff, or lose consciousness. Other patients simply pull bed covers over their heads. Once a catastrophic reaction has begun, it is difficult to stop. The best treatment is prevention by eliminating sources of stress, anxiety, and perceived potential of failure. Medical personnel can be injured by a violent patient, but there have been no reports in medical journals of death or injury to a patient because of a clinically diagnosed catastrophic reaction. However, major catastrophic reactions are certainly physically and psychologically stressful. Their proper management falls within minimum standards of care for physicians, speech-language pathologists, nurses, occupational and physical therapists, and other specialists who treat patients prone to them.

Some patients with neurogenic communication disorders have exaggerated emotions. Emotional lability is particularly common in those patients who have bilateral damage to the motor strips of the brain (and associated corticobulbar tracts). It is sometimes called pseudobulbar emotional lability and thus is common in patients who have spastic dysarthria. Patients with emotional lability appear to cry for no apparent reason or cry too much over little things. They can also laugh too easily, but because there is more to be sad about, emotional lability usually involves crying. Emotional lability can convey a false impression of dementia (Duffy, 1995). Patients with pseudobulbar emotional lability have lowered emotional thresholds; their reactions are exaggerated and not inappropriate. Emotional lability has also been considered as a manifestation of a catastrophic reaction in patients prone to crying (Gainotti, 1989).

Highly charged words, such as a family member's name or "nursing home," can set off bouts of emotional labile crying. Situational prompts, such as visiting relatives, can also precipitate them. Emotional labile crying can also be caused by negative thoughts, particularly about the patient's predicament. Like a catastrophic reaction, once an episode of emotional lability begins, it is difficult to stop.

Some authorities suggest that labile crying is simply the motor act and devoid of true feelings. Crying and laughing are disconnected true emotions in these patients. However, the existence of nonemotional crying (or laughing) in labile patients has not been confirmed by research and is conjecture at this point. In addition, some caretakers can view all emotional responses by labile patients as a manifestation of brain injury and not due to environmental factors. This misdiagnosis can cause improper management of the patient's psychological reactions to the neurogenic communication disorder.

Neurogenic communication disorders involve three dimensions of loss and the human reaction to them: the grief response. According to Code, Hemsley, and Herrmann (1999), the grief model is powerful in its ability to explain some of the emotional and psychosocial reactions seen in patients with neurogenic communication disorders, although more research is necessary. The three dimensions in which patients experience loss are self, person, and object, and they can be expected to go through predictable stages of grief as a result of those losses (Tanner, 2006; Tanner, 2003a; Tanner, 2003b; Tanner, 1999; Tanner and Gerstenberger, 1996; Tanner, 1980).

Loss of self occurs because of loss of the abilities such as walking, talking, dressing, and bowel and bladder control. Loss of person is the psychological separation the patient experiences from family and friends due to the communication disorder, and also because of physical placement in a nursing home or other type of extended care facility. Loss of object includes the use of a motor home, car, sewing machine, computer, or other valued object or pet due to physical and cognitive limitations and/or placement in a nursing home.

Aware patients can be expected to grieve over the above losses and pass through several stages of grief which ultimately lead to acceptance. Psychological attempts to overcome the losses can include denial, anger, and bargaining. Grieving depression occurs when attempts to overcome the losses have failed, and it may last for several months, depending on the value the patient placed on that which was lost. Finally, most patients reach a resolution of the losses and view the changes from a larger accepting perspective. Not all patients experience the grief response, nor do all individuals necessarily pass through all of the stages. Although difficult to quantify, loss in all three dimensions can be considered in compensation and assessing damages.

Perseveration is the tendency for a sensory or motor act to continue for a longer duration than is appropriate or warranted by the significance of the stimuli. The patient gets stuck in a mental set or behavior pattern and cannot shift to another one. There are two types of perseveratory behaviors. Verbal perseveration is when the patient repeats the same sound, word, or phrase over and over. It is sometimes called recurrent perseveration. The patient utters the same word repeatedly regardless of what question has been asked. When the patient repeats the last word or words spoken by someone else, the behavior is called echolalia. Echolalia is also a feature of many degenerative brain diseases (Benson and Ardila, 1996). Graphic perseveration is when the patient's writing consists of letters repeated over and over. The patient cannot shift his or her hand movements from one pattern to another. According to Kreisler, Godefory, Delmaire, Debachy, Leclercq, Pruvo, and Leys (2000), the caudate nucleus is a likely area of damage in perseveration. The caudate nucleus is a subcortical structure.

Organic depression occurs because of brain injury and the resulting imbalance of neurochemicals that control and regulate mood. Unlike grieving, where the depression is related to loss of self, person, or object, organic depression is a result of neurochemicals gone awry. Organic clinical depression is a direct result of the brain injury or indirectly related to the general altered chemistry caused by the stroke, traumatic brain injury, disease, and the medications used to treat them. In many cases, this type of depression is associated with anxiety. As a result of depression-anxiety, the patient may become anxious and preoccupied with body and mental changes. The "joie de vivre" is lost. For some depressed patients there is the possibility of suicide. Depression-anxiety is more common in patients with predominantly expressive aphasia. Although there are differing incidence estimates of depression-anxiety disorder in patients with neurogenic communication disorders, as many as 50 percent to 70 percent may suffer from it (Tanner, 2003a). Antidepressants have a high success rate of reducing the duration and extent of depression. For some patients, antidepressant medication will be permanently required, and for others they are only temporarily necessary until the brain readjusts its biochemistry. Table 9.3 shows the psychological concomitants of neurogenic communication disorders.

9.6 Neurogenic Communication Disorders Malpractice Litigation and Efficacy of Treatment

During neurogenic communication disorders malpractice litigation, attorneys, lawyers, and jurors may question the overall efficacy of aphasia treatment and the value of therapy with a particular patient. The question may arise: "Given that brain damage is irreversible, how can patients be expected to recover communication abilities?" This question is particularly relevant to aphasia given the phenomenon of spontaneous recovery.

Table 9.3
Major Psychological Concomitants of Neurogenic Communication Disorders

Psychological Reaction	Manifestation or Behavior
Catastrophic Reaction	Panic attack and the need to flee or fight
Emotional Lability	Exaggerated emotions; excessive crying or laughing
Response to Loss	Predictable stages of adjustment to unwanted change
Perseveration	Tendency for a thought or motor act to persist
Organic Depression	Chronic severe negative emotions as a result of a brain chemistry imbalance

Spontaneous recovery is where patients automatically and without the benefit of treatments and therapies regain some, or in rare instances all, of their communication abilities following strokes, head traumas, or other types of injuries to the brain and nervous system. Significant spontaneous recovery can occur for twelve months or longer but is more apparent early postonset. Spontaneous recovery of speech and language abilities has been attributed to a reduction of pressure in the brain, new or improved blood supply to affected areas, biochemical activities at the cellular level, adjacent areas of the brain assuming the functions of the damaged ones, the right brain hemisphere taking over functions from the damaged left one, and generally to the tendency of the human body to repair itself. Determining the benefit of any treatment or therapy is complicated by the presence of spontaneous recovery. During the middle of the last century, some scientists and physicians theorized that all gains in speech and language were the result of spontaneous recovery and not attributable to treatments and therapies.

As a response to the criticism, much research has been conducted on the efficacy of therapies and treatments for these communication disorders. Research includes large double-blind studies, single subject designs, and subjective reports from patients and their families (see Chapter 6). Some are done to learn whether a particular therapy or treatment results in significant gains for a specific type of disorder. With few exceptions, studies support the hypothesis that patients who receive therapies and treatment for their communication disorders benefit from those services. The gains they make go beyond what can be expected to occur from spontaneous recovery. Patients who receive treatments and therapies make more rapid gains and in broader dimensions than do control subjects. Unfortunately, as a

group, patients with global aphasia, also called complete or severe expressive-receptive aphasia, do not gain from treatments and therapies. Consequently, this type of aphasia is sometimes called irreversible aphasia syndrome (see Table 9.1).

Certain factors are related to prognoses for patients with neurogenic communication disorders. Studies have found that, as a rule, patients with mild impairments do better than those who suffer severe neurogenic disorders. The age of the patient is also important. Younger patients tend to do better than older ones. This also may be related to the types of injuries experienced by the young and old. Younger patients tend to be more prone to traumatic brain injuries, which also appear to have a better prognosis for some types of disabilities. Studies have shown that the earlier treatments and therapies are initiated, and the more intensive they are provided, the better the prognosis for some types of disorders. With regard to the type of treatments and therapies, patient gains go beyond the stimuli used in them. There is generalization to speech and language functions other than those targeted for rehabilitation. Several studies have shown that one of the greatest benefits of treatments and therapies is in the psychological domain and improvement in quality of life. Constructive family involvement also is associated with patient gains (Baker and Tanner, 1990).

9.7 Neurogenic Communication Disorders Malpractice Litigation and Evaluation Philosophy

During neurogenic communication disorders malpractice litigation, a particular patient's test results may become a central issue to the case. Consequently, attorneys, judges, and jurors may be confronted with diagnostic test scores and various interpretations of the test result. Before discussing factors to understanding test scores and their interpretation, reviewing the purpose of the evaluation is necessary.

There are four reasons for evaluating patients with neurogenic communication disorders. First, it is necessary to decide whether the patient has detectable aphasia, apraxia of speech, or the dysarthrias. Second, comprehensive testing is necessary to categorize, quantify, and describe the symptoms of the neurogenic communication disorders and to determine a prognosis for recovery with and without treatment and therapies. Third, evaluation of neurogenic communication disorders is done for therapeutic purposes, to set goals and design treatments and therapies to maximize the patient's recovery of speech and language abilities. Fourth, comprehensive speech and language evaluation may be required for litigation purposes.

The controversies discussed in Chapter 2 must be considered when reviewing diagnostic tests, methods, procedures, scores, and interpretation of results, particularly concerning expert testimony. Some experts view these disorders in the Darley tradition, while others do not separate motor speech from language disorders. In addition, some experts, especially neurologists, view neurogenic communication disorders primarily from a localizationist perspective. They diagnose symptoms and manifestations of the disorders based on the site and size of the damage to the brain and nervous system. Also, particularly with regard to aphasia, the language-thought controversy must be considered. Some authorities consider language only to reflect and express thought, while others believe language and thought are inseparable, particularly in adults. Many professionals and experts are eclectic in their approaches to neurogenic communication disorders, but their underlying philosophies about the brain, mind, language, and human thought affect their interpretations of results. Examples of screening tests for aphasia, apraxia of speech, and dysarthria are provided in Appendix A.

Speech and language testing can provide specific information about the overall presentation of symptoms. Each standardized test administered should be reviewed for validity, reliability, and potential for bias. Validity is the extent to which a test does what it purports to do. A test that is valid is one that measures what it says it does. Reliability is how dependable a test is; it is the consistency of the scores and results over repeated test administration. A reliable test is one that produces the same results when given to the same person at different times or by different forms of the same test. Particularly with regard to language testing, a test may be biased that does not reflect the ethnic and cultural background of a patient. For patients who are multilingual, testing using the language spoken in the home will give a more accurate appraisal of overall language strengths and weaknesses.

9.8 Neurogenic Communication Disorders and Malingering

Malingering is to pretend incapacity so as to avoid duty, work, or tasks considered unpleasant. Malingering is a type of factitious disorder where an illness is self-induced or falsified by the patient. In neurogenic communication disorders, malingering is the willful and deliberate feigning or exaggerating of a neurologically based speech and language disorder for a self-serving end. The self-serving end is usually financial but can also include exemption, attention, sympathy, drugs, or employment rewards. The true malingerer willfully and consciously feigns expressive and receptive speech and language impairments. "Functional" is used to refer to a communication disorder that is nonorganic and can be inclusive of malingering.

When investigating malingering and neurogenic communication disorders, the notion of conscious versus subconscious rewards must be addressed. For some patients, the rewards or exemption for loss of speech and language abilities may be subconscious. A conversion reaction is the loss of voluntary control over normal striated muscle movements or over the senses, resulting from interpersonal conflicts or environmental stress (Aronson, 1990). Conversion reactions and subsequent loss of speech, voice, and hearing have been well-documented in the psychiatric and psychological literature. Many authorities consider the loss of sensory or motor functioning, whether it is the sense of hearing or the ability to use the muscles of speech, to have symbolic importance. In communication disorders, these conversion reactions suggest interpersonal distress such as an unsatisfying or dangerous relationship. They symbolize the psychic trauma associated with the negative relationship. Many patients present with "la belle indifference," meaning "the beautiful indifference." The psychological mechanism underlying the conversion reaction gives the patient relief from distress and thus the blissful indifference. The case can be made that some malingerers are receiving subconscious psychological rewards. The rewards are subconscious; the patient is not fully aware of the self-serving end.

There is no single test to detect malingering in neurogenic communication disorders. However, there are several diagnostic and observational factors to consider. First, brain scans such as computed tomography (CT), magnetic resonance imaging (MRI), single photon tomography (SPECT), positron emission tomography (PET), and functional magnetic resonance imaging (fMRI) diagnostic tests can provide information about brain damage. Interpretation of these test results must allow for the fact that speech and language centers of the brain are not uniform and consistent for all people. According to Zemlin (1998) and Restak (1984), the left cerebral hemisphere is specialized for language, handedness, analytic thought processes, and certain types of memory in about 90 percent of right-handed people (See Chapter 2). Left hemisphere dominance is found in about 64 percent of left-handed people and right dominance in about 20 percent. In ambidextrous people, the left hemisphere is dominant in about 60 percent of the population. Both hemispheres are equally dominant in about 30 percent of people who are ambidextrous. In addition to brain scans, laboratory and other medical tests can confirm brain and nervous system injury.

The second factor to consider in detecting malingering is the speech and language test results and the patient's presentation of symptoms: Are they typical symptoms of aphasia, apraxia of speech, and the dysarthrias? Although there are unusual ways patients present neurogenic communication disorders, whether they are typical of the type, size, and location of alleged neurological injury can provide information about malingering.

The consistency of the speech and language symptoms presented by the patient suspected of malingering should also be reviewed. It is now recognized that most patients with neurogenic communication disorders evolve in their presentation of symptoms. This change in the patterns of speech and language deficits begins early postonset. Patients with one type of aphasia sometimes evolve into another type, and most patients with neurogenic communication disorders have early spontaneous improvement. This spontaneous improvement can be noticed as early as two or three days postonset. Even patients with progressive neuromuscular speech disorders, such as seen in multiple sclerosis, sometimes have remissions and exacerbations of symptoms. In Parkinson's disease, abrupt change in severity of the speech pathology is called the off-on phenomenon. Apraxia of speech is often present early in strokes and traumatic brain injuries, only to subside and even disappear later as the brain swelling subsides. Also, in apraxia of speech, there is the volitional-nonvolitional dichotomy. Some purposeful speech acts are impossible but can be spoken normally or nearly normally when little forethought is given to them.

Inconsistent voicing can suggest malingering. If a patient feigns aphonia, loss of voice, during speech, but can laugh, hum, or forcefully clear his or her throat, malingering may be present. Although there are rare exceptions, a patient who can laugh aloud, hum, or forcefully clear his or her throat has the neurological and muscular integrity to produce voice during speech; neurological and muscular diseases usually do not result in this voicing dichotomy. A patient who whispers during speech, yet can voice during nonspeech activities, has inconsistent presentation of symptoms and should be further evaluated for malingering.

Obviously, patients with global aphasia and severe neuromuscular disorders have less room for spontaneous recovery and changes in symptoms. However, careful examination of their speech and language abilities will often show minor spontaneous recovery and evolution of symptoms. Lack of spontaneous recovery and little change in speech and language symptoms over time suggests an unusual and atypical course of neurogenic communication disorders. Conversely, too much spontaneous recovery and evolution of symptoms also suggest an unusual and atypical course of neurogenic communication disorders. Certain medications, especially those that affect alertness and arousal, can also cause unusual shifts in the patient's presentation of symptoms. In addition, clinically depressed patients may experience a change in symptom presentation when the depression lifts.

Munchausen syndrome is where the patient feigns an illness to gain nurturing, attention, comfort, sympathy, and consolation from healthcare professionals. When applied to neurogenic communication disorders, patients displaying Munchausen syndrome will present with signs and symptoms of aphasia, apraxia of speech, or the dysarthrias primarily to satisfy the psychological need to revert to the role of a dependent person. Patients with Munchausen syndrome applied to neurogenic communication disorders are likely to show the most obvious symptoms such as slurred speech, weak voice, gross comprehension difficulty, and stuttering-like speech struggle. Patients with Munchausen syndrome have a mental disorder involving internal rewards that are separate from the external type of rewards or exemptions seen in patients with malingering.

Munchausen syndrome by proxy is a form of child abuse where a caregiver, usually the mother, purposefully creates an illness in a dependent, usually a child, to receive attention, sympathy, and comfort from healthcare professionals. Munchausen syndrome by proxy applied to neurogenic communication disorders may involve the parent insisting that the child has one or more signs of a neurogenic communication disorder in the absence of repeated tests confirming the presence of such disorders. In Munchausen syndrome by proxy, the parent may purposefully create situations at home that delay, retard, impede, or otherwise interfere with the child's normal speech and language development. The parent may also purposefully create medical conditions that include communication disorders in their manifestations. The parent may appear very attentive and knowledgeable about communication disorders and require a great deal of attention from special education or medical personnel.

9.9 Neurogenic Communication Disorders Malpractice Litigation: Assessing Standards of Care

The scopes of practice for speech-language pathologists (see Figure 4.1) and audiologists (see Figure 4.2) are detailed in Chapter 4. Litigation issues involving speech-language pathologists and audiologists with regard to patients with neurogenic communication disorders can include patient assessment and monitoring, reports documenting changes in condition, following hospital protocols, and delegation of responsibilities.

Standards of care for both speech-language pathologists and audiologists include competent assessment, diagnosis, treatment, referral, and follow-up services for people with communication disorders. Failure in any aspect of these areas of patient management can cause or contribute to negative patient outcomes. It is important that speech-language pathologists and audiologists report changes in the condition of the patient to responsible parties. This is particularly important with regard to swallowing disorders (see Chapter 8) because medical complications can be life threatening. Changes in symptoms and conditions of patients with neurogenic communication disorders can also indicate improper or insufficient medication regimens and neurological complications requiring prompt medical intervention. All substantial changes in patient conditions should be documented in the chart and verbal reports promptly made to responsible parties. Failure to follow the chain of command with regard to provision of services also can create negative patient outcomes. This is particularly true with regard to referrals to specialists and family counseling. Litigation issues can also involve improper delegation of clinical and professional responsibilities to speech-language pathology assistants and audiometrists.

Physicians, nurses, occupational therapists, and others involved with patients who have neurogenic communication disorders have an implied responsibility with regard to institutional quality of care and the potential for neglect and abuse. Because many of these patients cannot communicate basic wants and needs, special arrangements must me made to accommodate their communication disabilities. Many of these special considerations are covered in the 1990 Americans with Disabilities Act (ADA). This act is designed to prevent discrimination against individuals with disabilities

in employment, housing, public accommodations, education, transportation, communication, recreation, institutionalization, health services, voting, and access to public services (USDOJ, 2001).

The long-term and short-term goals and objectives, frequency, duration, and outcomes of treatment and therapies depend on the type and severity of the neurogenic communication disorder. Treatment and therapy regimens can be brief and occasional, or provided intensively for several months. Individual and group therapies are also provided. Inpatient hospital treatments typically are conducted once or twice daily, and outpatient and home health services provided one, two, or three times weekly. As long as the patient continues to profit from the experience, i.e., learn and the gains are functional, meaningful, and contributors to improved quality of life and/or vocation, services are justified. The Code of Ethics of the American Speech-Language-Hearing Association specifically prohibits providing services to patients who have no reasonable expectation of improvement. Managed care has changed the traditional provision of services for patients with neurogenic communication disorders. Many clinical and rehabilitation decisions once made by therapists and physicians now are made by managed care organizations based on financial guidelines. Medicare and other third-party insurers place caps on the monetary amounts that can be provided for a particular category of disorder. In addition, in hospitals, nursing homes, and home health agencies, for third-party payment the patient's physician must authorize the goals, objectives, and procedures monthly.

9.10 Neurogenic Communication Disorders Malpractice Litigation: Assessing Quality of Life

Although changes in quality of life may be issues in medical malpractice cases, there are few systematic ways of quantifying those changes. Lawton (1991) defines quality of life in a multidimensional framework. According to this model, there are four critical domains: (1) objective environment, (2) behavioral competence, (3) perceived quality of life, and (4) psychological well-being. Each of the domains interact with one another. Neurogenic communication disorders, especially severe ones, can have dramatic effects on a person's quality of life. They can affect all of the critical domains.

The first critical domain, objective environment, can have profound implications on the patient's quality of life. The environment must meet basic needs and supply the materials necessary to thrive and for self-actualization. The objective environment must provide the patient with food and shelter, opportunities for recreation, stimulation, exercise, meaningful interaction with others, and access to community services for the disabled.

The second critical domain, behavioral competence, involves the patient's ability to exercise basic control over his or her life. Behaviorally, the patient must be able to functionally interact with and control fundamental aspects of his or her environment. Both mobility and communication may be denied the patient with a neurogenic communication disorder. When assessing this aspect of quality of life, the patient's access to assistive devices for communication disorders should be considered. These include the Internet, video recorders, digital hearing aids, voice recognition devices, type-to-speech systems, cochlear implants, and other technologies. The availability of aides and volunteers and ease of mobility within the home, institution, and the community should also be considered.

The third dimension in Lawton's model, perceived quality of life, is the assessment the individual has about his or her existence. It is a subjective judgment about satisfaction with life overall. Quality of life for patients with neurogenic communication disorders can be affected by their preconceived notions and stereotypes about the nature of communication disorders and cooccurring physical disabilities. This aspect of quality of life is highly individual and what is considered an impoverished existence by some, others may consider rich and rewarding.

Finally, quality of life is dependent on the person's psychological well-being. The psychological concomitants in neurogenic communication disorders can range from euphoria to clinical depression. As noted previously, most patients who suffer serious, irreversible loss of the ability to communicate also feel a sense of loss. The losses may result in several adjustment stages, including depression (Tanner, 2003a; Tanner 2003b). Two Bill of Rights for aphasic patients address the four quality of life dimension. The *Aphasic Patient's Bill of Rights* (Tanner, 1999) details the aphasic patient's rights in a medical care facility and especially with regard to the patient-clinician relationship. The National Aphasia Association (2005) also provides the *Aphasia Bill of Rights* addressing the information and services needed for patients to move forward with their lives.

9.11 Issues in Neurogenic Communication Disorders Litigation: Disability Determination

There are three primary areas of disability litigation for patients with neurogenic communication disorders: vocational rehabilitation eligibility, antidiscrimination issues, and insurance-social welfare determination and compensation. Neurogenic communication disorders vary greatly with regard to severity, thus making litigating these issues highly case dependent.

Legislation covering vocational rehabilitation services began more than seventy-five years ago and has greatly expanded to provide services to address the employment and independent living needs of persons with disabilities (Bruyère and DeMarinis, 1999).

The legislative mandate requires that the order of selection for the provision of vocational rehabilitation services shall be determined on the basis of serving first those individuals with the most severe disabilities. Individuals with disabilities, including individuals with the most severe disabilities, are generally presumed to be capable of engaging in gainful employment, and the provision of individualized rehabilitation services is designed to improve their ability to become gainfully employed (Bruyère and DeMarinis, 1999, p. 681).

Many patients with neurogenic communication disorders are potentially employable and able to compete in the labor force. Vocational rehabilitation counselors make job-related disability determinations and arrange for therapies, adaptive devices training, and educational experiences to facilitate the patient's return to gainful employment. Litigation issues related to neurogenic communication disorders include determination of vocational rehabilitation potential and the appropriateness, adequacy, and duration of training programs.

The primary antidiscrimination statue is the Americans with Disabilities Act (ADA) of 1990. Title I of the act applies to private employers with at least fifteen employees and state and local governments. It protects qualified individuals with disabilities from discrimination (Bruyère and DeMarinis, 1999). This act requires employers to make reasonable accommodations to allow disabled persons to perform their jobs. Litigation issues in patients with neurogenic communication disorders involve what is considered reasonable accommodations, job applications and hiring procedures, training, wrongful discharge, and also the right of prisoners to speech therapy.

Insurance claims and social-welfare determinations with patients having neurogenic communication disorders range from quantifying levels of disabilities for damages to qualifications for social security disability payments. Litigation issues often revolve around assessing functional speech and language abilities and disabilities. See *Arneson v Heckler, 879 F2d 393 (8th Cir 1989)*

9.12 Issues in Neurogenic Communication Disorders Litigation: Determining Mental Competence

As a rule, patients with pure motor speech disorders are not compromised with regard to intelligence and cognition. Apraxia of speech and the dysarthrias are motor disorders, and although they can render a patient severely communication disabled or even mute, his or her intelligence and cognition can be unaffected. Therefore, patients with pure apraxia of speech, flaccid, spastic, ataxic, hypokinetic, hyperkinetic, and mixed-multiple dysarthrias are not necessarily compromised with regard to intelligence and cognition. For example, amyotrophic lateral sclerosis, Lou Gehrig's disease, can result in severe mixed dysarthria, and the patient may need an assistive device, such as a speech synthesizer, to communicate. If the patient is provided with an effective alternative communication device, he or she is mentally competent to understand, create, modify, and change a will or trust. Motor speech disorders, by themselves, and with proper accommodations, do not interfere with the ability to distinguish right from wrong, manage affairs, or to assist counsel in legal proceedings.

The competence of patients with aphasia depends on the severity and type of language impairment and the area of competency at issue. Some issues may involve basic abilities to process language, while others may involve complex use and understanding of language and mathematics. See *Holmes v. Texas A&M University, 145 F.3d 681 (5th Cir 1998)*. Benson and Ardila (1996, p. 339) address the complexity of determining aphasic patients' competence to sign checks, make wills, to manage business affairs, etc.:

> Many aphasic patients are fully capable of managing their own affairs; many others are obviously unable to make important decisions and deserve the protection of a conservator or guardian; another group of aphasic patients, intermediate to the first two, can prove troublesome for the clinician who is asked to provide judgment concerning their competency.

With regard to mental competence: "A sizable number of aphasic patients are far more intelligent than general appearances would indicate, and many are capable of making their own decisions in significant legal matters" (Benson and Ardila, 1996, p. 340).

Benson and Ardila (1996) note that when a legal act, such as executing a will or entering into a contract, is required of an aphasic person, the information should be provided on a bit-by-bit basis and that careful ongoing assessment of the patient's ability to comprehend written and spoken language is required. They go on to suggest videotaping the event, which can take several sessions, to document the processes followed and the patient's responses to them.

Receptive language impairment can significantly impede the patient's comprehension of legal and medical issues. Benson and Ardila (1996, p. 337) note that studies addressing intelligence and aphasia vary greatly in research design: "Most of these tests treat aphasia as a single, unitary disturbance, failing to note that intellectual dysfunction will vary tremendously, depending on the neuroanatomical locus of damage." They go on to opine that damage to the posterior area of the brain is more likely to interfere with intellectual competence than anterior brain damage. Anterior and posterior refer to speech and language centers lying in front or behind the fissure separating the frontal and parietal lobes. Receptive aphasia is associated with posterior brain damage. Graphic disturbances and acalculia can prevent the patient from understanding financial and business affairs. Loss of abstract attitude and the inability to communicate can create unsafe living environments. Driving competence is suspect for patients with moderate to severe aphasia because of alexia, agnosia, loss of abstract attitude, and the tendency to perseverate.

One particularly important issue regarding mental competence and patients with neurogenic communication disorders has to do with the accuracy of their yes/no responses. Verbal paraphasias are common word-retrieval behaviors in aphasic patients. A verbal paraphasia is the producing of a word that has a semantic relationship to the desired word: "car" for "truck," "pen" for "pencil," "up" for "down." They are associated semantically. Aphasic patients may erroneously report "yes" for "no," and vice versa, to questions because of semantic associations. Both "yes" and "no" are one word, closed-end responses. Consequently, for patients who are unaware of their word-finding errors and who are not self-corrective, their competence to accurately answer these types of questions is suspect. Additionally, the tendency for perseveration and echolalia compromises the accuracy of their verbal responses.

Intelligence testing is occasionally used to determine current mental competence in aphasic patients. Many cognitive psychologists operationally define intelligence simply as how well a person performs on IQ tests. Typically, an aphasic patient will do poorly on verbal aspects of intelligence tests and have normal or near normal performance subsections. "Formal test results, although of some usefulness as a base, are not capable of measuring the mental competency of an aphasic patient" (Benson and Ardila, p. 339). Informal observations can be useful in gauging an aphasic patient's intelligence. "Information concerning the patient's retention of social graces; the ability to count and/or make change; the exhibition of appropriate concern about family, business, and personal activities; competency in finding their way in the environment; the ability to socialize; and the presence of self-concern provide valuable indications of residual intelligence in the aphasic person" (Benson and Ardila, 1996, p. 338).

When an aphasic patient's current competence is at issue, videotaping the reading and executing of a document provides supporting evidence of the reliability and validity of the procedure, and several sessions should be devoted to demonstrating the patient's understanding of each aspect of the legal act. For example, if an aphasic patient is to sign a document relinquishing control of a business or to change a will, several steps should be followed. First, the patient's ability to understand simple auditory commands should be assessed. This can be done using subtests of several aphasia batteries or by using the Token Test, of which there are several varieties. The Token Test has the patient match differently colored and sized geometric forms from the examiner's verbal commands. Second, the patient's reading abilities should be assessed by having the patient follow one, two and three degree directional commands from written stimuli, e.g., "Point to the door," "Point to the door and then point to the ceiling." Third, the patient should show that he or she understands the implications of his or her signature. Many aphasic patients can only approximate their signatures. The patient should be provided with several opportunities to sign a request for goods or services, such as receiving water, being moved to a different side of the table, etc. Only when the patient signs for the goods or services does he or she obtain them. Fourth, the patient is asked about his or her understanding of the implications of signing the document. This should be done over more than one session. Questions should be asked in several ways about the implications of relinquishing business control or changing the will. These should be short questions such as "Do you want your son to run the business now?" "Do you want to quit the business?" and "Point to whom you want to run the business?" A picture or photograph of the business and parties in the agreement can also be shown to the patient and used during the questioning.

An important aspect of this determination is to ask the patient to sign a document that he or she obviously would not want to sign if the question and its implications were understood. A short document saying that his or her signature will give up a beloved pet or that his or her television will be destroyed should be placed before the patient. The patient refusing to sign such a document suggests a basic under-

standing of the pragmatic implications of his or her signature. After the patient has signed the document relinquishing business control or the change of a will or trust, he or she should be queried about the implications of the act. Does the patient now understand what has occurred, and is that what he or she wanted? These questions should be asked over several sessions. While the above procedure does not assure that the patient understood all of the implications of his or her signature on the legal document, it does provide evidence of an objective and comprehensive attempt to determine mental competence.

Retrospective competency involves whether a person was competent to read, understand, and sign a legal document, and/or write checks and to have made business management decisions. Retrospective competency may be an issue in family-owned businesses where the spouse and children were reluctant to deny business authority to a relative following a stroke or other illness. Retrospective competency determination can also occur in the above situation where the spouse and children were too zealous and unreasonable in denying business authority to a relative.

According to Benson and Ardila (1996), in a retrospective competency determination, a judgment is required about the aphasic patient's mental and language capabilities at or near the time he or she signed the document in question. In cases where there is no videotape of the reading and signing of the document, expert testimony can only be rendered based on reports and depositions from people witnessing the act, and medical records of the patient's status at the time of the signing. Benson and Ardila (1996) conclude that in cases of retrospective competency a firm decision about the patient's mental competence or specific desires at the time in question cannot be assured.

9.13 Case Study in Neurogenic Communication Disorders Litigation: Mental Competence Determination

A man in his early sixties suffered a stroke with resulting neurogenic communication disorders. He was the founder and owner of a family-run, beverage distributing business. The business began as a small delivery service and grew into a large distribution corporation with many employees, trucks, and warehouses and operated in several towns and cities. Over the years, his wife and children assumed various roles in the operation of the business although he maintained tight control over the day-to-day operations. He made decisions about expansion, supervised everything from forklift safety to union concerns, and personally signed payroll checks. When he suffered the stroke he had aphasia and apraxia of speech, and his ability to function in his previous capacity was at issue. The family sought professional advice about whether he would recover his communication abilities and be able to return to his previous role in the business. There were also disputes within his family about who should take responsibility for the business affairs in his absence.

Some family members believed that the patient could "understand everything" that was said. They believed that although the stroke had disrupted his ability to communicate it did not affect his mental abilities with regard to business operations and that all he needed was for people to accommodate his communication disorder. Other family members believed that the stroke had rendered him mentally incompetent and that he was no longer fit to assume even a minimal role in the operation of the business. During the dispute two pivotal questions arose about his ability to communicate subsequent to the stroke: 1) did he understand other people's speech and writing, and 2) did he appreciate the financial concerns he needed to address?

The tests showed that the patient was significantly impaired in all aspects of communication. Receptively he was unable to understand most single words spoken to him, and short phrases using simple words were beyond his comprehension. Although he nodded and appeared to understand what was spoken and written, objective tests showed profound auditory comprehension deficits, and his graphic impairments paralleled his verbal ones. Although some auditory comprehension typically returns spontaneously in the majority of aphasic patients, this individual did not experience appreciable return of communication abilities. To demonstrate the patient's communication abilities to the family members, the tests were explained to them prior to administration and given to the patient in their presence. Afterward, there was no question as to his functional communication abilities and inability to return to his previous position in the company.

9.14 Chapter Summary

Neurogenic communication disorders can be divided into motor speech disorders and language disturbances. This type of distinction provides a foundation to understanding the medical-legal and forensic aspects of these communication disorders. Typically, the language disorder of aphasia is further divided into predominantly expressive and receptive deficits which usually affect all modalities of communication. In aphasia, perceptual disorders and loss of abstract attitude also can occur. There are five major psychological

concomitants of neurogenic communication disorders: catastrophic reaction, emotional lability, grief response, perseveration, and organic depression. Medical-legal and forensic issues related to neurogenic communication disorders are complex and can involve any or all of the above issues.

Suggested Readings and Resources

Darley, F. (1982). *Aphasia*. Philadelphia: Saunders

Darley, F., Aronson, A., and Brown, J. (1975). *Motor speech disorders*. Philadelphia: Saunders.

The above listed books clearly delineate the motor speech disorders from the language disturbance of aphasia.

Tanner, D. (2007). *The family guide to surviving stroke and communication disorders* (2nd Edition.) Boston: Allyn & Bacon. This book examines aphasia, apraxia of speech, and the dysarthrias in easily understood terms and with examples and illustrations.

Tanner, D. (2003). *The psychology of neurogenic communication disorders: A primer for health care professionals*. Boston: Allyn & Bacon. This book explores three psychological factors associated with neurogenic communication disorders: organic precipitants, psychological conflict and defense, and the grief response.

Tanner, D. (2003). *Exploring communication disorders: A 21st century introduction through literature and media*. Boston: Allyn & Bacon. This book examines communication disorders using references to media and literature.

Tanner, D. (2006). *Case studies in communication sciences and disorders*. Upper Saddle River, N.J.: Pearson Merrill Prentice Hall. Several chapters examine neurogenic communication disorders and provides case studies regarding their etiology, diagnosis, and treatment.

Tanner, D. (2006). *An advanced course in communication sciences and disorders*. San Diego: Plural Publishing. This book examines the language-thought controversy and provides a history of the study of neurogenic communication disorders.

Zemlin, W. (1998). *Speech and hearing science* (4th ed.). Boston: Allyn & Bacon. This book is the definitive volume on speech and hearing sciences, particularly anatomy and physiology

References

Aronson, A. (1990). *Clinical voice disorders: An interdisciplinary approach (3rd ed.).* New York: Thieme.

Baker, M. and Tanner, D. (1990). Recovery from brain insult: Investigation of patient and family adaptation. A paper presented to the annual convention of the Canadian Association of Speech-Language Pathologists and Audiologists, Vancouver, BC.

Benson, D. and Ardila, A. (1996). *Aphasia.* New York: Oxford University Press.

Bruyère, S.M. and DeMarinis, R, K (1999). Legislation and rehabilitation service delivery. In *Medical aspects of disability: A handbook for the rehabilitation professional* (2nd ed.), M. Eisenberg, R. Glueckauf, and H. Zaretsky (Eds). New York: Springer.

Code, C., Hemsley, G., and Herrmann, M. (1999). The Emotional impact of aphasia. *Seminars in speech and language*, Volume 20, Number 1, Pp. 19-31.

Craig, A. and Cummings, J. (1995). Neuropsychiatric aspects of aphasia. In *Handbook of neurological speech and language disorders,* Kirshner, H. (Ed). New York: Marcel Dekker, Inc.

Darley, F. (1982). *Aphasia.* Philadelphia: Saunders

Darley, F., Aronson, A., and Brown, J. (1975). *Motor speech disorders.* Philadelphia: Saunders.

Davis, G. A. (2007). *Aphasiology: Disorders and clinical practice* (2nd ed.). Boston: Allyn & Bacon.

Duffy, J. (1995). *Motor speech disorders.* St. Louis: Mosby.

Eisenson, J. (1984). *Adult aphasia,* (2nd ed.). Englewood Cliffs, NJ: Prentice-Hall.

Gainotti, G. (1989). The meaning of emotional disturbances resulting from unilateral brain injury. In *Emotions and the dual brain,* G. Gainotti and C. Caltagirone (Eds). New York: Springer-Verlag.

Goldstein, K. (1948). *Language and language disturbances.* New York: Grune and Stratton.

Goldstein, K. (1952). The effects of brain damage on the personality. *Psychiatry*, 15: 245-260.

Goldstein, K. (1959). Functional disturbances in the brain. In *American handbook of psychiatry,* S. Arieti (Ed). New York: Basic Books.

Groenen, P., Maassen, B., Crul, T., and Thoonen, G. (1996, June). The specific relation between perception and production errors for place of articulation in developmental apraxia of speech. *Journal of Speech and Hearing Research*, Volume 39, 468-482.

Katz, W. F., Bharadwaj, S. V., and Carstens, B. (1999). Electromagnetic articulography treatment for an adult with Broca's aphasia and apraxia of speech. *Journal of Speech, Language, and Hearing Research*, Vol., 42, 1355-1366, December.

Kreisler, A., Godefory, O., Delmaire, C., Debachy, B., Leclercq, M., Pruvo, J.P., and Leys, D. (2000). The anatomy of aphasia revisited. *Neurology*, 54, March, pp. 1117-1123.

Lawton, M. (1991). A multidimensional view of quality of life in frail elders. In *The concept and measurement of quality of life in frail elders.* J. Birren (Ed). San Diego: Academic Press.

National Aphasia Association (2005). *Aphasia Bill of Rights.* Retrieved April 24, 2006 from the World Wide Web: http://www.psha.org/Handouts/Seminar13and24.pdf.

Owens, R., Metz, D., and Haas, A. (2000). *Introduction to communication disorders.* Boston: Allyn & Bacon.

Restak, R. (1984). *The Brain.* Toronto: Bantam Books.

Tanner, D. (1980). Loss and grief: Implications for the speech-language pathologist and audiologist. *Journal of the American Speech and Hearing Association*, 22:916-928.

Tanner, D. (1999). *The family guide to surviving stroke and communication disorders.* Austin: Pro-Ed.

Tanner, D. (2003a). *The psychology of neurogenic communication disorders: A primer for health care professionals.* Boston: Allyn & Bacon.

Tanner, D. (2003b, Winter). Eclectic perspectives on the psychology of aphasia. *J. Allied Health: 32:256-260.*

Tanner, D. (2006). *Case studies in communication sciences and disorders.* Upper Saddle River, N.J.: Pearson Merrill Prentice Hall.

Tanner, D. and Gerstenberger, D. (1996). Clinical Forum 9: The grief model in aphasia. In *Forums in clinical aphasiology*, C. Code (Ed.). London: Whurr Publishers

United States Department of Justice (2001). The American's with Disabilities Act. Retrieved September 17, 2001 from the World Wide Web: http://www.usdoj.gov/crt/ada/adahom1.htm

Wise, R.J.S., Greene, J., Büchel, C., and Scott, S.K. (1999). Brain regions involved in articulation. *Lancet*, 353: 1057-61.

Zemlin, W. (1998). *Speech and hearing science* (4th ed.). Boston: Allyn & Bacon.

Chapter 10

Medical-Legal and Forensic Aspects of Communication Disorders Resulting from Traumatic Brain Injury

10.1 Chapter Preview

This chapter examines communication disorders resulting from traumatic brain injuries with an emphasis on medical-legal and forensic aspects. Focalized and diffuse traumatic brain injuries are discussed and the effects they have on communication, orientation, memory, behavior, and metacognition. There is a discussion of posttraumatic dys-phagia and psychosis, pediatric head trauma, and audiologic concerns. Malingering, vocational rehabilitation, compensation, and mental competence legal issues are addressed in this chapter. There is also a case study involving a Native American with traumatic brain injury and special linguistic and cultural litigation issues that were addressed during the trial.

10.2 Traumatic Brain Injury As a Special Etiology of Neurogenic Communication Disorders

Traumatic brain injuries often result in neurogenic communication disorders. In Chapter 9, the primary neurogenic communication disorders—aphasia, apraxia of speech, and the dysarthrias—are discussed including litigation issues associated with them. In addition, traumatic brain injuries can also result in dysphagia, which is discussed in Chapter 8. The communication disorders resulting from traumatic brain injuries can be understood in terms of the neurological damage and whether or not it directly or indirectly affects the major speech and language centers and the tracts leading to and from them.

As Table 10.1 shows, the communication disorders resulting from traumatic brain injuries can be classified by the site(s) of the brain damage and whether speech and language centers of the brain, and the tracts leading to and from them, are damaged. Focalized traumatic brain injury can damage the major speech and language centers of the brain or spare them. There can also be diffuse and disbursed injury that includes damage to the speech and language centers of the brain. As discussed below, each type of traumatic brain injury can result in clusters of symptoms which have implications in disability and mental competence determination, medical malpractice, and other medical-legal issues.

Table 10.1
Type, Style, and Symptoms of Traumatic Brain Injuries

Focalized Traumatic Brain and Nervous System Damage Affecting the Major Speech and Language Centers/Tracts	Traumatic Brain Damage Not Affecting the Major Speech and Language Centers/Tracts	Diffuse Brain and Nervous System Damage Also Affecting the Major Speech and Language Centers/Tracts

Aphasia:
    Expressive
    Receptive
    Global
Apraxia of Speech
Dysarthria:
    Flaccid
    Spastic
    Ataxic
    Hypokinetic
    Hyperkinetic (slow)
    Hyperkinetic (quick)
    Mixed/Multiple
Dysphagia
	Impaired or Disrupted:
	    Self-Regulation
	    Orientation
	        Time
	        Place
	        Person
	        Situation
	    Memory
	        Long-Term
	        Short-Term
	    Disinhibition,
	Excitability, Indifference
	Dysphagia
		Aphasia, Apraxia of Speech, Dysarthria Compounded and Complicated by Impaired or Disrupted:
		    Self-Regulation
		    Orientation
		    Memory
		Disinhibition, Excitability, Indifference
		Dysphagia

Reduced or impaired consciousness is the common denominator in many patients with significant traumatic brain injuries. In traumatic brain injury, reduced or impaired consciousness is manifest in several ways, including coma, problems with self-regulation, orientation, memory, inhibition, and reality testing. However, in some patients with traumatic brain and nervous system injury, the focalized damage is limited to the speech and language centers of the brain and/or the tracts leading to and from them. These patients present with one or more classic neurogenic communication disorders typically seen in stroke patients. (This is not to say that some patients with strokes and neurogenic communication disorders do not also have problems with reduced and disordered consciousness.)

Other patients have traumatically induced brain damage but the major speech and language centers/tracts are unaffected. Although these patients may have problems communicating, the fabric of language and the integrity of the motor speech process remain intact. These patients primarily present with the self-regulation, orientation, memory, and inhibition problems associated with impaired or reduced consciousness.

Many patients with traumatic brain injuries have neurogenic communication disorders compounded and complicated by reduced or impaired consciousness. Because of the reduced or impaired consciousness, these patients present with unique symptoms of neurogenic communication disorders.

10.3 Incidence, Prevalence, and Economics of Traumatic Brain Injury

Over the past thirty years, there has been an increase in the number of patients with traumatic brain and neck injuries seen by rehabilitation specialists. This is because there has been a decrease in mortality and improved outcomes for patients with serious traumatic brain injury (Ghajar, 2000). Emergency transportation services now transport patients with traumatic brain and neck injuries to hospitals in time to save their lives. Current advances in head trauma management have increased the incident of nonfatal traumatic brain injuries as measured by discharge rates from hospitals to 180-220 per 100,000 population per year (Kraus and Sorenson, 1994). Douglas (2004) notes that the incidence estimates for the United States, Australia, and the United Kingdom are similar. Much of the improved success rates in treating traumatic brain injuries can be attributed to maintaining oxygenated blood supply through a swollen brain (Ghajar, 2000). Of course, there has been a general population increase in the United States, and we live in an increasingly violent society, which also accounts for the increase in the number of patients with traumatic head and neck injuries during the past three decades. Consequently, there has been an increase in litigation for survivors of traumatic brain injures seeking damages, compensation, accommodation, and rehabilitation.

Ylvisaker, Szekeres, and Feeney (2001) reviewed current and past traumatic brain injury incidence and prevalence rates. They found that there are approximately 500,000 traumatic brain injury hospitalizations per year, yielding a rate of 145 per 100,000 persons per year (slightly lower than the discharge rate from hospitals reported above). They note that statistics on incidence and prevalence may be questionable because of changing hospital admission standards, and that mild cases of traumatic brain injury may not be counted. They report studies showing that approximately 75,000 people die each year from traumatic brain injuries, and there are 50,000 to 80,000 people in the United States added to the roles of those with persistent TBI- related disabilities annually (they consider these statistics overestimates). "Furthermore, even the most optimistic incidence trends should not obscure frank recognition of the growing numbers of individuals living, often for several decades, with TBI-related disability requiring some degree of ongoing professional support and societal accommodation" (Ylvisaker, Szekeres, and Feeney, 2001, p. 746). Not counting the financial costs related to vocational limitations and ongoing support, direct medical costs associated with acute hospitalization and rehabilitation are $48.3 billion per year (Ylvisaker, Szekeres, and Feeney, 2001). Douglas (2004) reports that the care for a person with traumatic brain injuries can be enormous, upwards of $1.8 million, and does not include the economic burden to family, society, lost earnings, and social service programs.

Traumatic neck and spinal cord injuries often occur with traumatic brain injury which can also affect the ability to communicate. According to the National Institutes of Health, in the United States between 10,000 and 20,000 people sustain spinal-cord injures each year. Quadriplegia, paralysis of all four limbs, occurs in half of the cases (Eisenberg, Glueckauf, and Zaretski, 1999). Spinal cord injuries are classified by the neurologic level of damage, whether they are complete or incomplete or by impaired function and there are several spinal cord syndromes (Mackay, Chapman and Morgan, 1997). Spinal injuries are usually classified by the site of the fracture. For example, a C1-C2 fracture occurs at the junction of the first and second cervical vertebrae and is sometimes called the "hangman fracture" because when people are hanged the break in the vertebrae is often at the C1-C2 level.

10.4 The Traumatically Brain-Injured Person

Many studies have been conducted on people at risk for head injuries, and they have yielded consistent results. What has emerged is a consensus of the type of person who is prone to traumatic brain injuries. Certain factors are consistently associated with traumatic brain injury: gender, age, risk-taking behavior, income, drug and alcohol abuse, and recidivism.

All studies show that males are at least twice as likely to have traumatic brain injury than females. Most studies allude to the fact that males, especially older adolescents, tend to engage in more risk-taking behaviors than females and younger males. In addition, males tend to be employed in jobs that put them at risk for employment-related traumatic brain injuries. This is particularly true of some low-paying entry jobs in construction, mining, farming, mechanics, and the military.

Young people tend to be more at risk for traumatic head and neck injuries than older ones. The age group of fifteen to twenty-four is at the highest risk for traumatic brain injury (Kraus and Sorenson, 1994). This group of young people tend to engage in high-risk activities in sports, motorcycles, and automobiles. Children also suffer frequent falls and can be brain injured from abuse (see section on pediatric head trauma).

Males who have low socioeconomic status are at higher risk for traumatic brain injuries. This factor may be related to the fact that many high-risk jobs also pay poorly. Indirectly associated with this risk factor is a low level of formal education.

All studies on risk factors for traumatic brain injuries show a positive correlation with blood alcohol levels. Ylvisaker, Szekeres, and Feeney (2001) also include recreational drugs in this risk factor. Not only do alcohol and drug abuse have a positive correlation with risk for traumatic brain injury, some studies and clinical experience have shown that they are also negatively correlated with rehabilitation outcomes. People with addictions do as well in rehabilitation programs as patients without addictions.

Many studies have shown a high recidivism rate in people who suffer traumatic brain injuries. One of the predictors of a person having traumatic brain injury is the fact that he or she previously suffered one. Studies showing a high recidivism rate suggest that young people who suffer traumatic brain injuries maintain employment in high-risk jobs, return to dangerous activities, and continue to abuse alcohol and drugs.

Other factors which may be associated with traumatic brain injuries include being unmarried, poor social skills, impaired academic abilities, and a history of psychological maladjustment. These factors are less confirmed in the literature, and there are some research and clinical observations countering them.

The following is a profile of a typical traumatically brain injured person:

A young single male with poor education and academic skills, working in a job where the risk of accidental injury is great, earning below average income, who engages in risk-taking behaviors while using alcohol or recreational drugs, and who has previously been admitted to a hospital for a traumatic head and neck injury.

According to the Centers for Disease Control (1997) about half of traumatic brain injuries are transportation related, followed by accidental falls, assaults, and sports-related injuries. Traumatic brain injuries are more common during periods of war. It is also likely that the increase in gang violence skews the data on risk factors to certain sectors of the population.

10.5 The Mechanics of Traumatic Brain Injuries

Traumatic brain injuries are divided into two categories. First, traumatic brain injuries can be caused by objects penetrating the head. The objects that penetrate the head are called missiles or projectiles and cause open head traumas. In war, soldiers and civilians sometimes survive when bullets or shrapnel penetrate the brain. In modern warfare, the size and force of projectiles entering the brain are so great that surviving these injuries is less common than in the past. Open head injuries are also seen in gang wars and drive-by shootings. Sometimes a person can have an open head injury when he or she falls or is in an automobile accident and the impact causes an opening into the brain. Other causes of open head injuries include nail guns, projectiles thrown from lawn mowers and garden machines, and farming, mining, propeller, and blasting accidents.

The second category of traumatic brain injuries is caused by blunt blows to the head. This blunt blow impacts, accelerates, and decelerates the brain (Gillis and Pierce, 1996). Impact injuries occur when a moving object strikes the head, such as a thrown rock or when a slower moving or stationary object is struck by the head, e.g., the head impacts a sidewalk during a fall. Acceleration damage to the brain occurs when it is suddenly propelled by an external force, such as a club, fist, or bat, and deceleration injuries occur when the head abruptly stops when it hits a fixed object, such as the dashboard of a car. Gillis and Pierce (1996) note that the principal type of injury in closed head trauma is a result of diffuse axonal injury (DAI) where there is a shearing of axons during rotational acceleration of the brain. Bomb explosions can cause both acceleration and deceleration brain injuries.

Both types of head trauma can cause focalized and diffuse brain damage. Focalized damage is limited to one identifiable site of the brain whereas diffuse injuries involve damage to more than one site. Low velocity penetrating injuries usually cause focalized brain damage limited to the site of the penetration. Closed head trauma, bomb explosions, and high caliper-velocity penetrating injuries, damage the brain at the initial point of impact, which is called the *coup,* while *contra coup* injuries occur on the opposite of the initial point of impact. This is because of the recoil of the brain inside the skull. The laws of physics dictate that for every action (coup) there is an opposite and equal reaction (contra-coup). Physicists Young and Geller (2007, p. 232) describe momentum and the contra-coup effect: "The brain's large mass gives it considerable momentum. When the skull stops moving, the brain runs into it. Depending on how suddenly the skull slows down, this second, contre-coup blow to the brain can cause as much or more injury as the initial blow. Animals with less massive brains rarely suffer this type of injury." Open and closed traumatic brain injuries often, but not always, result in similar symptoms early postonset, but they diverge as time passes. The type of brain damage seen in open penetrating head injuries is also dependent on the nature of the penetrating missile. Hollow-point bullets and jagged tips create a shearing and tearing action which can cause differing types of brain injuries. The course of the penetrating missile through the brain can also be irregular.

According to Ylvisaker, Szekeres, and Feeney (2001), in traumatic head injuries, secondary brain damage is associated with slowly developing hemorrhages and localized or widespread swelling and edema. Ylvisaker, Szekeres, and Feeney go on to note that the hypoxic-ischemic injury, pathologic neurotransmitter surges, and consequent damage to the hippocampus can be especially ominous for young people because of the learning challenges they face in school and on the job. (The hippocampus is a structure in the brain which plays an important role in learning and memory.)

10.6 Traumatic Brain Injury, Consciousness, and Coma

The effect of reduced or impaired human consciousness is pivotal to describing many issues in traumatic brain injury litigation. Some traumatic brain injuries do not affect the patient's consciousness. However, most patients with significant traumatic brain injuries do have their consciousness affected, and when the major speech and language centers and the tracts leading to and from them are also damaged, they often have unusual symptoms of neurogenic communication disorders. Patients in various levels of coma have reduced or disordered consciousness.

The sensorium is the hypothetical *seat of consciousness* (organ of consciousness) and is sometimes used as a generic term for the intellectual and cognitive functions (Dirckx, 2001). Awareness and consciousness can be used synonymously. To be conscious is to have knowledge of oneself and the environment. It is memory and integration of the past, awareness and alertness to self and the environment, and a realistic appraisal of the future. Throughout history, human consciousness has been a major philosophical theme, and philosophers since Aristotle, Plato and Socrates have pondered its nature.

The clinical concept of consciousness refers to levels of wakefulness; a person in a deep coma is unconscious. To be unconscious is to be unresponsive to bodily needs and the environment and is measured by several coma tests and scales (see below). Consciousness also refers to awareness of thoughts and acts; there are subconscious thoughts and automatic acts. In the broadest sense, it can be said that all perceived experience affects awareness of self and the environment. For example, exposure to political or religious ideas can raise consciousness. By experiencing an injury or illness, one's consciousness will be heightened about disabilities. Psychologically, the number and nature of defense mechanisms affect consciousness. The more radical the defenses, and the more persistently they are employed, the less awareness a person has of himself or herself and the environment. For example, denial is a blocking of conscious awareness of threatening thoughts or events. There are several dissociation syndromes where a person separates and compartmentalizes his or her consciousness or identity to reduce anxiety. In this chapter, when referring to consciousness, the clinical definition of the concept is used. Unfortunately, there is no direct way of measuring consciousness; it can only be inferred by the patient's responses and actions.

A person in a deep coma is in a complete state of unconsciousness. Authorities differ on technical definitions of coma but agree that the person in a deep coma is unresponsive to internal or external stimulation and is incapable of voluntary acts. A person in a deep coma appears asleep, but the two states are vastly different. Studies of coma patients have found they also sleep but cannot be aroused. Encephalitis lethargia, sometimes called sleeping sickness, involves the patient displaying reduced or impaired consciousness caused by brain swelling. Sometimes a person in a coma is said to be in a vegetative state. The term vegetative state denotes a profound loss of consciousness, but life-sustaining functions continue. The term comes from vegetation life existing without consciousness. Eye-open vegetative state refers to a person in a coma, but his or her eyes are reflexively open.

Other, lesser states of reduced awareness are called stupor, delirium, and clouding of consciousness. A stuporous person has reduced and impaired consciousness and requires continued stimulation to show degrees of arousal and attention to the environment. A delirious person has reduced or disordered consciousness and is confused, disoriented, and usually agitated. Clouding of consciousness is the clinical term given to the least level of reduced awareness. A person with clouded consciousness has overall reduced awareness of internal needs and the external environment. He or she has mild levels of confusion and disorientation that may fluctuate over time.

The most widely used test to measure and evaluate coma is the Glasgow Coma Scale (Teasdale and Gennet, 1974). This test measures the patient's eye-opening, best motor response, and speech, and the scores range from three to fifteen. Severe head injury usually results in a score of eight or less. Another test used to measure cognitive functioning in head trauma patients is the Rancho Los Amigos Scale (Hagen, 1981). The scores range from "no response" to "purposeful, appropriate" ones. According to Mackay, Chapman, and Morgan (1997), Level I (No Response), Level II (Generalized Response), and Level III (Localized Response) are seen most often in intensive care units, and they describe varying levels of coma.

10.7 Traumatic Brain Injury and Disorientation

One of the most frequently occurring symptoms of traumatic brain injury is disorientation. Patients with significant traumatic brain injuries are often confused about their surroundings. Many patients are disoriented at some time during recovery from their head injuries, and for some it is a persistent problem. As discussed below, memory deficits and disorientation are usually coexisting problems, and they can be central litigation issues when addressing a patient's mental competence and level of disability.

Usually a person with a significant traumatic brain injury is disoriented, more or less, to all aspects of reality. He or she has generally lost his or her bearing. It may take detailed testing to discover the nature and degree to which the patient is disoriented, but most patients, to various degrees, are disoriented to time, place, person, and situation/predicament. In medical terminology a person completely disoriented is said to be "disoriented times four." Some patients are primarily disoriented to one aspect of reality. They may primarily be disoriented to person and place or only to situation. These patients are said to be disoriented times two or times one, respectively. As noted above, the four aspects of reality to which a person can be disoriented are time, place, person, and situation/predicament.

Clinical experience suggests that disorientation to time is the most common type of confusion experienced by patients with significant traumatic brain injury. There are two aspects to this type of disorientation. First, the patient may be confused about time events. He or she may not know days of the week, the season, or the year. The time for eating breakfast may be confused with dinner time. Second, the patient may not appreciate the passage of time. He or she may believe that fifteen minutes have transpired, when in fact an hour has gone by. For example, a patient may be brought to physical therapy and after only five minutes ask if the time for the hour session has expired. Time disorientation is a frequent symptom of significant traumatic brain injury because time is fleeting and intangible. Some patients, particularly those with right brain injuries, who have access to timepieces continue to make errors of time orientation (Pimental and Kingsbury, 1989). When patients are completely disoriented to time, it is as if the concept of time passage and events has been lost.

Patients disoriented to place confuse rooms, buildings, cities, states, and even countries. For example, when asked what city they are in they report one they lived in as a child or were moving to before an automobile accident. They may believe a library is a solarium or that a hospital room is an elevator. A patient disoriented to place may believe a hospital is a school or a police department. Some patients are so disoriented to place so as to be totally confused about their location within a hospital building. They are unable to find their rooms and cannot be trusted to go from one part of the building to another without supervision.

A patient disoriented to person has lost awareness of relationships. Although all types of disorientation are disconcerting to family and friends of the patient, disorientation to person significantly threatens relationships. The patient disoriented to person may selectively lose the awareness of a relationship with a particular family member or friend, or he or she may be globally confused about all relationships. In addition, the disorientation to person may be limited to some aspects of a particular relationship while sparing others. For example, a patient may remember the nature of the friendship shared with a coworker but be disorientated about the business aspects of their relationship.

Disorientation to person can also extend to loss of identity. Although not all authorities on traumatic brain injury consider this loss a part of disorientation to person, many consider loss of identity a subcategory of this type of confusion. Patients become confused about roles and ego boundaries, and some completely lose their identities. Gender disorientating has also been reported where a male patient reports that he is his father's favorite daughter, or a woman may talk about having a faithful wife. Many problems with identity involve vocations. Patients report that they are soldiers, attorneys, explorers, teachers, or doctors, when in fact they were never involved in those professions and activities.

Early writings on disorientation in head trauma patients only referred to three types of disorientation: time, place, and person. In the past two decades most references to disorientation now also include situation/predicament. Disorientation to situation/predicament is directly affected by the other types of disorientation. A person who is confused about his or her medical situation, e.g., that he or she is in a hospital because of an automobile accident, is also disoriented to place. Disorientation to situation/predicament includes lack of awareness or denial of disability. Some patients, because of organic factors, are not aware of their communication disorders, paralysis, paresis, etc. This lack of awareness can also be caused by the psychological defenses, especially denial, where perceptions of threatening thoughts or events are blocked from consciousness. Disorientation to situation/predicament can be chronic, temporary, complete, or only related to specific aspects of the patient's disabilities. Organic and non-organic memory loss are discussed later. Table 10.2 lists the types of disorientation and provides examples.

10.8 Accurate Diagnosis of Disorientation in Aphasic Patients

The above types of disorientation can often be discovered from verbal reports made by the patient. For example, a patient disoriented to time reports the wrong day; disorientation to place is seen when the patient says he or she is in the wrong city; and a patient calling his wife his mother is an indication of confusion about relationships. These verbal statements can be accurate indications of disorientation in patients with motor speech disorders. However, when a patient has the language disorder of aphasia, the accuracy of these reports is suspect.

Table 10.2
Types and Examples of Disorientation Seen in Patients with Traumatic Brain Injuries

Medical Distinction (Categories May Vary)	Type of Disorientation	Examples
Times One	Time	• Believing it is the fall season rather than winter • Believing an hour has transpired when, in fact, ten minutes have gone by
Times Two	Place	• Believing the hospital room is a sleeping compartment on a passenger train • Not knowing the state in which he or she resides
Times Three	Person	• A male patient confuses his mother for his wife • A female patient believes she is her father's favorite son
Times Four	Situation/Predicament	• A patient believes he is in the hospital for routine tests, rather than in rehabilitation for traumatic brain injury. • A patient denies the existence of a communication disorder

In Chapter 9, two types of naming errors were reported. First, when an aphasic patient is asked to name an object or tries to retrieve the name of a word in conversation, he or she may say a word that rhymes with the correct one. This is called a literal paraphasia or an approximation error. Second, when the aphasic patient says a word that has a semantic relationship with the desired word, he or she has produced a verbal paraphasia or an association error. The errors are associated semantically with the desired word, e.g., car for truck, run for walk, fork for knife, up for down, high for low, and yes for no. The presence of the later paraphasia can cause misdiagnosis of disorientation in some patients (Tanner, 2006a; Tanner, 1999; Culbertson, Tanner, Peck, and Hooper, 1998). This is particularly true when a patient is suspected of confabulation.

Confabulation is the tendency to remark about events without regard to the truthfulness of the statements. These are usually fluent and often bizarre verbal reports stated in disregard to facts and accuracy. Confabulation occurs in patients with traumatic brain injuries and appears to be related to the extent of memory defects. Confabulation may serve a

psychological function in that it comforts the patient. Confabulating patients seem to make-up stories and report them in an attempt to appear normal, or they are simply reporting fantasies that randomly occur to them. Pimental and Kingsbury (1989) call these inaccurate reports confabulated journeys and attribute them to damage to the right hemisphere of the brain. An example of disorientation to place and a confabulated journey occurred with a professor. He had a traumatic head injury subsequent to a motor vehicle accident and reported that he was traveling through Europe on a train and his hospital room was a sleeping compartment. His wife reported that he rarely traveled by train and had never been to Europe. For this patient, the train confabulation may have served as an escape fantasy. A patient from England confabulated stories about family life in an apartment flat and appeared to be reliving events that happened to her as a girl. Sometimes confabulation can be disquieting. One patient engaged in morbid confabulation and talked on and on about the food chain until the statements dealt with cannibalism, frightening her and causing her abruptly to stop the monologue (Tanner, 1977).

A patient's report of a real event can be confused with delusions because of verbal paraphasias (association errors). A young male with a traumatic brain injury resulting from a motor vehicle accident reported that he was taken from the nursing home and driven to a fire station early one morning. His report was denied by nursing staff, and there was no confirmation of it by others. It appeared that this was a confabulated journey until investigated. The investigation showed that the patient because of good behavior was allowed to sit in his wheelchair adjacent to the nurses' station, something he found rewarding. There was a fire hose in a glass container directly behind his position by the nurses' station. Through verbal paraphasias he was simply reporting that they took him from the nursing home (his room), and drove (wheeled) him to the fire station (next to the fire hose). What appeared to be confabulation was simply a report of a real event verbalized with paraphasia (Tanner, 2006a).

As can be seen by the examples above, when a patient with traumatic brain injury has damage to the speech and language centers, his or her verbal statements about time, place, person, and situation/predicament may lead to inaccurate conclusions about his or her orientation. The patient may be oriented, but because of naming errors, report the wrong time, place, person, or information about the situation/predicament. To determine levels of disorientation in patients with traumatic brain injury and aphasia, it is necessary to go beyond their verbal reports and test their beliefs and observe their behaviors. Does the patient believe he or she is in the wrong city? Does the patient act as if her husband is her father? It is necessary to observe the patient's behaviors for indications that his or her verbal reports are actual beliefs.

A traumatic brain-injured person's memory and orientation are fundamentally related, but clinicians often diagnose and treat them as separate entities. There are separate tests and treatments for memory and orientation, and few that integrate both psychological and cognitive functions. Many aspects of disorientation are functions of amnesia. For example, disorientation to place can be viewed as a form of amnesia; the patient cannot remember the city in which he or she resides. Disorientation to person involves forgetting people and relationships. A patient disoriented to time cannot properly remember time events. Disorientation to situation/predicament has, at its core, memory deficits involving the nature and severity of the patient's injuries. Certainly there is more to disorientation than just amnesia, but memory loss and disorientation are fundamentally related.

10.9 Retrograde and Anterograde Amnesia

The point in time of the traumatic brain injury is an important dividing line for assessing and treating amnesia. The memory loss seen in patients with traumatic brain injury can be separated into those occurring before and after the event causing it. Retrograde amnesia refers to loss of memory for events occurring before the traumatic brain injury, while anterograde amnesia refers to loss of memory occurring after the trauma. A patient with retrograde amnesia may have amnesia for all or part of a block of time before the injury. For example, he or she may not remember leaving on the trip, the car ride immediately before the accident, or the accident itself.

Few patients with serious traumatic brain injuries can remember the details of the incident that caused it. The block of time taken by the traumatic injury can be much more lengthy than several days. One patient had selective amnesia for almost a decade of his life and could not remember that a beloved brother had died several years ago. When told of his brother's death, the patient broke down as if the death had just occurred. For the patient, his grieving response was appropriate. Because of the amnesia he was being notified of the death of his brother for the first time. A woman who was in a multiple-vehicle accident could not remember many events associated with the birth of her youngest child. A young Japanese couple honeymooning in the United States were both head injured in a car accident, and the husband could not remember their marriage or their engagement. After months of rehabilitation, he was reintroduced to his wife. For many patients, there is a gradual return of past memories, but usually there is a vagueness about them and some events are permanently lost. For the memories that return, it is likely that for some patients they are simply remembering peoples' reports of events before the traumatic brain injury and not actually remembering the events themselves.

The first permanent memories a TBI patient may have are the visits by family members or experiencing procedures such as a brain scan or a session of therapy. There is often a gradual return of memory of some events that happened since the brain injury. Caregivers are often surprised that a patient cannot remember events from one day to the next. Some patients appear alert and cognizant of their surroundings, but later when quizzed about the events and activities of a previous day are completely unable to recall them. Anterograde amnesia involves problems with short-term and long-term abilities to retain and recall new information.

The reasons many patients have amnesia immediately before and after the event that caused the traumatic brain injury are both psychological and organic (Tanner, 2003). Certainly, traumatic brain injured patients suffer from memory loss due to brain damage. The hippocampus, located in the temporal lobe, is an important brain structure for memory. It is part of the limbic system which is involved with memory and emotion. Damage to this structure and other parts of the brain causes amnesia. The psychological defense of repression may also account for loss of memory associated with traumatic events. Repression is the involuntary exclusion of a painful thought or memory from awareness. Carlat (1999) describes repression as a stuffing of emotion out of conscious awareness. Because of the negativity and psychological distress associated with the event causing the traumatic brain injury, the patient represses memory of it. Repression is done unconsciously; the patient is unaware of doing it and is different from suppression, which is a conscious psychological coping style and defense. It is likely that both organic and psychological factors combine to account for many patients being unable to remember the events immediately before, during, and after the traumatic brain injury.

10.10 Components of Memory

Memory is integral to learning, orientation, and appropriate behavior. Learning new information is impossible without intact and functional memory. Disorientation has, at its core, a loss of memory for time, place, person, and situation/predicament. Appropriate behavior requires memory of societal admonitions about acceptable and unacceptable behaviors. Memory bridges the past, present, and future and provides the continuity of life experiences. For many patients, as would be expected, it is frightening to lose this continuity.

There are three components to unimpeded memory, and a breakdown in any aspect of the process can cause selective or global amnesia. Each component is evaluated and treated in rehabilitation programs for patients with traumatic brain injury. The patient's communication abilities are directly affected, individually and collectively, by all three components. A patient's ability to profit from experience, e.g., benefit from therapies, is dependent on memory and is the basis of determining prognosis for patients with traumatic brain injuries. Traumatic brain injuries can eliminate, impede, and block (1) attention, (2) storage, and (3) retrieval.

The first component to memory is attention. A person must be able to attend to and concentrate on himself or herself and the environment for normal memory. One aspect of attention is arousal, which is the general state of readiness to process sensory input (Gillis, 1996). The arousal level of a traumatic brain-injured patient must be sufficient for him or her to profit from experience. Obviously, a patient in a deep coma has profoundly reduced arousal and is unready to process sensory input. Patients in lesser degrees of coma have proportionally better arousal and thus are more likely to profit from experience and benefit from rehabilitation.

An experimental therapy provided to patients at some rehabilitation facilities is coma stimulation. The goal of this therapy is to increase the patient's arousal and ability to attend to himself or herself and the environment. The patient is given multisensory stimulation. The stimulation can include placing different odors and fragrances under the nose, applying contrasting temperature and textures to the skin, massages, range of motion exercises, and presenting speech and nonverbal sounds to alternate ears (Gillis, 1996). Some patients are read books, newspapers, and magazines.

There are clinicians who believe that coma stimulation therapy improves the TBI patient's arousal and general ability to attend to information. However, there are no definitive studies that clearly support it. Although it is well intentioned, coma stimulation therapy is an experimental treatment that has not been proven to benefit patients. Clinical research does not clearly show that it reduces the extent or duration of coma, nor does it significantly affect the patient's rehabilitation outcomes. On the positive side, it does provide the patient's family and friends with activities they can engage in for the comatose patient, thus reducing their feelings of helplessness. Unfortunately, coma stimulation therapy can also create false hope, unrealistic expectations, and interrupt the normal grieving process (Tanner, 2003). The cost-benefit of having professionals provide this therapy to comatose patients also must be weighed.

The concept of figure-ground is an important area of attention. Figure-ground involves separating that which is important and relevant from the unimportant or irrelevant, and it occurs in all senses. Figure-ground is sometimes likened to signal-noise, where the signal is the important aspect of the environmental information and the noise is unwanted and irrelevant. Patients with traumatic brain injuries sometimes have difficulty separating the figure or signal from the ground or the noise, and this is particularly important in the auditory sense. Their auditory selective attention is dysfunctional. Although there may be nothing wrong with the patient's hearing mechanism, he or she can have problems separating salient auditory information from background noise. A figure-ground problem involves perception rather than sensation.

Patients with traumatic brain injuries often cannot selectively attend to speech while ignoring background noise such as an overhead paging, vacuum cleaners, and the sounds of a television. Most people can selectively attend to speech sounds while minimizing their awareness of background noise. A structure in the brain called the thalamus is pivotal in auditory figure-ground perception. The thalamus is sometimes called the gatekeeper because it, along with other aspects of the brain, allows certain sense information to become conscious while keeping other input from awareness. To have an auditory figure-ground problem does not require that the thalamus be damaged by the traumatic brain injury; damage to the tracts leading to and from it and other cerebral structures can cause this selective attention deficit.

Visual figure-ground deficits can also occur in patients with traumatic brain injury. Although there may be nothing wrong with the patient's eyes, his or her perception of visual information can be impaired. For example, when looking at a written page the patient may be unable to attend and perceive the important shapes, letters, and words while ignoring the others. The patient may be unable visually to focus his or her attention on tracking and reading. When people enter the patient's hospital room, because of visual figure-ground difficulties, he or she may attend to the television, pictures on a wall, or a doorknob and not give the visitors the necessary attention.

Obviously, selective attention deficits can account for a patient's inability to remember information. A patient who cannot selectively attend, either visually or auditorially, to salient aspects of the environment will not be able to recall that information. Because the information is perceptually distorted or does not reach conscious awareness, the patient will experience amnesia for new information and consequently be unable to profit from experience. In head trauma rehabilitation, the patient's attention is the first aspect of the process of memory to be evaluated and treated because it is a requisite for unimpaired storage and retrieval of information.

The second component to memory is storage of information received through the senses. The salient information about the self and the environment is stored in short-term and long-term memory. Both types of memory storage occur for purposeful and incidental information. In short-term memory it is likely that there is a continuation of neural impulses, while long-term memory is a result of permanent chemical alterations in the brain. Short-term memory occurs for as long as the person rehearses the information, and long-term memory occurs when it has been internalized. As reported above, an important brain structure for memory is the hippocampus which is vulnerable in traumatic brain in-

juries. "Because of the extreme vulnerability of the hippocampus to post-injury anoxia, new learning problems are very common after TBI, despite potentially good recovery of pretraumatically acquired and effectively stored knowledge and skills" (Ylvisaker, Szekeres, and Feeney, 2001, p. 755).

Short-term memory is also called working memory. It occurs for as long as the person rehearses the information and is subject to rapid decay because of distraction and loss of attention to the task. Accurately measuring short-term memory capacity has proven difficult. Historically, short-term memory was measured by how long a person could hold the information in his or her memory while rehearsing it. Digits and icons were used for auditory and visual short-term memory assessment. Auditory short-term memory is seven plus or minus two digits, meaning the average person can retain seven digits with the range of normal being five through nine. Examiners have the patient repeat digits forward and backward and recall similar and dissimilar objects (Aronson, 2000). The length of local telephone numbers in the United States was determined by using the average of seven digits for normal short-term memory. Testing of short-term memory often yields inconsistent results because of chunking and the speed at which the numbers are presented to the patient. Chunking is remembering a series of related numbers, and digit memory is more efficient when said rapidly to the patient.

Storage in long-term memory occurs when the information can be recalled without rehearsal. As noted above, long-term memory involves a permanent change in brain chemistry rather than a continuation of nervous energy. In a person's mind, information stored in the long-term memory has been made personally relevant. It has been associated with other stored information and internalized. Long-term storage can be both purposeful and incidental. Extensive rehearsal can result in long-term storage as can the use of mnemonic devices which are purposeful associations. Incidental long-term storage occurs when memories are laid down without intentional associations.

Some authorities on human memory believe that all information attended to and stored is potentially available for retrieval. However, it is likely that as time passes there is a disintegration of some stored memories and the clarity of others is compromised. The strength of storage is also an important variable in how easily and completely they are recalled. Certain memories are stored with extreme clarity. They are called peak memory experiences and are associated with major events occurring in a person's life. For example, most people can remember what they were doing, who they were with, and the emotions associated with the news that Pearl Harbor was bombed by the Empire of Japan, President John F. Kennedy was assassinated, and the tragedy of September 11, 2001 occurred.

The third component to memory is retrieval. There are several types of retrieval problems that block the ability to retrieve stored information. Because of psychological or organic factors the memories cannot be retrieved. Psychological factors that can block memories include repression and suppression. As was discussed previously, some memories may be too disturbing and troubling to allow conscious awareness of them. The person may consciously keep them suppressed or unconsciously repress them. Many defense mechanisms have, at their core, exclusion of all or part of memories, motivations, and information. Traumatic brain injury and secondary brain damage can also block memories from retrieval. The mechanism by which this occurs is not understood but possibly includes synaptic dysfunctions, axon shearing, tearing, and traumatically induced neurochemical disruptions.

High levels of physical tension and mental anxiety can block information retrieval. College students sometimes have acute anxiety over examinations that interferes with successful test-taking behaviors. Their anxieties over the examination become so great that it is difficulty for them to recall information and think clearly. Several studies have shown that some aphasic patients recall words better during confrontation naming tasks when they have undergone relaxation exercises. Related to tension and anxiety is the fact that hypnosis often helps witnesses recall events surrounding a crime. Hypnosis is a state of suggestive relaxation, and the reduction in tension and anxiety allows for more thorough recall. There have been accounts of hypnotized adults remembering crimes that occurred in their youth. In addition, memories of remote events are more readily recalled just before a person falls asleep because of relaxation and lowered psychological defenses.

An important distinction about memory is the different requirement for recognition and recall. As a rule, recognition of information is easier than recall. In recognition, the patient is supplied with alternatives and simply chooses the correct answer. In recall, the patient is asked an open-ended question and must supply the correct information. Recognition supplies cues and alternatives to the patient, whereas in recall the patient must provide the entire the answer. An example of a recognition question is, "Which of the following are parts of your body?" and the patient is supplied with several options: pen, hand, car, banana. With recall, the patient is asked to answer the following question: "What part of the body do you write with?" With recognition, the patient simply chooses the correct response, while in recall he

or she must supply the answer. In word-retrieval testing, high scores in recognition and low scores in recall suggest intact receptive vocabulary and deficient expressive abilities.

Attention, storage, and retrieval are fundamental aspects of memory. A breakdown in one or more will result in the patient being unable to learn new information or recall old ones. With the traumatic brain-injured person, it is necessary to find out where the memory deficits occur, design appropriate treatments, and set up a therapy program involving family and members of the staff. Improved memory will result in gains in orientation, learning, behavior, and communication (see Figure 10.1). One common approach to the treatment of memory and orientation deficits is reality orientation.

Attention
    Arousal
    Figure-ground
    Signal-noise
Storage
    Short-term working
        Chunking
        Rate of presentation
    Long-term internalization
        Purposeful
        Incidental
Retrieval
    Recall versus recognition
    Repression, suppression
    Tension, anxiety

Figure 10.1 *Components and factors affecting memory*

10.11 Posttraumatic Amnesia and Loss of Consciousness As Indicators of Severity of Traumatic Brain Injury

Two of the most commonly used gauges of the severity of traumatic brain injury involve the length of time the patient was unconscious and his or her first memories following the event that caused it. According to Lucas (1998), the length of posttraumatic amnesia (PTA) is an accurate measure of predicting recovery of function. Lucas reports that patients with posttraumatic amnesia of less than one hour have mild head injuries. Moderate head injuries occur in those patients with posttraumatic amnesia of one to twenty-four hours, and severe injuries occur in patients with PTA longer than twenty-four hours. Other authorities have even more highly refined measurements of the severity of traumatic brain injury based on length of PTA. "These include very mild

(PTA less than 5 minutes), very severe (PTA for 1-4 weeks) injuries" (Lucas, 1998, p. 247). Davis (2007) notes that post traumatic amnesia lasts longer than one day in all severe head injuries.

According to Lucas (1998), the time it takes for the patient to regain consciousness is also predictive of the severity of the traumatic brain injury. Loss of consciousness occurring for fewer than thirty minutes results in mild head injury, while loss of consciousness occurring for longer than that period indicates moderate to severe head injury. Often, patients are not reliable informants of the length of time they are unconscious or the length of posttraumatic amnesia, so reports from witnesses must be used. According to Lucas (1998), the period the patient is unconscious is a less reliable predictor of severity of head injury than is the length of posttraumatic amnesia. Table 10.3 provides general indicators of the severity of traumatic brain injuries.

10.12 Personality Changes, Behavioral Problems, and Metacognition

Traumatic brain injuries often cause personality changes and behavioral problems, and can be sources of litigation involving mental competence and criminal acts perpetuated by the patient. To a limited degree, the nature and severity of the personality changes and behavioral problems depend on the site and extent of the neurological damage occurring to the patient. The patient's premorbid personality, coping styles, typical defense mechanisms, and environmental factors also influence personality and behavior following the traumatic brain injury. A combination of factors can predispose, precipitate, and perpetuate personality changes and behavioral problems in traumatic brain injury. Personality problems seen in moderate to severe traumatic brain injuries usually result from damage to the temporal and frontal lobes of the brain (Lucas, 1998).

Some authorities on traumatic brain injuries have correlated levels of recovery and typical personality changes and behavioral problems. Using the Rancho Los Amigos (RLA) Hospital Levels of Cognitive Functioning, Ylvisaker, Szekeres, and Feeney (2001) have developed three stages of recovery from TBI. The Early Stage begins with the first generalized responses to environmental stimuli and includes visual tacking, localizing to sound, recognition of common objects, and the comprehension of some commands. The Middle Stage includes heightened alertness and increased activity. Initially, there are confusion, disorientation, and agitation unrelated to provocation. Behavioral problems include impulsivity, lack of initiation, and difficulty planning and organizing complex tasks. The Late Stage of recovery from head trauma includes superficial and fragile orientation and, in many patients, functional disabilities in real-world settings. "These levels begin with an adequate, though perhaps superficial and fragile orientation to important aspects of life and end with the individual's ultimate level of neurologic improvement, which may or may not include cognitive and communicative impairments that are functionally disabling" (Ylvisaker, Szekeres, and Feeney, 2001, p. 752).

Table 10.3
Indicators of Severity of Traumatic Brain Injury

Length of Unconsciousness	Mild Traumatic Brain Injury	Fewer Than Thirty Minutes
Length of Unconsciousness	Moderate to Severe Brain Injury	Longer than Thirty Minutes
Length of Posttraumatic Amnesia	Very Mild Traumatic Brain Injury	Less Than Five Minutes
Length of Posttraumatic Amnesia	Mild Traumatic Brain Injury	Less Than One Hour
Length of Posttraumatic Amnesia	Moderate Traumatic Brain Injury	One to Twenty-Four Hours
Length of Posttraumatic Amnesia	Severe Traumatic Brain Injury	Twenty-Four Hours to One Week
Length of Posttraumatic Amnesia	Very Severe Traumatic Brain Injury	One to Five Weeks

(Source: Lucas, 1999)

Many personality changes and behavioral problems seen in traumatic head injuries can be classified under the headings of impaired mental executive functioning and disruptions with metacognition. They involve the patient's ability to regulate, plan, execute, and monitor acts, and they often occur from damage to the frontal lobes of the brain. These deficits are part of frontal lobe syndrome. According to Lucas (1998), the changes in personality attributable to frontal lobe syndrome include excitability or reduced activation. Excitability can be manifested by impulsivity, emotional lability, and mood swings. There also may be socially inappropriate behaviors or childishness. Reduced activation can include apathy, flat affect, decreased spontaneity, lack of interest, and emotional blunting. Abulia, the chronic inability to make decisions and engage in voluntary acts, may also occur in frontal lobe syndrome.

Metacognition is a more encompassing term than executive functioning and is "thinking about thinking." The term refers to knowledge about all cognitive processes, their products, and anything related to them (Gillis, 1996). According to Gillis, metacognition is monitoring of cognitive process and includes how and when to attend and knowing how, when, and what to remember. On a higher cognitive level, it includes knowing when problems exist and what processes and strategies exist for solving them.

The personality changes and behavioral problems seen in traumatic brain injuries can be classified in the following categories: social disinhibition, aggressiveness, and indifference and flat affect. They can occur in all patients with significant traumatic brain injury, and at various stages of recovery. For some patients they are temporary and necessary aspects of recovery, while for others they are chronic personality changes and behavioral problems. Although generalities are made about brain localization, e.g., the site and size of the brain damage and specific personality and behavioral problems, they may occur independently of assumed specific brain lesions. A patient's communication disabilities often dictate how these personality changes and behavioral problems are presented.

Social disinhibition can be seen in several personality changes and behavioral problems. Many issues related to social disinhibition involve communication intent and appropriateness. Some patients act too friendly around strangers. They behave as if there is a preexisting relationship with total strangers. Social disinhibition can also include crying at inappropriate times, which may or may not be related to pseudobulbar emotional lability (see Chapter 9), boasting, talking too loudly, and walking naked in public places. Many patients are disinhibited regarding social conventions and sex. In traditional Freudian terms, the super-

ego has lost the ability to regulate the personality. Sexual drives are uninhibited, and the patient makes inappropriate comments and engages in inappropriate actions. Many patients proposition strangers and make sexually suggestive remarks. They may inappropriately touch people in elevators or halls and grope visitors to their rooms. They may touch their genitals in public and masturbate. Socially, patients are disinhibited about societal mores. They violate expected social norms and appear oblivious to social customs. They act as if they are amoral sexually.

Patients with traumatic brain injuries may physically strike out and injure staff, family, and friends. Although violent behaviors may be inhibited by physical limitations associated with paralysis and paresis, many patients are capable of unprovoked attacks. They may attempt to strike people with their quad canes or fists, spit, yell, scratch, and throw food trays. They show low tolerance for frustration and act out physically. Verbal aggressiveness is seen in conversations where the patient refuses to engage in socially acceptable turn-taking. They disregard other people's communication and are dismissive toward staff, family, and friends. Aggressiveness is often related to their perceived territorial needs. They may refuse to allow other patients to eat at a dinner table with them and take objects not belonging to them. Aggressiveness is also seen sexually, with patients demanding sexual favors. Some patients are hypersexual and are aggressive with their urges.

Although some patients are excitable and hyperactive, others have reduced mood, emotion, feeling, and temperament, which is called flat affect. The patient with flat affect displays little concern about his or her predicament and seems emotionally removed from the situation. There is a general indifference to self, people, and things. Family members report that the patient does not seem to be himself or herself and is emotionally distant and removed from them.

Response delay is the tendency for a patient to be delayed in responses to questions, commands, and other stimuli. It often occurs in traumatic head-injured patients with reduced activation. Response delay contributes to perceptions of flat affect because the patient may take excessive time to respond to emotional stimuli, and this gives the appearance of indifference. Muscular spasticity also affects response delay. Frontal lobe damage can include the motor strips of the brain and cause spasticity. The muscles have increased tone. They are rigid and tight and resistant to easy body movements. Thus, the patient with reduced activation may have his or her response delay exacerbated by rigid and tight muscles. For the patient it is more difficult to respond physically and verbally because of the spasticity, and this contributes to the response delay and consequent perceptions of indifference. Other verbal indications of indifference and flat affect include reduced emphasis, monoloudness, and monopitch.

The patient's indifference may extend to activities of daily living (ADLs). Some patients with traumatic brain injuries neglect to bathe, clean their rooms, brush their teeth, change stained and dirty clothing, shave, or comb their hair. They do not appear concerned about hygiene nor do they want to expend the energy to keep themselves or their rooms clean. Many behaviors displayed by traumatically brain-injured patients are seen in severely depressed individuals, and the indifference, apathy, and response delay may also be symptoms of underlying depression.

For many patients with decreased activation, there is an apparent loss of will, difficulty making decisions, poor attention, and impaired concentration. Combined, these deficits result in the patient having decreased assertiveness. They will not assert themselves and become passive, dependent patients. Motivation to improve is reduced and, for many patients, results in a poor prognosis to benefit from rehabilitation. Most therapies require a degree of motivation and responsiveness to benefit from them.

For some patients, particularly those with mild head traumas, many of the above orientation, memory, and behavioral problems resolve over time. However, for the majority of patients with appreciable head traumas, there are persistent problems. Personality changes, behavioral problems, and memory deficits are the most persistent long-term deficits experienced by patients with significant traumatic brain injuries. Table 10.4 shows the personality changes, behavioral problems, and some communicative acts seen in some patients with traumatic brain injuries.

10.13 Posttraumatic Psychosis

Psychosis is a severe mental and behavioral disorder affecting the capacity to recognize reality, communicate, and relate to others, and which interferes with the ability to cope with everyday life (Dirckx, 2001). It is a problem of recognizing and testing reality. Posttraumatic psychosis is a generic label for psychotic illness in a person with brain injury (Smeltzer, Nasrallah, and Miller, 1994). In patients with traumatic brain injuries, psychosis is difficult to diagnose due to patients' communication disorders. Smeltzer, Nasrallah, and Miller (1994) note that data on the incidence of psychosis in traumatic brain-injured persons are highly variable. Some studies show as many as 20 percent of traumatic brain-injured patients may be classified as psychotic, while more than 50 percent have signs and symptoms of problems with reality testing. Hallucinations and delusions are signs and symptoms of posttraumatic psychosis.

Table 10.4
Personality Changes, Behavioral Problems and Communicative Acts in Traumatic Brain Injuries

Social Disinhibition	Acting Too Friendly Crying at Inappropriate Times Boasting Talking Too Loudly Suggestive Sexual Remarks
Aggressiveness	Refusal to Verbally Take Turns Disregard Others' Communication Dismissive Statements Rapid Speech
Indifference and Flat Affect	Verbal Response Delay Reduced Emphasis Monoloudness Monopitch Slow Speech

Hallucinations are false perceptions of sensory information. They can occur in all of the senses, but visual and auditory are the most commonly reported. A visual hallucination is the misinterpreting of visual stimuli, or seeing people and things that do not exist. An auditory hallucination is hearing voices and environmental sounds that do not exist, or having misperceptions of real voices and environmental sounds. Obviously, organically induced auditory perceptual disorders and auditory hallucinations overlap regarding classifications and symptoms. Several auditory perceptual disorders share common attributes with auditory hallucinations. Auditory and acoustic agnosia are perceptual disorders in which the patient misperceives or is unable to recognize salient perceptual information. Visual agnosia and visual hallucinations also overlap regarding classifications and symptoms. Visual agnosia is a perceptual disorder where the patient misperceives or is unable to recognize salient perceptual information. In traumatic brain-injured patients, auditory and visual hallucinations may be related to organically or psychotically induced misperceptions.

A delusion is a false idea or belief rigidly held in spite of proof to the contrary. Delusions and hallucinations often go hand in hand. There are several types of delusions, including somatic, grandeur, and persecutory (paranoid). A patient with a somatic delusion has a false belief about his or her body. He or she is convinced a disease or impairment exists when in fact there is no clinical support for the belief. Extreme hypochondriacs may be psychotic in nature, and people with anorexia nervosa may have delusional beliefs about body image. A patient with a delusion of grandeur believes he or she is a superior human or supernatural savior of the world. He or she may have the delusional belief that he or she has powerful insights and is gifted with supernatural abilities to be used to save the world. A patient with a delusion of persecution believes that he or she is in extreme danger or at the mercy of powerful forces. Patients with persecutory delusions sometimes wear metal hats to protect themselves from dangerous invisible forces. As with hallucinations, delusions are difficult to detect in patients with major neurogenic communication disorders because they cannot report or discuss them.

With patients who are noncommunicative, the only indications of hallucinations and delusions are unusual and bizarre behaviors. A patient having tactile hallucinations about spiders crawling on his or her body may scratch and pull at body parts. A patient having auditory hallucinations may respond to imaginary verbal requests by unexpectedly attempting to move from one location to another. A patient who appears to be having difficulty visually attending to a task may in fact be having a visual hallucination about angels on a bookcase, or a visit from a long-deceased relative. Many bizarre behaviors seen in patients with traumatic head injuries have at their core delusional thoughts. In some patients the difference between an inaccurate belief and a delusional thought can be tested by determining whether they rigidly believe them despite proof to the contrary. Patients with delusions are persistent in their beliefs even when provided with repeated proof to the contrary.

10.14 Classifying Traumatically Induced Neurogenic Communication Disorders

Traumatic brain injuries cross the spectrum of neurogenic communication disorders with regard to type and severity of the symptoms presented. For example, a patient in a deep coma is verbally, graphically, and gesturally unresponsive and presumably unable to comprehend speech. (There are accounts of patients who reported being able to comprehend speech during their comas, but empirical support is lacking regarding intact auditory comprehension in coma patients.) At the other end of the type and severity continuum, patients with postconcussive syndromes may have impaired attention, reduced concentration, and amnesia early postonset, but most are symptom free by twelve months (McAllister, 1994). Patients with mild traumatic brain injuries may have the symptoms resolve early postonset or be plagued by long-term communication disorders.

There is no universally accepted classification system for the communication disorders accompanying traumatic brain injuries. Classifying communication disorders seen in traumatic brain injuries is fraught with vague terminology, nondescript categories, and poor or nonexistant supporting research. This is because professionals from a variety of disciplines study, diagnose, and treat patients who have extremely divergent traumatically induced communication disorders. Because of this lack of consensus, litigating head trauma cases requires a logical and systematic method of addressing the myriad of terminology, theories, perspectives, and philosophies about the communication disorders. The following system provides a logical basis and easily understood system by which attorneys, judges, and jurors can understand the communication disorders seen in traumatic brain injuries. It also can accommodate the wide variety of philosophical perspectives of expert witnesses. As was noted at the first of the chapter, the communication disorders seen in traumatic brain-injured patients can be classified by whether the speech and language centers and the major tracts leading to and from them have been damaged or spared.

In Chapter 9, it was reported that aphasia is a language disorder affecting all modalities of expressive and receptive communication. Apraxia of speech is a motor speech programming disorder, and the dysarthrias are a group of neuromuscular disorders caused by muscle paralysis, paresis, or movement irregularities. These disorders can occur alone or in combination with each other and are classified under the category of neurogenic communication disorders. They are called the "big three" neurogenic communication disorders.

Ylvisaker, Szekeres, and Feeney (2001) state that classical aphasic syndromes are relatively uncommon in traumatic brain injuries. The types of aphasia reported in Chapter 9, those language disturbances seen in patients who have suffered strokes affecting the major speech and language centers and the tracts leading to and from them, are relatively rare in traumatic brain injuries. Typical language disorders seen in stroke-caused anterior, motor, nonfluent, Broca's, posterior, sensory, fluent, Wernicke's, and global aphasia are rare, especially in moderate to severe traumatic brain injuries. This is because major head traumas usually damage or destroy large areas of the brain and connecting fibers. Mild head injuries are more likely to damage only the speech and language centers of the brain and consequently cause symptoms of classical aphasic syndromes. Ylvisaker, Szekeres, and Feeney (2001) and others suggest that anomia is likely to be the primary residual aphasic symptom in the absence of general cognitive disruptions. Anomia is the inability to recall the names of people, things, and ideas. Naming is the core deficit in aphasia and appears to be represented throughout the brain (Ryalls and Behrens, 2000).

Classic verbal, oral, and limb apraxias typically seen in stroke patients also occur infrequently in patients with major traumatic brain injuries. The patient's voluntary intent affects these motor planning and programming abilities, and the disinhibition seen in many traumatically brain-injured patients results in a low occurrence of classic apraxia symptoms. However, ideational apraxia, where intent of the complex motor behaviors cannot be planned, is often seen in patients with traumatic brain injuries, especially early on. Ideational apraxia is the loss of the power to formulate the ideational concepts necessary for movements. The patient cannot grasp or retain the idea of the desired act, especially for complicated movements.

Spastic, ataxic, hyperkinetic, hypokinetic, flaccid, and mixed-multiple dysarthrias occur in traumatic brain injuries depending on the level and type of neurologic damage. As is the case in the classic dysarthrias, mixed and multiple varieties are the most common. Spastic and ataxic dysarthria

are presumably the most common individual types to occur as a consequence of the frontal lobe and cerebellar damage to the brain.

When traumatic brain injury spares the major speech and language centers and the tracts leading to and from them, patients present with self-regulation, orientation, memory, and inhibition problems. Although communication may be disordered, the fabric of language and the motor speech processes are largely unaffected. A label applied to the speech and language of these patients is the language of confusion. These patients present with disordered and impaired communication that reflect the memory deficits, disorientation, inhibition problems, and impaired self-regulation. Ylvisaker, J. Feeney, and T. Feeney (1999) categorize some of the symptoms of the language of confusion as frontolimbic injury and executive system impairment. Specifically included in this classification are reduced awareness of personal strengths and weakness, difficulty setting goals, planning, organizing, initiating, inhibiting, and monitoring behaviors. There are also general inflexibility and concreteness in thinking, talking, and acting.

The most common type of communication disorder seen in significant traumatic brain injuries involves aphasia, apraxia of speech, and the dysarthrias compounded and complicated by reduced or impaired consciousness. Here, patients present with one or more of the above neurogenic communication disorders, and the symptoms are affected by inhibition, memory, orientation, and self-regulation problems. The American Speech-Language-Hearing Association (1988) classifies these disorders as cognitive-communicative impairments. Ylvisaker, J. Feeney and T. Feeney (1999) include in this blended category, which they call frontolimbic injury and cognitive-communication impairments, disorganized, poorly controlled discourse, paucity of spoken and written discourse, inefficient comprehension of language, imprecise language, word-retrieval problems, and impaired verbal learning.

When aphasia, apraxia of speech, and the dysarthrias are compounded and complicated by reduced or impaired consciousness, the patient's speech and language symptoms are highly variable. Many patients are often unaware of their word-finding errors and do not attempt self-corrections. Higher level language disorders abound and include problems with verbal reasoning, proverb interpretation, categorizing, problem-solving, and generalizations. Apraxia of speech is often produced with less struggle and fewer complication errors because of the reduced propositionality by the patient. The distorted speech sounds of dysarthria are often produced with less intelligibility than warranted by neurological damage because patients are unconcerned, indifferent or unaware of these disorders. Many aspects of the pragmatics of language are usually lost to the patient, and he or she is inappropriate, aggressive, and disinhibited with regard to communication.

10.15 Human Communication: Brain Hemisphere and Lobe Localization Generalities

Expert witness testimony often involves localization issues concerning communication abilities. Expert witnesses, particularly neuropsychologists and neurologists, frequently opine about the site of brain damage and expected communication disorders. Localizing specific sites in the brain, particularly those involved with communication, is far from an exact science because there is high individual variability and difficulty measuring functional speech and language abilities and correlating them with damaged tracts of neurons. According to Tetnowski (2003, p. 2):

If we knew all there was to know about human behaviors, modern brain imaging techniques would

be the sole tool required to identify symptoms, strengths, and weaknesses of our patients with neurogenically based communication disorders. Obviously much more is needed. I have personally witnessed patients perform a given task that clinical tools of the trade indicated were physically impossible. The opposite is also true.

Localizing motor and sensory aspects of the brain, and certain areas important to perception, memory, and learning, is far more precise than localizing areas of the brain responsible for verbal thought and higher level language functions. In addition, in many generalities about brain localization, it is more accurate to note that certain areas are important to a particular speech and language function rather than to opine that an entire function is located in a particular area (Tanner, 2006b; Tanner, 2006c). The brain operates as a whole, especially about human communication. No better support for this exists than the fact that language cannot be localized in the left hemisphere for all people.

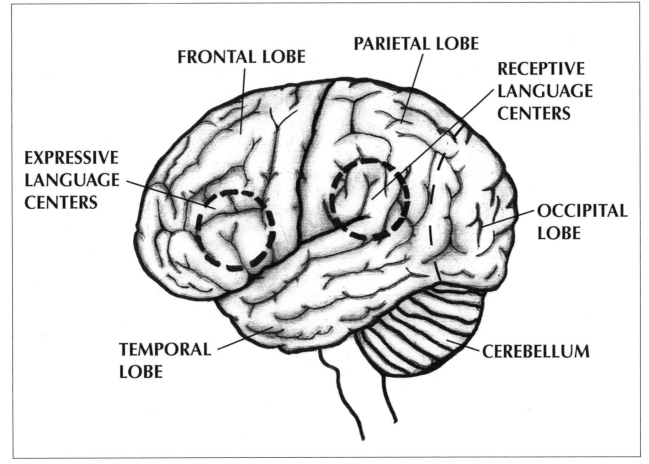

Figure 10.2 The lobes of the left hemisphere of the brain

The right hemisphere of the brain is sometimes errone-ously called the silent hemisphere. The right hemisphere is far from silent regarding communication. As reported pre-viously, in a considerable segment of the population, the major speech and language functions are located in the right hemisphere. And in left dominate individuals, the right hemisphere also has verbal functions. The right hemisphere of the brain is specialized for rhythm, melody, gestures, fa-cial expression, and intonation. It is important to the expres-sion, comprehension, and interpretation of verbal intent and emotion.

Neuropsychologists and neurologists also often discuss the lobes of the brain in terms of speech and language func-tioning. The lobes of the brain are anatomical designations. Functional generalizations about their roles in communica-tion are far from precise and absolute. However, broad gen-eralities can be made. Lovell and Franzen (1994) list com-mon sequelae of traumatic brain injury relative to the lobes of the brain which are damaged. Damage to the temporal lobes causes verbal memory deficits, auditory agnosia, and Wernicke's aphasia. Damage to the parietal lobes results in right-left confusion, acalculia, alexia, apraxia, and denial of illness. These are also called visuospatial impairments. Damage to the occipital lobes results in impaired reading and writing, cortical blindness, and homonymous hemian-opsia (blindness in one half of the fields of both eyes). Lovell and Franzen (1994) list other sequela related to the site of brain damage, but the ones listed above are primarily associated with speaking, reading, writing, and understand-ing the speech of others. Again, the above are generalities for large groups of people, and there are considerable indi-vidual variations. Figure 10.2 shows the lobes and speech and language centers of the human brain.

10.16 Pediatric Traumatic Brain Injury

"Closed-head trauma in children is a major public health problem. It is a leading cause of death among youth and re-sults in substantial neurobehavioral morbidity for survi-vors" (Yeates, 2000, p. 92). Davis (2007) observes that young people with closed head trauma have deficits of at-tention, episodic memory, behavioral organization, and learning new information. Communication disorders in children often have different symptoms and outcomes than those seen in adults. This is particularly true when the com-munication disorder occurs before the child is approxi-mately eight years old. Although there is high variability in the rate normal children acquire speech and language, by the time a child is approximately eight years old, he or she should have acquired the fundamental aspects of speech and language (Tanner, Culbertson, and Secord, 1997; Tan-

ner, Lamb, and Secord, 1997). Language structure and function are essentially established, except for continued semantic learning, at a young age. People learn the mean-ings of words and how to use them in appropriate contexts throughout their lives. However, the fundamental aspects of grammar, syntax, and the acquisition of sounds are essen-tially complete by the time most children are eight years old. Consequently, a child with a traumatic brain injury oc-curring before or during the peak speech and language de-velopment period often presents with different symptoms than what is seen in an adult. In addition, children are still developing socially, physically, and emotionally, which can cause different symptoms and outcomes than what occurs in adults.

It has been said that at birth the human brain is a blank slate. The younger the child, the more flexible and plastic is his or her brain. As a human matures, more and more of the brain becomes committed, e.g., memories, emotions, asso-ciations, concepts, learning strategies, and physical abilities are established. Consequently, children with damage to ma-jor speech and language centers and the tracts leading to and from them are more likely than adults to have adjacent areas of the brain and/or the nondominate hemisphere as-sume the functions previously performed by the damaged areas. This has led to the general belief that children with traumatic brain injuries tend to have a better prognosis for speech and language recovery than adults with similar brain damage. On the negative side, whereas adults have estab-lished learning styles and a history of successful learning, children with traumatic brain injuries may be more nega-tively affected by the disruptions in learning and memory.

Many of the risk factors associated with traumatic brain injuries in adults also apply to children. The number one cause of traumatic brain injuries in children is high-speed automobile accidents (Snow and Hooper, 1994). Other causes of traumatic brain injuries in children include bicycle, motorcycle, car-pedestrian accidents, falls, and child abuse. The shaken child syndrome occurs when an adult violently shakes the child to stop him or her from cry-ing, to cease other behaviors, or when shaking is used as a punishment. The same mechanical factors seen in closed head injuries are involved in the shaken child syndrome and other types of child abuse. Brain rotational acceleration, impact, and deceleration can cause diffuse axonal shearing and tearing. The spinal cord can also be damaged. The type of injury, medical complications, severity of the trauma, premorbid functioning of the child and family, and the ef-fects of rehabilitation all influence the outcomes in children with traumatic brain injuries (Snow and Hooper, 1994).

Habilitation and rehabilitation of pediatric traumatic brain injury involve transition and return to school. The school must adapt teaching and learning strategies to the child's cognitive, physical, and emotional changes brought about by the traumatic brain injury. Most children with significant traumatic brain injuries are involved in special education programs. Individualized education plans (IEPs) are created by parents, teachers, counselors, and therapists to address the disabilities caused by the traumatic brain injuries.

10.17 Traumatic Brain Injuries, Hearing Loss, and Deafness

"Ideally, all patients admitted with a diagnosis of traumatic brain injury should undergo some type of risk assessment screening to establish the likelihood of damage to auditory structures" (Mackay, Chapman, and Morgan, 1997, p. 483). Open and closed traumatic head injuries can damage the hearing mechanism, and testing is necessary to determine the patient's hearing acuity and perception. It is particularly important to assess hearing before speech and language testing. Hearing loss and deafness must be ruled out before a determination can be made as to a patient's auditory comprehension, orientation, and memory. This is because testing of speech and language often involves auditory input, e.g., asking questions and giving directions. A patient with damage to the hearing mechanism may fail to respond or respond incorrectly, not because of language, cognition, or other brain injury problems, but because of the hearing loss or deafness.

Traumatic head injuries can damage or tear off the pinna (external ear) and disrupt the functions of the middle ear. Consequently, external and middle ear damage can cause conductive hearing losses. Bleeding in the middle ear or disruption of the ossicular chain can create a maximal 60dB conductive hearing loss (Northern and Downs, 1991). The inner ear can be damaged by the force of impact. According to Northern and Downs (1991), permanent sensorineural hearing loss can be caused by even moderate trauma to the skull. Sensorineural hearing loss is caused by damage to the cochlea and/or the auditory-vestibular cranial nerve. According to Mackay, Chapman, and Morgan (1997), injury to the auditory-vestibular cranial nerve occurs because of acceleration and deceleration forces during the traumatic event. Additionally, secondary brain damage associated with slowly developing hemorrhages, infections, and localized or widespread swelling and edema can also damage the hearing mechanism. Northern and Downs (1991) note that meningitis, a cause of deafness, may be a late complication of temporal bone fracture.

When traumatic brain injuries damage the hearing mechanism, there are several surgeries and therapies available to reduce the effects on the patient. Amplification with hearing aids and other devices can help the patient compensate for the hearing loss. Modern digital hearing aids are helpful because they typically do not result in the auditory feedback problems that plagued older amplification devices. Unwanted auditory feedback can be particularly detrimental to traumatic head trauma patients with orientation and concentration problems. Also, the quality of amplification with digital hearing aids is greater than with previous ones. Most conductive hearing deficits can be surgically corrected. With a few exceptions, damage to the structures of the external or middle ear can be addressed by surgeons. Even sensorineural hearing loss can be addressed with cochlear implants which in recent years have dramatically improved. Central auditory dysfunctions and acoustic and auditory agnosia overlap as diagnostic categories. They are addressed with auditory training and aural rehabilitation when conducted by audiologists or as perceptual disorders when treated by speech-language pathologists.

10.18 Traumatic Brain Injury and Dysphagia

Dysphagia is discussed in Chapter 8, including the stages of a normal swallow, diagnostic and treatment procedures, and factors related to litigation. The broad definition of dysphagia includes the patient's psychological responses to the smell of food and liquid, his or her cognitive abilities to recognize and understand what to do with them, and the motor and sensory aspects of moving substances from the mouth to the stomach. There are two factors to consider when litigating cases involving dysphagia secondary to traumatic brain injuries: sensory-motor deficits and cognitive impairments.

The sensory-motor deficits seen in some patients with traumatic brain injury are discussed in Chapter 8. Particularly in patients with focalized brain and nervous system damage, the three stages of the swallow may be disrupted primarily by sensory-motor deficits. At the oral stage, the patient may have trouble chewing and containing food substances, creating a bolus, and moving it to the back of the mouth by the sensation deficits and muscular paralysis or paresis. Velopharyngeal closure, the closing of the vocal folds as a protective action, initiation of laryngeal elevation and anterior movement, and the covering of the glottis by the epiglottis can also be disrupted by sensation deficits and muscular paralysis or paresis. The completed swallow, including the esophageal-laryngeal activities, can be impaired by sensation deficits and muscular paralysis or paresis. Diagnosis and treatments are similar to what is done for patients without cognitive impairment.

The second factor to consider in dysphagia secondary to traumatic brain injury involves patients with impaired orientation, memory, behavior, and other factors related to mental executive functioning. These patients may present with dysphagia though their oral, pharyngeal and laryngeal sensory-motor functioning are unimpaired. They may be impulsive about eating and show poor judgment about food portion size. Some patients may not recognize certain foods and liquids. Many patients attempt to talk during the swallow and pose choking and related aspiration risks. Agitation, memory, and orientation deficits can prevent them from participating in instrumental swallowing studies and profiting from the therapeutic experience. In addition, patients with traumatic brain injuries can have motor and sensory swallowing deficits compounded by their cognitive impairments. Choking and aspiration risks are greater for these patients than what is seen in patients with other sensory motor swallowing disorders. Additionally, medications used to combat behavioral problems can sedate the patient, contributing to the dysphagia. Cognitively impaired patients can also pull NG tubes and IV lines and must be restrained from doing so.

10.19 Rehabilitation of the Head-Injured Person

A program of reality orientation is offered by most hospitals, rehabilitation facilities, and nursing homes for their head-trauma patients. Reality orientation is a concerted effort by all rehabilitation professionals to improve the patient's memory, orientation, and behavior. The goals and objectives of the particular reality orientation program are established during the rehabilitation team meetings, which typically occur weekly. Although reality orientation programs differ with the facility and the particular patient, they all have the goal of regularly giving the patient relevant, important information. Each rehabilitation professional provides input into the patient's deficiencies, and the team reaches a consensus about short-term and long-term goals, and methods of achieving them. Typically in a reality orientation program, all who come into daily contact with the patient state information about orientation. These are statements about time, place, person, and situation/predicament. They can also include goals and objectives about behavior management. In the patient's room are familiar pictures of family and friends, pets, home, and other aspects related to the patient's life. A large print calendar is placed in easy view of the patient, and the days are marked off. The patient's daily schedule is usually written on a black board

so that he or she can see it. Familiar music and television programs are made available to the patient. Consistency is the most important aspect of reality orientation. Orientation information and new learning are consistently presented to the patient by all staff members who come in contact with him or her.

A common statement made about the treatment of traumatic brain injuries is "Rehabilitation begins at the scene of the accident." An early start with treatments and therapies insures that all that can be done is done for the patient with a traumatic brain injury. As for speech and language therapy, studies are conclusive in showing that those patients who get an early start in rehabilitation, and whose therapies are provided intensively, do better in the recovery of their communication abilities. With few exceptions those patients whose therapies begin early postonset, and who have them provided intensively, make more rapid recovery and in broader dimensions than those whose treatments are delayed or provided less intensively. (The questionable benefits of coma stimulation therapy were addressed above.) Studies have also shown that the treatments and therapies should, where practicable, be relevant to the patient's premorbid personality and interests and focus on real-life issues and problems. The stimuli used in treatments and therapies should be based on the patient's gender, education, vocational, psychological, and social history.

No better example exists of the benefits of the medical team approach than what is seen in the rehabilitation of traumatic brain-injured persons. The rehabilitation of the traumatic brain-injured person involves professionals from medicine, including several specialities, nursing, psychology, rehabilitation counseling, audiology, social work, food and nutrition sciences, dentistry, occupational, physical, and speech services, and others. For children with traumatic brain injuries, teachers and special education professionals are also involved. The patient's family members are pivotal members of the rehabilitation team. Because of the diverse training, education, and rehabilitation focus, regular and effective communication between these professionals, and with the patient and his or her family, is essential. Standards of practice in the treatment of traumatic brain-injured patients require regular team meetings, often on a weekly basis, and additional formal and informal communication among professionals and family members as situations require. Because of the disorientation, memory problems, behavioral deficits, and learning problems often seen in traumatic brain-injured patients, the rehabilitation team, including family members and friends of the patient, should have regular, open, and unimpeded communication. This team approach emphasizing the importance of communication is particularly relevant in treating impaired executive functions. A clinician's primary responsibility is to help people with brain injuries achieve goals and live satisfying lives (Ylvisaker and Feeney, 1998). To help meet that responsibility, Ylvisaker and Feeney (1998, p. 53) have proposed that the treatment of executive functions address the following:

- Self-awareness of strengths and limitations, and associated understanding of the difficulty level of tasks;

- Ability to set reasonable goals;

- Ability to plan and organize behavior designed to achieve the goals;

- Ability to initiate behavior toward achieving goals and inhibit behavior incompatible with achieving those goals;

- Ability to monitor and evaluate performance in relation to the goals; and

- Ability to flexibly revise plans and strategically solve problems in the event of difficulty or failure.

10.20 Traumatic Brain Injury Litigation: Determining Current and Retrospective Mental Competence

Some patients with traumatic brain injuries have motor speech disorders, but their language and cognitive communicative abilities are unaffected. Patients whose neurological damage is limited to apraxia of speech and the dysarthrias do not have compromised mental competence. Though these patients may be severely communication disabled or even mute, their intelligence and cognition are not affected by the motor speech disorders. Apraxia of speech and the dysarthrias are motor speech disorders and are not likely to call a patient's current or retrospective mental competence into question. Patients with neck and spinal injuries are also unaffected cognitively and intellectually by their injuries. Depression and other psychological reactions may cloud their legal judgment, but the disorders themselves do not necessarily affect intelligence and cognition.

Rarely does a traumatic brain injury result in focalized damage to the language centers and the tracts leading to and from them. However, when this does occur and patients suffer from language disorders, several factors must be considered when determining their current or retrospective mental competence. Accuracy of yes/no responses, interpretation of intelligence tests, graphic disturbances, agnosia, loss of abstract attitude, perseveration, and acalculia must be addressed in mental competence determinations. These issues, and others related to language disorders, are discussed in Chapter 9. They are relevant to patients with traumatic brain injuries when the neurogenic communication disorder is limited to the aphasia.

There are several factors that can complicate current and retrospective mental competence determinations in patients who have traumatic brain injuries not affecting their speech and language centers. These patients, to various degrees, may have impaired or disrupted self-regulation, orientation, memory deficits, disinhibition, excitability, and/or indifference. Though the fabric of language is intact, and there are no motor speech deficits, these patients' mental competence is largely dependent on the degree of mental executive functioning impairments and their ability to engage in metacognition. Each cognitive communicative function must be tested and evaluated separately concerning the likelihood that the individual patient can competently engage in and understand the implications of participating in legal defense, signing checks, making or changing wills, drive, live independently, care for children, manage business affairs, etc. Because of the high degree of individual variability of deficits in self-regulation, orientation, memory, inhibition, excitability and/or indifference among traumatic brain-injured patients, a case-by-case determination must be made based on test results. Neuropsychologists have a battery of tests for assessing these deficits (Snyder and Nussbaum, 1998).

For forensic purposes, it is extremely difficult to determine current or retrospective competence of patients with significant diffuse brain and nervous system damage that also affects the major speech and language centers of the brain and the tracts leading to and from them. When patients have aphasia, apraxia of speech, and dysarthria compounded and complicated by impaired or disrupted metacognition and executive function impairments, mental competence is suspect. Certainly, there are some patients with these combinations of disorders that are mentally competent, but demonstrating it is difficult if not impossible. This is especially true in patients with aphasia complicated by impaired or disrupted metacognition and executive functions impairments. The multimodality nature of aphasia affects the testing of the cognitive communicative deficits to the extent that the reliability and validity of the results are suspect. There must be at least one unimpeded expressive and receptive modality available to assess accurately the extent of the cognitive communicative disorders.

10.21 Traumatic Brain Injury, Vocational Rehabilitation, Antidiscrimination, and Insurance-Social Welfare Determination and Compensation

The legal issues in patients with traumatic brain injuries are similar to the ones discussed in Chapter 9. They include vocational rehabilitation eligibility, antidiscrimination issues, and insurance-social welfare determination and compensation. Dixon and Layton (1999) reviewed studies on postinjury employment rates and patients with traumatic brain injuries and found that the severity of the TBI has predictive value in determining the likelihood of vocational success. They found that approximately 80 percent of persons with severe traumatic brain injuries were employed prior to their injuries, but only 30 percent were able to resume working. With moderate to severe traumatic brain injury (in urban areas), the preemployment rate was 51 percent and declined to 25 percent postinjury. Motivation is sometimes an issue in traumatic brain injury and neurogenic communication disorders. See *Groeper v Sullivan*, 932 F2d 1234 (8th Cir 1991).

Dixon and Layton (1999) note three distinctive characteristics about traumatic brain injury which differ from many other disabling conditions. First, unlike many other disabling conditions, patients with traumatic brain injury usually have intellectual and emotional limitations that can interfere with adaptation. Second, unlike developmental cognitive and intellectual disabilities such as are seen in mental impairment-mental retardation, people with traumatic brain injuries have abruptly diminished social and vocational roles where there were no preexisting limited expectations for productivity. Third, unlike visible disabilities such as limb amputation and paraplegia, the cognitive communicative disorders in traumatic brain injury are invisible on casual inspection. Each of the above can affect vocational rehabilitation eligibility, antidiscrimination issues, and insurance-social welfare determination and compensation.

Several personality, emotional, and cognitive disorders associated with traumatic brain injury can profoundly impede vocational rehabilitation. Even in patients who regain functional communication abilities, the memory deficits, confabulation, response delay, disorientation, and a host of behavioral problems can result in poor vocational rehabilitation potential. For moderately to severely involved TBI patients who have significant residual communication disorders, the potential to reenter the workforce is bleak. For patients who were previously employed in jobs and careers with high status and earning potential, the traumatic brain injury can cause frustration and anger. The psychological reactions to neurogenic communication disorders discussed in Chapter 9 can also occur in patients with traumatic brain injury. These include anxiety, depression, and the grief response. According to Dixon and Layton (1999), other factors that play a role in employment for TBI patients include transportation, access to rehabilitation services, employer attitude toward disability, and job availability. Tanner and Martin (1986) note that Native Americans with communication disorders may have disproportional difficulty finding employment especially on Indian reservations where the unemployment rate can be 70 percent or higher. "Many people with TBI who are able to return to work may have to change jobs in order to accommodate impaired abilities; job changes of this nature entail reductions in pay and status and engender resistance, anger, and feelings of loss" (Dixon and Layton, 1999, p. 116). Statistics from the U.S. Equal Employment Opportunity Commission show that in a five-year period in the mid-1990s, over half of the charges filed related to alleged unlawful discharge (Bruye're and DeMarinis, 1999).

Patients with traumatic brain injuries, as a group, pose greater difficulties in determining vocational rehabilitation eligibility than any other category of communication disorder. The severity and complexity of the TBI symptoms can also cloud issues in discrimination in housing, public accommodations, education, communication, transportation, voting, and other factors addressed by the Americans with Disabilities Act. Difficulties quantifying the cognitive, communicative, and social deficits as seen in many patients with moderate to severe traumatically induced disabilities can create major issues in insurance-social welfare determination and compensation.

10.22 Traumatic Brain Injury and Malingering

As it is used in this chapter, malingering is the willful and deliberate feigning or exaggerating of traumatic brain injury symptoms for exemption, attention, sympathy, academic, and/or employment rewards, or for financial gain. Malingering was discussed in Chapter 9 where patients with aphasia, apraxia of speech, and dysarthria fake or exaggerate symptoms for a self-serving end. In patients with traumatic brain injuries, malingering usually involves exaggeration of symptoms and deficits. Malingering patients are more likely to exaggerate existing symptoms and deficits rather than make up nonexistent ones. Regarding communication disorders, malingering patients may exaggerate dysarthric output by producing less distinct phonemes than what they are capable. Apraxia of speech may be produced with more struggle and complication than necessary. Malingering patients may exaggerate language deficits in all modalities. They may write less legibly, speak with more anomia, read with poor comprehension, and feign difficulty understanding questions and following instructions. In the cognitive communication realm, patients may exaggerate memory and orientation deficits. They will do poorly on memory and orientation tests to exaggerate symptoms.

Computed tomography (CT), magnetic resonance imaging (MRI), single photon tomography (SPECT), positron emission tomography (PET), and functional magnetic resonance imaging (fMRI) and other brain scanning diagnostic tests can provide evidence of malingering in patients who create nonexistent impairments. Unfortunately, as for communication disorders, they cannot provide definitive evidence of malingering because of the variability of localization of speech and language in the human brain. As has been reported previously, speech and language are not dominant in the left hemisphere for a considerable percentage of the normal population, especially among left-handed individuals. Current brain scan technology is also ineffective for quantifying and qualifying patient communication disorders symptoms based on the site and size of lesions. For example, damage to the hippocampus can suggest memory, orientation, and learning impairments, but brain scans cannot quantify or qualify the nature and extent of the amnesia presented by the patient with any degree of accuracy. In addition, nonmalingering patients with normal brain scans can have orientation and memory problems. Davis (2007) notes that studies are being planned using the fMRI as a predictor of traumatic brain injury outcomes.

A TBI patient's real-world functioning is a better indicator of his or her disabilities than are brain scans or psychometric tests. For example, family reports of how well a patient remembers directions at home is better evidence of memory functioning than the patient's performance on psychometric tests or the results of brain scans. Consistency is also important when litigating suspected malingering. Although spontaneous recovery does occur, and there is a gradual evolution of symptoms over time, the natural course of recovery from traumatic brain injury has been well documented. Ninety percent of people with traumatic brain injury attain their ultimate outcome classification within six months (Dixon and Layton, 1999). This is not to say that some patients do not have an unusual course of recovery. However, from deep coma to maximal recovery there is a typical and usual presentation of symptoms for most patients with traumatic brain injury. Deviation from this normal course of recovery, and lack of consistency of symptoms, suggests unusual outcomes and possibly malingering.

10.23 Case Study in Traumatic Brain Injury Litigation

A male Native American college student was involved in a truck-automobile accident and suffered a mild closed head injury. Following the motor vehicle accident, he claimed communication disorders, impaired memory, and difficulty learning new information. He also claimed that because of the head injury his ability to succeed in college was compromised. The student showed declining grades in undergraduate courses, and he ultimately dropped out of college.

Two issues concerning communication disorders were pivotal in this case. First, describing and quantifying the claimant's loss of communication abilities, memory, and ability to learn new information were required for compensation purposes. Second, the role of the alleged disabilities in his failure to succeed in college needed to be established. If there were significant chronic communication, memory, and learning deficits, did they result in or contribute to the claimants inability to succeed in college?

Several psychometric diagnostic tests were administered to describe and quantify the claimant's loss of communication, memory, and learning abilities. As is often the case when testing for memory loss, disorientation, and language disorders in Native Americans, the validity and reliability of standardized aphasia and neuropsychological tests were called into question. Few language, orientation, and aphasia tests are standardized on Native American populations. The validity and reliability of these tests are often suspect, especially with individuals whose language spoken in the home is one other than English. In addition, the results of testing must also be tempered by whether the patient is a traditional, nontraditional, urban, or rural Native American and whether English is a second language for him or her. When translators are used, the accuracy of their translation may be suspect because they often are not literal word-for-word reports.

An example of the cultural difficulties in aphasia testing with some Native American individuals involves tests for anomia. Anomia is loss of the meaning of words: an inability to remember names. Many tests and subtests for anomia require the patient to say the name of a person, place, or thing when requested either verbally or graphically by the examiner. During the assessment, an examiner may ask the patient to provide the name of a relative when pointing to a picture. The patient's failure to report that the person in the picture is a cousin or sibling, for example, suggests anomia and/or disorientation to person. However, some Navajo respondents, particularly traditionalists, will state the relationship of the person in the picture to their family and clan rather than report the proper name, e.g., my cousin, sister, or aunt. To further complicate orientation and aphasia testing, many pictorial stimuli used for Navajo speakers are culturally biased. For some rural, traditional Navajo speakers, who may live in a hogan without electricity, pictorial stimuli of blenders, vacuums, and washing machines are likely to be more foreign to them than pictures of feathers, sheep, and horses. Consequently, their scores on those tests are not true measures of language comprehension or expression.

Linking communication disorders to academic failure also involves many variables. Mild to moderate motor speech disorders pose few barriers to studying, attending lectures, participating in study groups, etc. However, anomia and memory deficits, even mild ones, are major barriers to successful academic performance. Obviously, naming and verbal recall impede test taking, even when the lecture and written information have been stored in memory. Other factors associated with frontal lobe damage also impede academic performance. Failure to turn in assignments on due dates and missing classes can be attributed to traumatic brain injury, especially when the patient had not displayed those behaviors before the accident. The patient's self-esteem also plays a part in successful academic performance.

The patient's knowledge that he has suffered brain damage may also interfere with academic confidence and contribute to posttraumatic brain injury ego weakness and subsequent ego restriction. Ego weakness is the reduced strength of the aspect of the personality involved in evaluating, directing, and controlling actions in response to reality. Ego restriction is a type of avoidance behavior used to protect the person from threats to self-esteem. The person using ego restriction refuses or abandons an activity because of pathological feelings of inferiority and readily turns to another activity rather than risk the possibility of failure and the resulting loss of self-esteem. Ego restriction is seen in some patients with traumatic brain injury as a defense mechanism and coping style (Tanner, 2003).

Given the learning, memory, and communication abilities necessary for successful academic performance, the patient's failure in college was at least partially attributable to the traumatic brain injury. Although a direct link to academic failure and the mild global learning and memory problems could not be established, the patient's academic deterioration was indirectly related to those deficits. The anomia was directly responsible for poor performance on examinations.

10.24 Chapter Summary

Today, more people survive major traumatic brain injuries albeit often with communication disorders. Some traumatic brain-injured survivors may have the fabric of speech and language undamaged, but experience problems with metacognition including memory, orientation, and behavioral problems. Others may have the site of brain damage limited to the major speech and language centers and present with classic aphasia, apraxia of speech, and the dysarthrias. Many patients have their speech and language centers damaged, and the symptoms are complicated and compounded by metacognition deficits. Traumatic brain-injured persons pose several unique litigation problems including factors related to mental competence, compensation, antidiscrimination issues, vocational rehabilitation, and determining malingering.

Suggested Readings and Resources

American Speech-Language-Hearing Association (1988, March). *The role of speech-language pathologists in the identification, diagnosis, and treatment of individuals with cognitive-communicative impairments.* This position paper by the American Speech-Language-Hearing Association details the professional expectations for speech-language pathologists in diagnosing and treating patients with traumatic brain injuries.

Snyder, P.J. and Nussbaum, P.D. (1998). *Clinical Neuropsychology: a Pocket Handbook for Assessment.* Washington, D.C.: American Psychological Association. This handbook provides comprehensive neuropsychological assessment information, including specific tests, brain localization information, and neuropsychological philosophies. There is a chapter specifically devoted to traumatic brain injuries.

Tanner, D. (2003). *The Psychology of Neurogenic Communication Disorders: A Primer for Health Care Professionals.* Boston: Allyn & Bacon. This book addresses the psychology of neurogenic communication disorders including traumatic brain injuries.

Ylvisaker, M., Szekeres, S.F., and Feeney, T. (2001). Communication disorders associated with traumatic brain injury. In *Language Intervention Strategies in Aphasia and Related Neurogenic Communication Disorders* (4th ed.), R. Chapey (Ed) (pp. 745-808). Philadelphia: Lippincott Williams & Wilkins. This is a comprehensive exploration of traumatic brain injuries and neurogenic communication disorders.

References

American Speech-Language-Hearing Association (1988, March). The role of speech-language pathologists in the identification, diagnosis, and treatment of individuals with cognitive-communicative impairments, ASHA, 30, 79, Author.

Aronson, A.E. (2000). *Aronson's neurosciences pocket lectures: Speech, language, voice.* San Diego: Singular.

Bruye're, S. M. and DeMarinis, R. K. (1999). Legislation and rehabilitation service delivery. In M. Eisenberg, R. Glueckauf, and H. Zaretski (Eds) (pp. 679-695) *Medical aspects of disabilities: A handbook for the rehabilitation professional.* New York: Springer.

Carlat, D. (1999). *The psychiatric interview.* Philadelphia: Lippincott, Williams & Wilkins.

Centers for Disease Control (1997). Traumatic brain injury- Colorado, Missouri, Oklahoma, & Utah, 1990-1993. *MMWR, 46,* 8-11.

Culbertson, W., Tanner, D., Peck, A., and Hooper, A. (1998). Orientation testing and responses of brain injured subjects. *Journal of Medical Speech-Language Pathology,* Vol 6. No 2.

Davis, G. A. (2007). *Aphasiology: Disorders and clinical practice* (2nd ed.). Boston: Allyn & Bacon.

Dirckx, J. H. (2001). *Stedman's concise medical dictionary for the health professions* (4th ed). Philadelphia: Lippincott Williams & Wilkins.

Dixon, T.M. and Layton, B.S. (1999). Traumatic brain injury. In M. Eisenberg, R. Glueckauf, and H. Zaretski (Eds.) (pp. 98-120) *Medical aspects of disabilities: A handbook for the rehabilitation professional.* New York: Springer.

Douglas, J. (2004). The Evidence Base for the Cognitive-Communicative Disorders after Traumatic Brain Injury in Adults. In *Evidence based practice in speech pathology,* S. Reilly, J. Douglas, and J. Oates (Eds). London: Whurr Publishers.

Eisenberg, M., Glueckauf, R. and Zaretski, H. (1999). Preface. In M. Eisenberg, R. Glueckauf, and H. Zaretski (Eds) (p. xix) *Medical aspects of disabilities: A handbook for the rehabilitation professional.* New York: Springer.

Ghajar, J. (2000 September 9). Traumatic brain injury. *Lancet, 356*: 923-29.

Gillis, R., and Pierce, J. (1996). Mechanism of traumatic brain injury and the pathophysiologic consequences. In R. Gillis (Ed), *Traumatic brain injury rehabilitation for speech-language pathologists.* Boston: Butterworth-Heinemann.

Gillis, R. (1996). *Traumatic brain injury rehabilitation for speech-language pathologists.* Boston: Butterworth-Heinemann.

Hagen, C. (1981). Language disorders secondary to closed head injury: Diagnosis and management. *Top Lang Disord., 1*: 73-87.

Kraus, J. and Sorenson, S. (1994). Epidemiology. In J. Silver, S. Yudofsky, and R. Hales (Eds) *Neuropsychiatry of traumatic brain injury.* Washington, DC: American Psychiatric Press.

Lovell, M. and Franzen, M. (1994). Neuropsychological assessment. In J. Silver, S. Yudofsky, and R. Hales (Eds), *Neuropsychiatry of traumatic brain injury* Washington, DC: American Psychiatric Press.

Lucas, J.A. (1998). Traumatic brain injury. In P. Snyder and P.D. Nussbaum (Eds), *Clinical neuropsychology: A pocket handbook for assessment* (pp. 243-265). American Psychological Association: Author.

Mackay, L., Chapman, P., and Morgan, A. (1997). *Maximizing brain injury recovery: Integrating critical care and early rehabilitation.* Gaithersburg, MD: Aspen.

McAllister, T. (1994). Mild traumatic brain injury and the postconcussive syndrome. In J. Silver, S. Yudofsky, and R. Hales (Eds), *Neuropsychiatry of traumatic brain injury.* Washington, DC: American Psychiatric Press.

Northern, J., and Downs, M. (1991). *Hearing in children* (4th ed.). Philadelphia: Lippincott Williams & Wilkins.

Pimental, P. and Kingsbury, N. (1989). *Neuropsychological aspects of right brain injury.* Austin: ProEd.

Ryalls, J. and Behrens, S. (2000). *Introduction to speech sciences.* Boston: Allyn & Bacon.

Smeltzer, D., Nasrallah, H., and Miller, S. (1994). Psychotic disorders. In J. Silver, S. Yudofsky, and R. Hales (Eds) *Neuropsychiatry of traumatic brain injury.* Washington, DC: American Psychiatric Press.

Snow, J. and Hooper, S. (1994). *Pediatric traumatic brain injury.* Thousand Oaks, CA: Sage.

Snyder, P.J. and Nussbaum, P.D. (1998). *Clinical neuropsychology: A pocket handbook for assessment.* Washington, D.C.: American Psychological Association.

Szekeres, S., Ylvisaker, M., and Cohen, S. (1987). A framework for cognitive rehabilitation therapy. In M. Ylvisaker and E. Gobble (Eds), *Community re-entry for head injured adults.* Boston: College Hill Press/Little, Brown.

Tanner, D. and Martin, W. (1986). Services and training needs in communicative problems and disorders for rehabilitation professionals serving Native Americans. *Journal of Rehabilitation Administration*, Volume 10, Number 4, p. 117-123.

Tanner, D., Lamb, W., and Secord, W. (1997). *Cognitive, Linguistic and Social Communication Scales (CLASS)* (2nd ed.). Oceanside, CA: Academic Communication Associates.

Tanner, D., Culbertson, W., and Secord, W. (1997). *Developmental Articulation and Phonology Profile (DAPP).* Oceanside, CA: Academic Communication Associates.

Tanner, D. (1977). Differential diagnosis of organic brain syndrome. A paper presented to the Annual Convention of the Arizona Speech and Hearing Association, Tucson.

Tanner, D. (1999). *The family guide to surviving stroke and communication disorders.* Boston: Allyn & Bacon.

Tanner, D. (2003). *The psychology of neurogenic communication disorders: A primer for health care professionals.* Boston: Allyn & Bacon.

Tanner, D. (2006a). *Case studies in communication sciences and disorders.* Upper Saddle River, N.J.: Pearson Merrill Prentice Hall.

Tanner, D. (2006b). *An advanced course in communication sciences and disorders.* San Diego: Plural Publishing.

Tanner, D. (2006c). Redefining Wernicke's area: Receptive language and discourse semantics. (Accepted for Publication in the *Journal of Allied Health*).

Teasdale, G., and Jennett, B. (1974). Assessment of coma and impaired consciousness: A practical guide. *Lancet, 13*: 81-84.

Tetnowski, J. (2003). Foreword. In D. Tanner, *The psychology of neurogenic communication disorders: A primer for health care professionals.* Boston: Allyn & Bacon.

Yeates, K. (2000). Closed-head injury. In K. Yeates, M. Ris, and H. Taylor (Eds.), *Pediatric neuropsychology.* New York: Guilford Press.

Ylvisaker, M., Feeney, J., and Feeney, T. (1999). An everyday approach to long-term rehabilitation after traumatic brain injury. In B. Cornett (Ed), *Clinical practice management in speech-language pathology: Principles and practacalities* (pp.117-162). Gaithersburg, MD: Aspen.

Ylvisaker, M. and Feeney, T. (1998). *Collaborative brain injury intervention.* San Diego: Singular.

Ylvisaker, M., Szekeres, S.F., and Feeney, T. (2001). Communication disorders associated with traumatic brain injury. In *Language intervention strategies in aphasia and related neurogenic communication disorders* (4th ed.), R. Chapey, (Ed) (pp. 745-808). Philadelphia: Lippincott Williams & Wilkins.

Young, H. and Geller, R. (2007). *Sears & Zemansky's college physics* (8th ed.). San Francisco: Pearson, Addison Wesley.

Chapter 11

Medical-Legal and Forensic Aspects of Voice and Resonance Disorders

11.1 Chapter Preview

This chapter reviews the human sound-source resonating system and the myriad disorders that can disrupt and impair it. Included are historical reviews of the advances in voice science, the relationship of respiration to voice production, and a comprehensive overview of the neurology, anatomy, physiology, and acoustics of voice production. The myo-elastic-aerodynamic principle of voice production is discussed as are pitch, loudness, and voice quality. Also addressed are medical-legal and forensic issues related to malingering, clinician proficiency, vocational rehabilitation, and damage-compensation determination. There is also a case study involving a voice disorder resulting from burn injuries.

11.2 The Sound-Source Resonating System

The human voice is more than the vibratory sound produced by the larynx; it is also resonance. Speech resonance is the modification of the vibratory sound produced in the larynx by passage through the resonating chambers of the neck and head. Respiration provides the driving force for vocal fold vibration, and the sound is modified, either amplified or damped, by the resonating chambers of the head and neck. Respiration provides compressed air to the vocal folds, which is the source of the vibratory sound, and the head and neck resonating chambers modify that energy to create voiced speech sounds, giving a person his or her distinct voice quality. Acoustically, the human voice is a double Helmholtz resonator, approximately 17 cm in length, and its function can be likened to a brass instrument.

In a brass instrument, the vibration created by the lips in the mouthpiece is modified, amplified and damped, by the shape, texture, valving, and length of the horn. Comparably, voice is the interplay between the biological pump of respiration, the laryngeal sound source, and the acoustic properties of resonance. It is a sound-source resonating system. Voice disorders occur across the age spectrum and can be minor nuisances or devastating disabilities affecting vocational alternatives, job performance, and quality of life. Singing careers and professions can be destroyed by improper diagnosis and treatment of voice disorders, and they can be saved by proper medical intervention.

11.3 Historical Perspectives

In the past two decades, voice science has advanced dramatically, particularly in speaker recognition technology. Today, through voice pattern recognition technology, speakers can be identified with a high degree of reliability. Digital telephones now allow dialing by voice commands, and there are speech-to-type devices for disabled individuals and for commercial use. Medically, technology now permits direct viewing of the larynx for early diagnosis of diseases and disorders. For more information about the above read *Part III: The Forensic Aspects of Voice Prints*.

The treatment of voice disorders has improved from the gross and radical treatments of the past. Laryngectomy, the surgical removal of the larynx, has been the principal treatment for laryngeal cancer for decades, and scalpel surgery on the delicate tissue of the vocal folds to remove benign tumors has often resulted in chronic voice problems. Today, although laryngectomies are sometimes necessary, advances in surgery, chemotherapy, and radiation cancer therapies have reduced the necessity of total laryngectomy. Laser surgery of the vocal folds has reduced the complications to patients' voices caused by scalpel surgery. Oates (2004) observes that during the nineteenth century, the treatment of voice disorders was the general responsibility of medical practitioners. Since the 1970s, the management of voice disorders by speech-language pathologists has become less of an art and more of a science.

Historically, viewing the workings of the larynx has been difficult and inexact for several reasons. First, the larynx is difficult to study because it is deep in the throat and out of direct view. Second, viewing the larynx is difficult because the muscles and structures are hidden by darkness and an artificial light source is necessary for illumination. Third, the movements of the vocal folds, and the muscles and cartilages responsible for pitch and loudness, are small and happen very rapidly; they are too small and fast to be observed meaningfully by the naked eye. There are several methods of laryngoscopy, the process of viewing the larynx.

Indirect laryngoscopy was invented in the early 1800s and was the procedure of choice until recently. In indirect laryngoscopy, a mirror is held to the back of the patient's throat and an eye-mirror (a mirror with a small hole in it) reflects a light source from over the patient's shoulder. The light is directed from the eye-mirror to a dental mirror at the back of the throat, and down to the larynx. This procedure was commonplace. Until recently, pictures and illustrations of physicians often showed them with the eye-mirror on their heads; it was integral to the public image of the doctor.

Other methods of viewing the larynx used in the past included transillumination (where a bright light was placed on the surface of the neck), high-speed photography, ultrasound, stroboscopy, X-rays, and other types of magnetic and computed scans. Today, a common method of viewing the larynx is through endoscopy where a fiberoptic tube with a light source is directed down a patient's throat. Stroboscopy uses a flashing light to illuminate the vocal folds' periodic movements. This procedure is known as laryngeal video stroboscopy (LVS).

11.4 Respiration and Voice Production

Respiration serves as the driving force for the production of voice. Litigating cases involving voice disorders can include issues related to a patient having compromised respi-

ration. Because respiration is the driving force for voice production, many actions of the larynx are dependent on respiratory support. Compromised respiration causes impaired voice—dysphonia—or the complete loss of voice—aphonia. Respiratory support is important in pitch and loudness control, emphasis, quality of voice, and the mechanics of setting the vocal folds into vibration. Although the primary function of respiration is to exchange gases to and from the environment for life-sustaining purposes, it is also a method of compressing air for making speech sounds, a biologically overlaid function. The respiratory mechanism is a biological pump.

There are two phases of respiration: inspiration (inhalation) and expiration (exhalation). Inspiration is air flowing into the lungs, and expiration is the outward flow of air. During expiration, speech sounds are made. During speech, the expiration phase usually lasts longer than inspiration as the compressed air is shaped into individual phonemes (speech sounds). Boyle's Law and the Kinetic Theory of Gases explain the workings of this biological pump.

Air is pumped in and out of the body by changing the size of the thorax. The thorax is the upper part of the torso containing the heart, lungs, and ribs. When the thorax expands, the pressure inside the lungs decreases relative to the outside air. During inspiration, air rushes from the region of higher atmospheric pressure to the lower pressure in the lungs. During expiration, higher pressure in the lungs is created by the muscles of respiration reducing the size of the thorax. The biological pump works because the muscles of respiration change the size of the thorax causing the pressure in the lungs to be greater or lesser than the atmospheric pressure. This causes the movement of gas from regions of higher to lower pressure.

The respiratory biological pump affects several physiological pressures and lung capacities (See Figure 11.1). The pressure in the lungs is the alveolar pressure. Pleural pressure is pressure within the thorax but outside the lungs. Abdominal pressure is the pressure in the abdomen. Tidal capacity is the total volume of air expired during each normal respiratory cycle and can be likened to the oceans' tides. The maximum volume of air that can be inspired and expired beyond the end of a normal tidal expiration is called supplemental air or expiratory reserve. Complemental air is the maximum volume of air that can be inspired beyond normal inhalation. It is also called inspiratory reserve. Vital capacity is the total volume of measurable air within the lungs. It includes the sum of tidal capacity, complemental air, and supplemental air. Measurements of vital capacity do not include residual air. Residual air is the volume of air in the lungs that is never expelled, for they would collapse.

Alveolar pressure:	Pressure in the lungs
Pleural pressure:	Pressure within the thorax, but outside the lungs
Abdominal pressure:	Pressure in the abdomen
Tidal capacity:	Total volume of air expired during each normal respiratory cycle
Expiratory reserve:	Volume of air expired beyond normal tidal expiration
Inspiratory reserve:	Volume of air inspired beyond normal tidal inhalation
Vital capacity:	Total volume of measurable air within the lungs
Residual:	Volume of air in the lungs that is never expelled

Figure 11.1 Respiratory pressures and capacities

The volume and flow of air involved in respiration are measured by spirometers and manometers. There are several types of spirometers and manometers, but they all involve the patient blowing into a tube and air volume and flow are figured out. Respiratory rates vary with age and activity. With an increase in age there is a decrease in respiratory rate. In certain stages of sleep, the respiratory rate can decrease by as much as 25 percent. Even standing requires a greater respiratory rate than does sitting or reclining.

The most important muscle of respiration is the diaphragm. The diaphragm is a dome-shaped muscle separating the thorax from the abdomen. In inspiration, when the diaphragm contracts, it moves downward and compresses the contents of the abdomen. It, with other muscles, particularly the external intercostals, expands the thorax to increase its size thus reducing the alveolar pressure and causing air to flow into the lungs. During expiration, the muscles gradually relax, the size of the thorax decreases, thoracic pressure increases relative to the atmospheric pressure, and air rushes outward. During relaxation of the muscles, air in the lungs is compressed primarily by elastic recoil of pulmonary tissue. There is also forced expiration involving muscular contractions. The muscles important to expiration are the internal intercostals, rectus abdominis, external oblique, and latissimus dorsi. Breathing is both conscious and unconscious. Respiration is mediated by the medulla oblongata in the brain stem and also controlled by higher centers of the brain. The cervical and thoracic peripheral nerves are involved in inspiration and expiration.

11.5 The Anatomy, Physiology, Neurology, and Physics of Voice Production

Sometimes called the voice box, the larynx is the primary anatomical location for the production of human voice. The larynx is considered a part of the pharynx. The pharynx is divided into the nasopharynx, oropharynx, and laryngopharynx. The vocal folds are found in the larynx. The opening at the level of the larynx is called the glottis and is the source of voiced sound. Phonation (voicing) refers to any type of vibratory sound produced at the level of the larynx. Whispering is also a function of partially contacting the vocal folds. The larynx can be viewed as a valve that opens for the passage of air and closes when food or liquid enters the throat. Biologically, the laryngeal valve also closes to create a column of compressed air for strenuous activities such as lifting weights, giving birth, and defecating. As discussed in the chapter on dysphagia, it also protects the lower airways from food and liquids entering them. The evolutionary basis for the larynx is open to speculation, but it likely permitted underwater protection of the lungs while the mouth was opened. The larynx also served a survival imperative by permitting shouted warnings, loud call signals, and speech.

The larynx consists of nine cartilages of which three are paired (there are two of them). A cartilage is a firm connective tissue that is softer than a bone. The unpaired cartilages are the thyroid, cricoid, and epiglottis. The thyroid cartilage is the largest. The "Adam's apple" is part of the thyroid cartilage and is more prominent in some males. The cricoid cartilage resembles a signet ring and is below the thyroid cartilage. The epiglottis has a free end projecting upward and closes over the larynx during swallowing as a protective action. It is important, but not essential, to a safe swallow.

The paired cartilages are the arytenoids, corniculates, and cuneiforms. The cuneiforms are wedge shaped, and the corniculates are small cartilages attached to the upper part (apex) of the arytenoid. The arytenoids are shaped like a pyramid and are fundamental to pitch and loudness control. The vocal folds are attached to the arytenoids. The arytenoids slide, rock, and rotate resulting in abduction and adduction of the vocal folds. Abduction is the opening of the glottis, and adduction is the closing of it. The movements of the arytenoids and vocal folds are caused by changes in subglottal air pressure and precise movements of the laryngeal muscles. The pitch of a person's voice depends on the rate of vocal fold vibration, and loudness is influenced by how hard or intensely they contact each other.

The muscles of the larynx are divided into extrinsic and intrinsic groups. Extrinsic laryngeal muscles have one connection outside the larynx, while intrinsic muscles have both their origin and insertion (attachment) within the larynx. Extrinsic laryngeal muscles are largely responsible for support of the larynx and holding it in position. The larynx does not rest on a bone and thus is held in position by muscles. Extrinsic muscles also elevate and depress the larynx during speech and swallowing. Anatomically, the extrinsic muscles may further be divided into suprahyoid and infrahyoid. The hyoid bone is a horseshoe-shaped bone that supports the tongue, and helps hold the larynx in place. Extrinsic laryngeal muscles are sometimes called neck strap muscles.

Intrinsic muscles are divided into four categories: abductor, adductors, tensors, and relaxers. Only one muscle functions to open the vocal folds: the posterior cricoarytenoid. There are several adductor muscles that close the vocal folds for phonation and during swallowing. Tensors elongate and tighten the folds, while relaxers shorten them. See Figure 11.2 for several views of the larynx.

The cranial nerve X, also known as the vagus nerve, enervates the muscles that abduct (open) and close (adduct) the vocal folds. Primarily, the recurrent branch of cranial nerve X, and to a lesser extent the superior branch, enervates the posterior cricoarytenoid (abductor muscle), vocalis, lateral cricoarytenoid, cricothyroid, and the interarytenoid (primary adductor) muscles. Medial compression of the vocal folds is done primarily by the lateral cricoarytenoid. Together, the vagus nerve and above muscles are responsible for the muscular movements that open and close the vocal folds in conjunction with aerodynamic factors. Respiration must be adjusted for increased or decreased resistance in the larynx. When the laryngeal valve is completely or partially occluded, the respiratory muscles must adjust for the increased resistance to the flow of air. The brain and nervous system sense the resistance and automatically adjust for the changes in resistance to air flow, thus allowing speech to be produced normally.

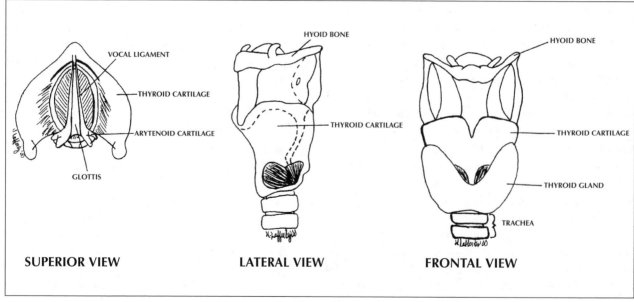

Figure 11.2 *Several views of the larynx*

Because of the difficulties in viewing the larynx, understanding the mechanics of phonation did not happen rapidly. Confusion and questions about vocal fold functioning persisted until the latter part of the 18th century. An early myth about voicing was that each cycle of vibration was caused by a separate neurological impulse to the vocal folds. This erroneous belief was known as the Neurochronaxic Theory of Vocal Fold Vibration. Disproving this theory illustrates important aspects of laryngeal functioning.

Separate neurological impulses could not result in vocal fold vibration for three reasons. First, for the vocal folds to vibrate at normal frequencies (cycles-per-second), the neurological impulses would have to occur at speeds that human neurology is incapable of producing. Second, the vocal muscles would fatigue during connected speech. They could not contract and relax during the thousands of vocal fold vibrations occurring during speech. The third reason this theory could not account for vocal fold vibration concerns the laryngeal nerve. Because of the position of the heart, the left recurrent laryngeal nerve is about 10 cm longer than the right. If separate neurological impulses caused vocal fold vibrations, the impulses would reach the muscles of the larynx out of phase. The vocal folds would not consistently meet at midline. A theory of vocal fold vibration that supplanted the Neurochronaxic Theory of Vocal Fold Vibration is the Myoelastic-Aerodynamic Theory of Voice Production. Actually, this is now considered the principle of phonation and is no longer theoretical.

Attorneys, judges, and jurors may address loss of voice due to reduced respiratory support and compromised neuromuscular functioning. Both muscular and aerodynamic principles combine to create vocal fold vibration. The muscular forces include the elasticity of tissue and movements of cartilages that adjust the tension and position of the vocal folds. Elasticity is the tendency of a substance to resume its original shape after being distended. The vocal folds are blown apart, and this elasticity partially accounts for their return to an adducted (closed) position. The aerodynamic force that closes the vocal folds is the Bernoulli principle. It is named after a Swiss mathematician who discovered that the velocity of the flow of air through a tube is inversely related to its pressure against the sides of the tube. When air flows through the glottis, negative pressure is created and the vocal folds are sucked together. Once they contact each other, the suction is stopped and they are blown apart again. The next cycle of vibration occurs when the air pressure

below the vocal folds builds to an extent sufficient to blow them apart, again permitting the flow of air followed by contact with each other and cessation of air flow, and another cycle begins.

The pitch of a person's voice is a function of the rate of vocal fold vibrations. There are several respiratory and laryngeal physiological factors related to pitch control. The mass per unit length of the vocal folds is a convenient way of examining the physiology of frequency and pitch. Mass refers to the thickness of the vocal folds, and length is related to the degree they are stretched. The arytenoids, which are attached to the vocal folds, are important in affecting their mass per unit length. The arytenoids slide, rock, and rotate, thus affecting several physiological factors of voice production. When the mass of the vocal folds is increased relative to their length, frequency of vibration decreases. Conversely, when the mass of the vocal folds decreases relative to their length, frequency of vibration increases. Pitch, the psychological perception of frequency of vibration, goes up or down depending on the mass per unit length of the vocal folds. Although pitch and frequency of vocal fold vibration have a positive relationship, it is not linear. There is not a 1:1 relationship between pitch and frequency. A unit increase in frequency does not necessarily have a corresponding unit increase in pitch, and vice versa.

Other physiological factors related to pitch control include the vocalis muscle, ligament tension, and subglottal air pressure (Psub). The vocalis muscle and ligament together primarily make up the vocal folds. When the vocal folds are stretched, thus increasing tension, frequency of vibration and the subsequent psychological perception of pitch increases. Conversely, when they are lax, frequency and pitch decrease. There is controversy about the independent contraction of the vocalis muscles. It is likely that contraction of it results in lowered frequency and pitch because the bulk of the folds is increased. However, contraction also likely increases longitudinal tension, thus contributing to increased frequency and pitch.

Subglottal pressure, Psub, the air pressure below the vocal folds, plays a role in pitch control. Subglottal air pressure is also called glottal pressure. As subglottal pressure increases, so does the frequency of vocal fold vibration and the psychological perception of pitch. This is true if all other physiological factors remain equal. Conversely, if subglottal pressure decreases, pitch decreases (see Figure 11.3).

Increase in mass/unit length of vocal folds	Decrease pitch
Decrease in mass/unit length of vocal folds	Increase pitch
Increase in vocal fold tension	Increase pitch
Decrease in vocal fold tension	Decrease pitch
Independent contraction of vocalis muscle	Effects on pitch not conclusively known
Increase in subglottal air pressure	Increase pitch
Decrease in subglottal air pressure	Decrease pitch

Figure 11.3 Physiological variables and their effects on pitch

A discussion of pitch is not complete unless falsetto and glottal fry are addressed. These are two separate modes of vocal fold vibration. Falsetto is a high-pitched voice produced by vibration of only part of the vocal folds; they are tightly adducted, and only part of them, approximately one-third, vibrate. Glottal fry, sometimes called creak voice or vocal fry, is a result of relaxed intrinsic vocal muscles, while extrinsic ones may be hypertense. Glottal fry is a low-pitched pulsating voice.

Loudness of voice varies with how intensely or forcefully the vocal folds contact each other. Subglottal air pressure also increases to produce increased loudness. Increased loudness results from the vocal folds contacting with more force. The maximum point of contact pressure is at the juncture of the middle and anterior one-third of the vocal folds.

Voice quality is related to the spectral characteristics of the speech signal. To initiate phonation, the vocal folds go from an abducted position to a partially adducted one. This is called the prephonation phase. The attack phase, when the vocal folds actually begin vibration, sets the foundation for voice quality. There are three general types of phonatory attacks. First, simultaneous attack occurs when respiratory air flow begins at approximately the same time of vocal fold vibration. Second, breathy attack involves air escaping before the vocal folds begin to vibrate, and/or a high ratio of air escape during vibration. Third, hard glottal attack, the opposite of breathy attack, involves the vocal folds contacting with more force during the initial aspects of the phonatory event and a low amount of air escape during vibration. Voice quality is related to the frequency of vocal fold vibration, the resonance of the vocal tract, and the pattern or mode of glottal attack.

Lay people describe voice quality by several terms: masculine, feminine, strong, weak, tinny, raspy, nasal, forceful, throaty, and so on. These terms are usually ill defined and useless in a scientific or clinical sense. Scientifi-

cally and clinically, there are nine established terms used for voice quality. As previously discussed, breathy is when the vocal folds do not completely close or the period of closure is very brief. Vocal/glottal fry is a pulsating low pitch. Hard glottal attack is a harsh voice with excessive force primarily on initial sounds. Harsh is a result of the vocal folds closing with excessive force. Hoarse voice is uneven closure of the vocal folds. Hoarse voice is a combination of breathy and harsh qualities. Hypernasal is too much nasality on non-nasal sounds, and hyponasal is too little nasal resonance. Two other clinically recognized voice qualities, strangled and wet strained-strangled, are a result of rigid muscles seen in certain neurological diseases such as multiple sclerosis and amyotrophic lateral sclerosis. Strangled voice quality is like the sound is being forced through tight muscles. Wet strained-strangled is a harsh quality with a liquid buildup in the oral tract (see Table 11.1).

Humans use voice quality as nonverbal communication tools. It has been estimated that as much as 90 percent of the information imparted during communication is nonverbal. Nonverbal communication involves an information exchange that goes beyond the meaning of the words spoken. For example, the clothing worn by a speaker sends information about socioeconomic status, education, and vocation. Pitch, loudness, and voice quality also tell much about a speaker's status and intentions. Although the spoken words give information, the nonverbal cues can speak volumes about how the speaker feels regarding what has been spoken. No better example of this exists than when a speaker utters "no" with a tentative voice, pitch rise at the end (signaling a question about resolve), and a contradictory head nod. Although "no" is a negative, the nonverbal cues can express opposite intentions by the speaker. When a listener is confronted with a conflict between verbal and nonverbal information, he or she will usually believe the latter. This underlying communication is often called the nonverbal agenda.

Table 11.1
Voice Quality

Term	Definition
Breathy	Vocal cords do not completely close or the period of closure is very brief
Hard glottal attack	Harsh voice with excessive force primarily on initial sounds
Harsh	Vocal cords close with excessive force
Hoarse	Uneven closure of the vocal folds (breathy and harsh)
Hypernasal	Too much nasality on non-nasal sounds
Hyponasal	Too little nasal resonance
Strangled	Voice being forced through tight muscles
Vocal/glottal fry	Pulsating low pitch
Wet strained-strangled	Harsh with liquid buildup in the oral tract

People also draw conclusions about an individual's personality based on voice quality. Some men with breathy voice qualities are considered sinister and evil, whereas women with the same voice quality are considered sexy and alluring. According to Kent (1997), women, besides having a higher pitch, tend to have a breathy voice quality. Breathy voice quality in some women has been called the bedroom voice. A harsh voice with both men and women signals aggressiveness and impatience. A voice that tremors sends cues that the speaker is emotional or tentative in his or her convictions. A high-pitched voice for a male suggests effeminate traits. A low-pitched voice on a woman can suggest masculine traits and, in some women, a sensuous allure.

Voice register is loosely defined as a series of succeeding sounds of equal quality and produced the same way. There are three general voice registers: head, neck, and mixed. Mixed is also known as middle voice register. Understanding and using voice registers are important in vocal instructions and singing, but from a speech science perspective, the concept is irrelevant. Acoustically, sounds of equal quality and produced the same way are identical sounds, regardless of the speaker's projection of speech energy.

When referring to voice, the fundamental frequency is the rate of vocal fold vibration. It is the number of times they contact each other during vibration. This frequency is the tone produced by the vocal folds before the effects of resonance. The average female has a fundamental frequency of 250 cycles-per-second (Hz) and males vibrate their vocal folds at approximately 130 cycles-per-second (Hz). Fundamental frequency of vocal fold vibration for both males and females are averages, and different phonemes have different average frequency of vibrations. Individuals have different fundamental frequencies and at different times in their lives. According to Kent (1997), from about age four to ten years, fundamental frequency is stable and typically the same for both boys and girls. At about age twelve, male fundamental frequency changes and remains about one octave below that of the female. With advanced age, male fundamental frequency typically increases, while in women it decreases.

A strong, pleasing voice is the result, in part, of the human resonance system operating effectively. In addition, because the vocal folds vibrate rapidly, many physiological factors can cause or contribute to their injury. There is evidence of an optimal pitch, a frequency of vocal fold vibration, which is particularly suitable for each individual. All structures, including body parts, have an optimal frequency of vibration, a frequency of vibration that is most natural to a structure, one that results in the maximum amplitude of vibration with the least expenditure of energy. The optimal frequency of vocal fold vibration is where they vibrate with the least amount of effort and create maximal loudness. This optimal pitch is sometimes called the natural frequency.

A person's optimal pitch is about one-quarter of his or her total pitch range, including falsetto. There are several ways of determining optimal pitch. Most involve the person demonstrating his or her total pitch range and then repeating the process and prolonging the note computed to be approximately one-quarter of the total range. Another method of learning optimal pitch is to have the person swell the loudness of several notes and decide which one is produced with the greatest loudness and clarity. Yawning and sighing can also provide information about a person's optimal pitch.

The habitual pitch is the one used most frequently by the person. It is a learned behavior. Some individuals, for a variety of reasons, habitually use a pitch that is not optimal for them. Some radio and television announcers, public speakers, and young male adolescents may use pitches that are unnatural. Radio and television announcers and public speakers often use pitches that are lower than their optimal ones. This is to give their on-air or public voices more power and authority. Young male adolescents sometimes use lower pitches than what is optimal to sound more masculine. As discussed later, in some people, the greater the difference between habitual and optimal pitch, the more likely there is a voice pathology.

11.6 Cleft Lip and Palate

Cleft lip and palate are the primary disorders of resonance and are part of a larger group of speech pathologies related to craniofacial abnormalities. These disorders result from impaired or incomplete fusion of the cranium and face and may be unilateral or bilateral. A slang term for a cleft lip is "harelip" and refers to the two vertical slits on both sides of midline in rabbits. A cleft palate is a congenial fissure, which may or may not extend through the soft palate (velum) and uvula. The incidence of cleft lip and palate is about one in 700 live births (Williams, Sandy, Thomas, Sell, and Sterne, 1999). Clefts limited only to the lip occur in fewer than 5 percent of the cases (Shprintzen, 1997). A submucous cleft palate is not visible because the intact soft tissue in the roof of the mouth covers it. A bifid uvula is a cleft of the muscle that hangs down from the back of the throat. A deviated uvula leans to one side, usually because of muscular weakness.

Craniofacial abnormalities cause several speech pathologies depending on their type and severity. Clefts of the lip and the dental process can cause articulation disorders. Hypernasality and nasal air emission, a sniffing sound, occur in cleft palate because there is a hole in the roof of the mouth and the nasal cavity cannot be effectively separated from the oral cavity. Hypernasality can also be caused by velopharyngeal incompetence where the soft palate is unable to adequately approximate the posterior pharyngeal wall. This can be a result of muscular weakness or structural limitations. In many cases of cleft palate, the eustachian tube is impaired in its ability to equalize pressure between the middle ear and the surrounding atmosphere, causing conductive hearing losses. Children with clefts are also

slower in their language development (Weiss, Gordon, and Lillywhite, 1987). Delayed language in these children is likely a result of both organic and environmental factors.

"In the hands of a competent surgeon, approximately 80–90 percent of patients who undergo primary repair of the palate (primary palatoplasty) will have adequate velopharyngeal closure. The other 10–20 percent may need to undergo secondary physical management" (Dalston, 2000, p. 273–274). Reconstructive surgeries begin at an early age, usually before the child's first birthday, and involve the creation of flaps to improve velopharyngeal closure and to close clefts. The effectiveness of the reconstructive surgeries greatly influences the child's ultimate ability to have normal speech. There is only so much therapies can do to improve articulation and resonance if the tissues are insufficient. Some children with craniofacial abnormalities are provided with prostheses. These are appliances such as bulbs, palatal lifts, and dentures that aid speech production. Together, surgeries, prostheses, and therapies are provided to these children usually through a team approach known as the cleft palate team. The cleft palate team usually consists of a reconstructive surgeon, orthodontist, pediatrician, audiologist, medical social worker, speech-language pathologist, the child's parents, and other specialists that may also be called on depending on case specific factors (see Figure 11.4).

Reconstructive surgeon
Orthodontist
Pediatrician
Audiologist
Speech-language pathologist
Medical social worker
Child's parents
Other medical, dental, and rehabilitation specialists
    as necessary

Figure 11.4 *Primary members of a cleft palate team*

11.7 Cancer of the Larynx

By far, the most serious voice disorder is cancer of the larynx. Tumors of the larynx may be malignant or benign. (Benign tumors are discussed in the section addressing noxious chemicals, vocal strain and abuse.) Malignant tumors are confirmed with a biopsy which is the taking of tissue and examining it for diagnostic purposes. If malignant laryngeal tumors are not diagnosed and treated, they may metastasize (spread) to other parts of the body. Traditionally, the primary treatment for laryngeal cancer was a laryngectomy, the surgical removal of the larynx. A complete laryngectomy is the removal of the entire larynx. Partial laryngectomy is the removal of a section of the larynx, such as a vocal fold. A radical laryngectomy is the surgical removal of the larynx and adjacent glands, muscles, and other tissue. A person who has undergone a laryngectomy is called a laryngectomee. Laryngectomees breathe through a hole in the neck called a stoma. Because of the surgery, the patient no longer breathes through his or her mouth and nose. There is a permanent opening from the respiratory tract to the atmosphere through the neck. Obviously, the laryngectomee loses the ability to speak, smell, blow his or her nose, lift heavy weights, and filter and warm the outside air. Swimming and bathing require special accommodations. Recent advances in the medical management of laryngeal cancer, especially chemotherapy, have reduced the need for laryngectomies. However, it is sometimes necessary, and once the larynx is removed, the patient must be provided with alternative methods of communication or alaryngeal speech. There are three alaryngeal speech options: surgery, electronic devices, and esophageal speech.

Surgery involves creating a pseudo glottis, an artificially created pair of vocal folds. The patient still uses the lungs to provide air support for vibration. There are several variations of surgery to produce the pseudo glottis and at least one documented case of a laryngeal transplant. However, some patients prefer not to undergo surgery, and in others there are medical contraindications. Some pneumatic devices work by directing the air through the speech mechanism by plugging the stoma.

An electrolarynx is a hand-held vibrating device that projects the sound through the neck and head of the patient. It is composed of a vibrating diaphragm that when placed on the neck radiates the energy upward through the speech tract while the patient mouths words. The electrolarynx becomes a substitute sound source, and energy is radiated upward through the neck and head resonators. There are several models, including those with more than one frequency of vibration and those that use a vibrating tube placed in the side of the patient's mouth. The advantage of an electrolarynx is that most patients can easily use it. The disadvantages are that speech is produced with a mechanical buzz and one hand must be used to hold it against the neck.

Esophageal speech is also known as belch talking. Actually, "belch" is not an accurate description of this type of speech. The air for speech does not come from the stomach; it is pistoned partially down the esophagus and allowed to be released gradually. During the release, the patient shapes the sound into speech. The advantages of esophageal speech are that the patient, with therapy and practice, can produce near-normal speech and does not need to hold a vi-

brating device to the neck. The disadvantages are that not all patients can learn to produce esophageal speech and for some there are physiological limitations to the amount of air they can inject into the esophagus.

Some laryngectomees are unwilling or unable to use the above methods of alaryngeal speech. They can still communicate with writing, gesturing, and by mouthing words. Other patients simply refrain from communication. However, to show the value patients place on communication, MacNeil, et al. (1981), in a study addressing laryngeal cancer and treatment options, found that the majority of subjects would be willing to trade life expectancy in order to retain the ability to speak. Most patients are motivated for alaryngeal speech of some type.

11.8 Vocal Fold Paralysis

Strokes, diseases, and injuries can cause vocal fold paralysis and weakness (paresis) and can be unilateral or bilateral. If the diseases and injuries affect the ability of one vocal fold to open, the voice pathology is called unilateral abductor paralysis or paresis. Bilateral abductor paralysis, or paresis, is when both vocal folds are impaired in their abilities to open. Unilateral and bilateral adductor paralysis and paresis occur when one side or both vocal folds are impaired or unable to close and contact (approximate) each other.

The type of stroke-related paralysis or paresis depends on the site of the vascular disturbance. Dysarthria affecting the respiratory and phonatory systems results from damage to the motor cortex and below (Davis, 2007). Trauma to the vagus nerve (X) may cause unilateral paralysis or paresis. The trauma can be caused by a missile or projectile, surgical error, or a blunt blow. Many diseases such as cancer, multiple sclerosis, amyotrophic lateral sclerosis, and Parkinson's disease, to name a few, can result in vocal fold paralysis or paresis and affect the ability of the vocal folds to open or close. Post-polio syndrome, characterized by vocal muscle fatigue and weakness, has been a source of litigation. Minor changes in voice production may signal the early onset of several progressive diseases because normal voice is produced with fine adjustments of the respiratory and laryngeal muscles. Minor unwanted changes in pitch, loudness, and quality may signal the beginning stages of amyotrophic lateral sclerosis, Parkinson's disease, multiple sclerosis, cancer, and other diseases.

The objective of therapy for adductor paralysis or paresis is to get the nonparalyzed or stronger vocal fold to approximate the impaired vocal fold by crossing midline, thus compensating for the functional impairment. Midline is the center part of the glottal opening. This approximation is done by combining phonation with strenuous activities such as isometric exercises, lifting heavy objects, and pushups. There are medications for the chemical deficiencies at the myoneural junction. The myoneural junction is the site where the nerve and muscle come together. Solutions can also be injected into the paralyzed vocal fold to make it thicker, thus improving the ability of the non-paralyzed fold to approximate it. Physicians avoid this treatment if the patient has compromised respiratory function.

11.9 Disorders Related to Vocal Strain and Abuse

Disorders related to vocal strain and abuse include nodules, polyps, and contact ulcers. They may occur on one or both vocal folds. They are common in people who do a lot of talking or singing and who otherwise strain their vocal folds. Teachers and cheerleaders are particularly vulnerable to them. More than one-third of the teachers with voice disorders report that the voice problems interfered with their ability to teach effectively (Sapir, Keidar, and Mathers-Schmidt, 1993). Famous people can be involved in voice disorder litigation. In 1999, actress and singer Julie Andrews filed a malpractice suit against a hospital and two physicians. She alleged that they ruined her ability to sing due to unnecessary surgery to remove noncancerous tumors on her vocal folds. According to the suit, she was not informed of the risk of permanent irreversible loss of voice quality. In November 2000, Julie Andrews was awarded $20 million in damages for the loss of her singing voice (See Tanner, 2003).

There are two types of vocal polyps, i.e., fluid-filled blisters occurring on the vocal folds: sessile and pedunculated. A sessile polyp is broad based and occurs along a large segment of the vocal fold. A pedunculated polyp is one hanging down from a stem. These types of blisters can be caused by one-time abuse such as a shouting match, screaming, cheering a sports team to victory, or because of a loud argument. Asthma and allergies may also be causative factors in the development of vocal polyps (Hall, Oyer, and Haas, 2001).

Contact ulcers are abrasions of the vocal folds. Although they can be caused by excessive talking, screaming, shouting, and other types of vocal abuse, they are also linked to exposure to noxious chemicals. Excessive smoking and alcohol abuse, as well as exposure to industrial chemicals, have been linked to vocal ulcers. Some contact ulcers are granulated and have a rough ridge. Contact ulcers

are more common in men. Prolonged stress and gastric reflux may also be causal agents.

Vocal nodules occur more often in women, particularly those who do much talking. They have been called teachers', screamers', singers', and preachers' nodes. Vocal nodules are about the size of a peppercorn. Physicians label some vocal nodules and polyps precancerous. Because these growths can be malignant, it is standard practice for speech-language pathologists to refer these patients to a physician, usually a laryngologist. Therapy is not conducted until a physician has ruled out malignancy.

Some people are more likely to develop and have recurrence of vocal nodules, polyps, and contact ulcers, although there are no clear genetic predisposing factors. Research is conclusive that even when surgery removes them, they recur because the underlying cause has not been eliminated. These voice disorders are symptoms of vocal strain and abuse and other factors. In addition, research and clinical experiences have shown that when the underlying causes are eliminated, in some cases, the vocal nodules, polyps, and contact ulcers disappear without the benefit of surgery.

There are several predisposing, precipitating, and perpetuating factors in vocal nodules, polyps, and contact ulcers. As discussed above, screaming, shouting, excessive smoking and drinking, hard glottal attacks, improper singing, frequent throat clearing, and exposure to noxious chemicals are associated with the development of vocal nodules, polyps, and contact ulcers. Some patients also overreact to temporary voice imperfection. They hear changes in their voice and feel an irritation in the throat. To eliminate them, they overcompensate by forcing voice. They have a low tolerance of temporary voice imperfections, and they overreact. Their reactions to impaired vocal functioning involve speaking with excessive muscular force. This results in increased laryngeal tension and irritation eventually increasing the severity of the voice pathology. A cycle of impaired voice and overcompensation is the result (Tanner, 1990).

Excessive tension of the respiratory muscles and the extrinsic and intrinsic laryngeal muscles account for the hard and abusive contact of the vocal folds. Many patients can benefit from systematic muscle relaxation exercises to reduce the muscle tension and to create conditions where the vocal folds vibrate with less abusive force. These exercises include autohypnosis, progressive muscle relaxation, and meditation and can be provided in an audio recording format (Tanner, 1990).

Having a habitual pitch that is significantly above or below a person's optimal one can also result in vocal pathologies. Because the vocal folds vibrate rapidly, chronically speaking in a frequency that is unnatural can cause harmful contact of the vocal folds. The vocal folds may contact with too much force and vibrate in a disharmonious manner. Over time, the sensitive tissue of the vocal folds become damaged.

Patients who appear to have a significant gap between their optimal and habitual pitch are shown the correct pitch and taught to use it. Determining optimal pitch in a patient with a growth on the vocal folds is difficult because the growth increases the mass per unit length. It is clinically inappropriate to use standard tests of optimal pitch for a patient who has an existing pathology. Only after surgery or therapies reduce or eliminate their size can optimal pitch be tested with any degree of accuracy. The patient's premorbid voice obtained from an answering machine or other taped sample can provide a basis for determining optimal versus habitual pitch and for a baseline during other litigation involving changes in the voice. The treatment of disorders related to vocal strain and abuse includes addressing specific speech behaviors. For example, vocally abusive patterns of behavior such as talking too long, too loud, and with too many hard glottal attacks are identified and patients counseled to reduce or eliminate them. Sometimes patients are placed on voice rest where they do not talk for several weeks, giving the vocal pathology time to heal itself. Complete voice rest is often unsuccessful because patients cannot maintain it. People who develop vocal nodules, polyps, and contact ulcers are, by nature, talkative and voice rest is unnatural and foreign to them. In addition, their jobs and professions often preclude voice rest. Some patients resort to whispering as a misguided attempt to reduce the amount of vocal damage. For many patients, whispering is more abusive than voiced speech because of the strain associated with it. The role of smoking and excessive job-related talking has been a legal point of contention. See *Fincannon v Eastern Airlines*, 611 So 2d 28 (Fla App 1 Dist 1992).

11.10 Psychogenic Voice Disorders

Psychogenic dysphonia is impaired voice of psychological origin and not due to physical or organic causes. It can include chronic or temporary problems with maintaining loudness, quality changes, pitch breaks, and occasional whispering. Psychogenic aphonia is the complete loss of voice of psychological origin where the patient consistently whispers during speech. Psychogenic voice disorders are usually the result of a conversion reaction where there is a loss of voluntary control over normal striated muscle move-

ments or over the senses, resulting from environmental stress or interpersonal conflict (Aronson, 1990). A psychological conflict or trauma is transformed into a physical disorder. There is an inner conflict, usually the need to express a thought, feeling, or attitude, and fear or anxiety in doing so. The trauma can be related to a violent act or event witnessed by the patient. Psychogenic voice disorders are more common in females and are sometimes called hysterical aphonia/dysphonia.

Most authorities on psychogenic voice disorders observe that the loss of voice symbolizes the nature of the emotional upheaval. Psychiatrists note that there is a symptom choice, where the patient chooses the manifestation of the psychological conflict or trauma. When communication is impaired, the disorder may represent a lack of meaningful relationships or an empty and unsatisfying one. It can also symbolize a dangerous relationship. The symbolic expression may relieve the patient from the distress, and some patients present with "la belle indifference." They have little if any concern for their lost or impaired voice and actually appear relieved or even pleased at having lost it.

Testing whether the voice disorder is caused by psychogenic factors is relatively simple with cooperative patients. Although patients with psychogenic voice disorders whisper during speech, when they laugh or hum, true voicing occurs. When a patient can voice during nonspeech activities and whisper during speech, the pathology is likely nonorganic in nature. Procedures for obtaining voiced speech are also relatively straightforward with cooperative patients. For example, they can regain their voices by transitioning from singing and humming to voiced speech.

Psychogenic voice disorders are symptoms of underlying psychological traumas and conflicts. Consequently, psychiatric or psychological referrals are required to address their underlying causes. Establishing normal voice without addressing the psychological factors is contraindicated. Psychogenic voice disorders are "flares sent into the air" by the patient to seek psychological treatment. It would be negligent to avoid addressing the underlying causes of the psychogenic voice disorder.

11.11 Voice Disorders Litigation and Malingering

Some patients willfully and deliberately feign or exaggerate a voice disorder for exemption, attention, sympathy, academic, and/or employment rewards or for financial gain. They pretend to have aphonia or dysphonia for a self-serving end, and the distinction between conscious and subconscious is not always easily made. (See the above section on psychogenic voice disorders.) At issue is whether the patient willfully and deliberately feigns or exaggerates a voice disorder or if the attempts at personal gain are subconscious. If the loss or impaired voice is from interpersonal conflicts or environmental stress, the patient technically is not malingering; he or she is suffering from a conversion reaction. But in voice disorders, this distinction is not always clear and it is certainly difficult to prove.

It can be said that most voice disorders related to strain and abuse have at their core a psychological component. A person who is under environmental stress and/or suffering from interpersonal conflicts resulting in voice pathologies such as nodules and polyps has a maladaptive coping style and/or immature psychological defenses. He or she is feeling either the effects of excessive stress, pushing too hard with regard to vocation, or ill equipped to cope with normal daily stressors. Consequently, the development of a voice disorder related to vocal strain and abuse is at least partially psychological in origin and it can be argued is also an attempt at personal gain, i.e., to repair or eliminate the stressors and conflicts. They may be used as attention-getting devices. These motives may be conscious, partially conscious, or completely subconscious.

Consistency of symptom presentation is important when investigating malingering in voice disorders. Patients should have consistent symptoms. Although patients may have periods of normal voice, loss or impaired phonation should be related to specific stimuli. For example, a successful accountant would lose his voice during tax season and particularly when using the telephone. His loss of voice was related to the stresses associated with tax accounting and the temporal urgencies associated with tax deadlines. Another patient experienced dysphonia only when talking to her husband, and the problem disappeared when they divorced. Many patients lose their voice only in the evenings.

As discussed above, patients who can voice normally while humming, singing, and laughing, only to be aphonic during speech, likely have a nonorganic pathology. When this discrepancy occurs, it signals a psychological etiology or malingering. The presence of an indifferent attitude about lost or impaired voice is also an indicator of a psychological etiology. At issue are motives and whether the patient is conscious of them. A case-by-case examination of conscious versus subconscious motives is necessary. Figure 11.5 lists factors to consider when investigating malingering.

11.12 Voice Disorders Malpractice Litigation and Clinician Proficiency

The American Speech-Language-Hearing Association requires that certified speech-language pathologists be proficient in diagnosis and treatment of voice disorders. This in-

cludes instrumental, structural, and functional assessment of laryngeal muscles and structures. Many of the guidelines and requirements for dysphagia management apply to voice disorders, including assessment of airway protection and administration and interpretation of instrumental tests (see Chapter 8). Clinicians should be proficient in laryngeal video stroboscopy (LVS).

Consistency of symptoms
Impaired phonation related to specific stimuli
"La belle indifference"
Humming, singing, and laughing with phonation
Associated with psychological trauma or conflict
Symbolic of relationship deficiencies or distress

Figure 11.5 *Factors to consider when investigating malingering in voice disorders*

An important clinical proficiency is the proper referral for voice-disordered patients. Most patients who come to speech and hearing clinics, private practitioners, schools, and hospital speech and hearing departments complaining of voice changes have benign growths or ulcerations of the vocal folds. They have voice changes due to prenodules, nodules, polyps, edema, ulceration, or strained vocal folds. The most common term used by lay persons and professionals for voice quality changes is laryngitis. Laryngitis means swelling of the mucous membrane of the larynx and it is a clinically nondescript term. However, in some the cases, the changes in voice are due to malignant, not benign, alterations of the vocal folds. Consequently, standards of practice require that a referral be made to a physician for evaluation before initiating therapy. Most insurance companies and HMOs require that the initial referral be made to the patient's primary care physician and that he or she refer the patient to a specialist such as an otolaryngologist or laryngologist. Only after a physician has ruled out malignancy can the speech-language pathologist initiate treatment. This standard of practice is not only for malignancies; medical evaluation can also detect webbing, wart-like growths, and disease processes not related to vocal strain and abuse that can compromise breathing.

The treatment of voice disorders requires regular and effective communication between the speech-language pathologist and the physician. "Many adults and some children are referred to the speech pathologist by their physician for voice disorders resulting from medical difficulties or surgical intervention" (Haynes and Pindzola, 2004, p. 275). Voice therapies are done in conjunction with surgeries and medications provided by medical specialists. To a significant extent, the results of therapy for voice and resonance disorders are dependent on surgeries and medications, thus requiring regular and effective professional communication.

11.13 Voice Disorders, Vocational Rehabilitation, Antidiscrimination, and Insurance-Social Welfare Determination and Compensation Issues

Vocational rehabilitation, antidiscrimination, and insurance-social welfare determination and compensation can be issues in all significant voice disorders, but they are particularly relevant to laryngectomy, vocal fold paralysis, and chronic loss or impaired voice due to vocal strain and abuse. Because of the surgical removal of the larynx or the impaired ability to produce voiced speech due to paralysis or chronic vocal strain and abuse, some patients may sue for compensation and vocational rehabilitation.

Patients with a laryngectomy are eligible for vocational rehabilitation to train for jobs that can accommodate the alaryngeal speech and other complications due to the loss of the larynx. Because the larynx is important in stabilizing the body for strenuous activities, most laryngectomy patients can no longer engage in heavy physical labor. In addition, those who use an electrolarynx must have one hand free to communicate verbally. Because of the stoma, an open hole from the respiratory tract to the atmosphere, jobs in extreme cold or that are dusty are contraindicated. Although bibs are available to cover the stoma (the opening in the neck), air is no longer filtered and warmed by the nose, mouth, and upper airway. In addition, the loudness of speech is compromised, and most patients must be retrained to work in jobs where there is little ambient noise or where sound amplification is available. Compensation may address the effects of the laryngectomy on quality of life, changes in vocation, and loss of self issues.

Patients with bilateral adductor paralysis have a poor prognosis for obtaining functional phonation. Consequently, vocational rehabilitation involves obtaining jobs where voiced speech is not required. With therapy, patients with unilateral adductor paralysis can usually obtain voiced speech, albeit with reduced volume, narrowed pitch, and a breathy quality. Compensation may address the quality and extent of phonation available after treatment and the effect the voice disorder has on interpersonal relationships and vocation. Loss of self issues discussed in Chapter 9 may also be relevant.

Patients who have chronic or recurrent vocal nodules, polyps, and contact ulcers and who do not respond to thera-

pies are also candidates for vocational rehabilitation. Many of these patients are in vocations requiring excessive verbal communication, such as sales and teaching. Vocations that involve little or no verbal speech, such as word processing and bookkeeping, are alternatives to those occupations. Compensation issues are related to reductions in salary and advancement and the costs of retraining.

11.14 Issues in Orofacial Anomalies Litigation

Two factors are relevant to cleft lip and palate and other orofacial anomalies litigation. First, at issue may be the adequacy of reconstructive surgeries and therapies in obtaining normal and unobtrusive speech production. Therapies to obtain normal speech production are dependent on the adequacy of the reconstructive surgeries. There are no therapies available to eliminate hypernasality, nasal emission, or distorted articulation in patients who have inadequate speech structures, tissue, and muscles. The improvement in speech production is dependent on surgeons creating enough tissue, movement, structural integrity, and dentition for velopharyngeal closure and production of dental and other speech sounds. There are therapies and prostheses that can reduce the amount of hypernasality in patients with insufficient velopharyngeal closure but not eliminate it. For example, if the fundamental frequency is altered, it can reduce, but not eliminate, the perception of hypernasality. If the patient is taught to produce speech sounds with a more opened oral cavity, the perception of nasal emission is reduced. Compensatory place of articulation can be taught to adapt to jumbled or missing teeth. When reconstructive surgeries are successful in creating adequate speech structure and function, it is reasonable to expect normal or nearly normal speech production because of competent therapies.

The second factor related to cleft lip and palate and other orofacial anomalies involves eligibility for special education programs and medical insurance coverage. Eligibility for special education is addressed in Chapter 12. The costly medical treatments associated with cleft lip and palate and other orofacial anomalies and syndromes are covered by most insurance companies or county, state, and federal social welfare programs. Most children with cleft lip and palate, other orofacial anomalies, birth defects, and syndromes are seen through children's hospitals, child rehabilitation facilities, or crippled children programs, and costs for services are routinely covered by them. There are also several philanthropic organizations that cover direct expenses for treatment and research.

11.15 Case Study Involving a Voice Disorder Resulting from Burn Injuries

A male college student experienced burns to his upper airways and lungs in a kiln accident. He was working unsupervised during the weekend on a course project at a university kiln. He dumped a bucket of sawdust on a ceramic pot to affect its temperature and cooling rate. Apparently, the sawdust was not treated with a chemical agent to prevent it from igniting, and the result was a flash fire. He sued the university for the burn injuries he sustained.

The student sustained severe damage to his lungs. During the flash fire, as a reflexive reaction, he inspired the hot air. Consequently, according to medical reports, he sustained scarring that diminished his respiratory function. He required supplemental oxygen and a portable oxygen tank. He alleged that the flash fire also damaged his ability to produce voice.

The student received outpatient voice therapy for several months. Initially he was aphonic, but gradually some voice returned. At the conclusion of the outpatient therapy the student presented with reduced volume, a breathy voice quality, restricted pitch range, and difficulty initiating phonation. His voice also fatigued toward the end of the day, rendering him aphonic.

During the trial, a point of contention was whether the student was malingering with regard to impaired voice. One of the issues was whether the lung damage and diminished respiratory flow and pressure could cause the type of voice disorder presented by the patient. In this case, the voice disorder was probably not related to the reduced air pressure and flow from the damaged lungs. Although evidence was provided that there were reduced pressure and flow, the amount of the reduction was not sufficient to impair the myoelastic and aerodynamic forces required for vocal fold vibration.

The student's voice disorder was probably caused by burn damage and scarring occurring to sensitive tissue of the larynx. The burn damage probably impaired the attack phase of phonation, causing the vocal folds to be compromised in their ability to initiate phonation. The breathy voice quality probably resulted from the tissue changes affecting the borders of the vocal folds and their vibratory mode. Pitch restriction and volume reductions also probably resulted from the burn damage to the vocal process.

The student presented with consistent symptoms. His problems with pitch and loudness, initiating of phonation, and voice quality were typical and consistent of the types of voice problems seen in burn damage. There were no indications that he was exaggerating the symptoms or feigning nonexistent ones. The fact that he benefitted from outpatient voice therapy and was able to improve his voice further supported the organic nature of his pathology.

11.16 Chapter Summary

A person's unique voice is a combination of the vibratory sound coming from the larynx and resonance occurring in the neck and head. Respiration is the driving force for speech sounds and provides the air pressure and flow for setting the vocal folds into vibration. Pitch, loudness, and voice quality are affected by minor movements of the muscles and structures of the larynx. Nasality is affected by the soft palate approximating the posterior pharyngeal wall. Litigation may involve several voice and resonance disorders, including cleft lip and palate, vocal fold paralysis, cancer of the larynx, voice disorders of psychological origin, and those related to vocal strain and abuse.

Suggested Readings and Resources

Aronson, A. (1990). *Clinical Voice Disorders: An Interdisciplinary Approach* (3rd ed.) New York: Thieme. This book has a comprehensive review of voice disorders.

Kent, R. D. (1997). *The Speech Sciences*. San Diego: Singular. This book provides a basic review of voice science and anatomical illustrations of the larynx.

Tanner, D. (2006). *An Advanced Course in Communication Sciences and Disorders*. San Diego: Plural Publishing. Chapters 7 and 8 address the anatomy, physiology, and acoustics of voice production.

References

Aronson, A. (1990). *Clinical voice disorders: An interdisciplinary approach* (3rd ed). New York: Thieme.

Dalston, R.M. (2000). Cleft lip and palate. In R. Gillam, T. Marquardt, and F. Martin (Eds) *Communication sciences and disorders*. San Diego: Singular.

Davis, G. A. (2007). *Aphasiology: Disorders and clinical practice* (2nd ed.). Boston: Allyn & Bacon.

Hall, B.J., Oyer, H.J., and Haas, W.H. (2001). *Speech, language, and hearing disorders: A guide for the teacher.* Boston: Allyn & Bacon.

Haynes, W.O. and Pindzola, R. (2004). *Diagnosis and evaluation in speech pathology.* Boston: Allyn & Bacon.

Kent, R. D. (1997). *The speech sciences.* San Diego: Singular.

MacNeil, B., Weischselbaum, R., and Pauker, S. (1981). Tradeoffs between quality and quality of life in laryngeal cancer. *New England Journal of Medicine,* 305: 983-987.

Oates, J. (2004). The Evidence Base for the Management of Individuals with Voice Disorders. In *Evidence based practice in speech pathology*, S. Reilly, J. Douglas, and J. Oates (Eds). London: Whurr Publishers.

Sapir, S., Keidar, A., and Mathers-Schmidt, B. (1993). Vocal attrition in teachers: Survey findings. *European Journal of Disorders of Communication, 27*: 129-135.

Shprintzen, R.J. (1997). *Genetics, syndromes, and communication disorders.* San Diego: Singular.

Tanner, D. (2003). *Exploring communication disorders: A 21st century introduction through literature and media.* Boston: Allyn & Bacon.

Tanner, D. (1990). *Tanner muscular relaxation program for voice disorders.* Oceanside, CA: Academic Communication Associates.

Weiss, C.E., Gordon, M.E., and Lillywhite, H.S. (1987). *Clinical management of articulatory and phonologic disorders* (2nd ed.). Baltimore: Williams & Wilkins.

Williams, A.C., Sandy, J.R., Thomas, S., Sell, D., and Sterne, J.A.C. (1999, November). Influence of surgeon's experience on speech outcome in cleft lip and palate. *Lancet, 354*: 1697-1698.

Chapter 12

Medical-Legal and Forensic Aspects of Childhood Communication Disorders

12.1 Chapter Preview

In this chapter, there is a review of childhood language, articulation, and fluency disorders. Language and articulation disorders are discussed including those associated with mental impairment-mental retardation, isolation from others during the speech and language development period, improper or impaired learning, autism, fetal alcohol and other syndromes. Stuttering and cluttering are also reviewed. The Individuals with Disabilities Education Act (IDEA) is examined including parent consent and Individual Education Plans (IEPs). Legal issues in childhood communication disorders are discussed including misdiagnoses, disputes, due process, and mediation.

12.2 The Primary Childhood Communication Disorders

The National Institute of Neurological and Communicative Disorders and Stroke (1988) reports that childhood speech and language disorders affect about 10 percent to 15 percent of school-aged children. This percentage range is the accepted prevalence rate for childhood communication disorders in the United States. Language, articulation, and fluency disorders are the principal childhood communication disorders. Although there are several other childhood communication disorders, the ones discussed in this chapter are commonly seen in schools and, as such, are often at issue in determining eligibility for special education. Language, articulation, and fluency disorders may also be factors when litigating medical malpractice cases. Less common childhood communication disorders are discussed in appropriate chapters of this book. (See the index for references to specific childhood communication disorders not addressed herein.)

Language, articulation, and fluency disorders involve loss or disruptions of several fundamental aspects of the ability to communicate. Language is the most complex component of communication. It is the multimodality ability to encode, decode, and manipulate symbols for the purposes of verbal thought and/or communication. It is a rule-governed, socially shared code for representing ideas with symbols. Articulation is shaping compressed air from the lungs into individual speech sounds. It is the act of moving the vocal tract structures so that speech sounds are produced. Fluency is the smooth and effortless flow of connected speech and stuttering is the primary fluency disrupting disorder. When children are impaired in these aspects of communication, they are usually seen by several professionals, and school districts are responsible for the costs of these special education services.

The Individuals with Disabilities Education Act (Public Law 101-476) is a continuation and refinement of Public Law 94-142 enacted in 1975. Public Law 94-142 was the first national legislation guaranteeing students with disabilities the right to free and appropriate public education. It and several other laws enacted in the past five decades specify the nature and type of services that can be provided to disabled individuals, including those with language, articulation, and fluency disorders.

During trials and depositions, lawyers and judges may be at a loss for a politically correct label for individuals with reduced intelligence. Unfortunately, there is no consensus for a word or words to refer to people with mental deficiency. "Retarded," "mentally disabled," "mentally deficient," "challenged," "differently abled," "mentally handicapped," and "alternately abled" are used in different contexts for individuals with reduced intelligence. To show the confusion and emotion about this issue, during a book acquisition and development review process, Tanner (2003) notes that reviewers complained, often zealously, about labels for people with low intelligence. The reviewers commented that there are negative connotations associated with them. In this book, mentally impaired-mentally retarded is used as to refer to people with low intelligence. Mentally retarded is commonly used by the public, and the nature and symptoms of the disorder referred to by the label are generally recognized and understood. Mentally impaired is a clinically descriptive label to refer to a person with abnormal mentation. To avoid offending and distracting jurors and others, it may be advantageous to address the issue of labels and connotations initially during litigation of communication disorders related to mental impairment-mental retardation.

12.3 Childhood Language Delay and Disorders

The reasons children are disordered or delayed in their acquisition of language range from environmental depravation to profound mental impairment-mental retardation. Language disorders in children can be a part of a specific learning disability and limited to minor reading, writing, or auditory processing abilities, or they can be all-pervasive and render the child mute. Before addressing the types of language disorders seen in children, it is necessary to define the term "language." The definition of a particular communication disorder can be central to litigation, and there are five necessary aspects to any language definition.

First, language is a socially shared code for representing ideas, events, things, and feelings, and the speakers of it—a language community—have agreed to the system of communication. Second, language is symbolic, where the word represents some aspect of reality. The symbol, and that to which it refers, is called the symbol-referent relationship. Third, language symbols are arbitrary, with no set rules dictating the creation of words and what they mean. Fourth, language is rule governed regarding combining and structuring the symbols. Finally, there are several modalities of language, i.e., avenues of expression and reception. The expressive language modalities are speech, writing, and gestures. On the receiving end, there are reading and comprehension of speech and expressive gestures. Of course, there are other forms of communication that meet some of the aspects of a language. Painting, musical compositions, and mathematics are also forms of language.

During depositions and trials, the concept of a child's linguistic competence and performance may emerge. Linguistic competence is the knowledge of the rules of language. A child with linguistic competence understands the rules of his or her language. Grammar is an all-encompassing term for the rules of the form and usage of a language. Syntax refers to the rules for arranging language, especially word order. Phonology is the way sounds are combined into words. Linguistic performance is how the child uses linguistic competence. It is his or her ability to use language effectively and efficiently to meet needs, interact with the environment, and influence events. Pragmatics refers to the set of sociolinguistic rules which include the speech act but also govern the discourse structures in which speech acts are embedded (Norris, 1998). Pragmatics deals with the communicative context and the environment in which language occurs. The pragmatics of language is the way language communicates the needs, desires, feelings, and ideas of the communicator. In this book, social-communication and pragmatics are used interchangeably.

12.4 Language Development

The language development period is a remarkable time of cognitive, physical, and neurological growth. By the time a child is six or seven years old, he or she has mastered most of the structure and form of language. Vocabulary continues to develop through adulthood, but by the time a child enters school, he or she will have mastered most aspects of language. With language development there are common sequential stages most normal children go through and a profile for diagnostic and therapeutic purposes can be created (Tanner, Lamb, and Secord, 1997; Tanner and Lamb, 1984). These stages are well documented and can be classified into cognitive, linguistic, and social-communication milestones.

In this chapter, the cognitive milestones are the thought processes that underlie language. A child acquires language based on these cognitive prerequisites. The cognitive prerequisites involve the child's gradual understanding of how things relate to each other, the use of symbols, and refinements in problem solving. Some of these milestones include finding hidden toys, knowing how to wind a toy to make it run, or realizing that by pulling a string a doll will talk. The ability to understand cause and effect, categorize, place things in rank order, engage in symbolic play, and abstract involves maturation in the cognitive prerequisites of language development. Only when the cognitive prerequisites are mastered can children acquire higher linguistic and social-communication functions.

Linguistic development is the acquisition of the structure and form of language. It involves the child learning to combine sounds into words and the creation, organization, and understanding of sentences. As a general rule, at about one year of age, most children produce one-word utterances. At two years of age, most normal children can put two words together, and at three they produce three or more words in meaningful, grammatically correct sentences. By twenty to thirty months of age the preschooler has a vocabulary of about 100 words and can comprehend most adults (Van Riper and Erickson, 1996). The child gradually learns to use tenses and contractions correctly. Receptive, he or she develops the ability to follow complex commands. By the time the child is six or seven he or she uses and understands adult linguistic structures.

Social-communication (pragmatic language processes) is learning and using the functional processes that underlie language. During this aspect of language acquisition, the child learns to use words to express needs, desires, ideas, and feelings. Acquisition in this dimension is observed in how the child plays with others and interacts with his or her parents. He or she ultimately learns to use language to engage in cooperative and symbolic play. See Appendix C for a comprehensive list, description, and examples of cognitive, linguistic, and social-communication milestones seen in preschool children and approximate acquisition ages (Tanner, Lamb, and Secord, 1997).

From preschool to school-aged children, the focus changes from semantics and pragmatics to written language, and the acquisition rate of language learning slows (Owens, 1998). Refinement of the syntactical, grammatical, and phonological aspects of language continues through adulthood. Older adults continue to refine their use of language as they learn new rules of construction and correct or refine ones learned incorrectly. Adults also continue to learn how language communicates needs, desires, feelings, and ideas.

12.5 Mental Impairment-Mental Retardation

In Chapter 2, the language-thought controversy was discussed. Does language simply express thought, or is language itself a fundamental aspect of thinking? As previously reported, language is a fundamental aspect of intelligence in adults. In young children, language probably only expresses concrete thoughts. Traditional intelligence tests have "verbal" sections, where the person's language abilities are computed to give a verbal intelligence score. In children with language disorders, their scores on performance sections are compared with their verbal scores when determining the effects of a language disorder on overall intelligence. A child's expressive and receptive vocabulary has a strong positive correlation with verbal intelligence. In most definitions of mental impairment-mental retardation, children must have significantly reduced intelligence scores, usually defined as two standard deviations below the mean.

The American Association on Mental Retardation (2006) provides a working definition of mental retardation as a disability, originating before age eighteen, and characterized by significant limitations both in intellectual functioning and in adaptive behavior as expressed in conceptual, social, and practical adaptive skills. The severity of mental impairment-mental retardation ranges from mild to profound. Owens (1995) and Grossmand (1983) provide statistics regarding percentages and degrees of limitation caused by mental impairment-mental retardation. People who are mildly disabled account for 89 percent of the mentally impaired-mentally retarded population. Mild mental impairment-mental retardation does not necessarily preclude independent living and successful job performance. About 6 percent of mentally impaired-mentally retarded people have moderate impairments. They are usually capable of semi-independence at work and in residence. Those with severe mental impairment-mental retardation are capable of learning some self-care skills and are not totally dependent on others. They account for about 3.5 percent of the mentally impaired-mentally retardation population. Profoundly mentally impaired-mentally retarded people are capable of learning some basic living skills but require continual care and supervision. They often have multiple disabilities and represent 1.5 percent of the mentally impaired-mentally retarded population.

Borderline mental impairment-mental retardation is sometimes used to describe people with mild impairments. Borderline refers to the I.Q. test score being close to the range of normal. Educable mental impairment-mental retardation refers to the child's ability to benefit from special and other education programs. Children with educable mental impairment-mental retardation presumably can learn aspects of language and academics. Trainable mental impairment-mental retardation refers to the child being able to be behaviorally modified and trained in basic self-help skills. People with this degree of mental impairment-mental retardation presumably cannot be taught higher level language or academics. Custodial mental impairment-mental retardation refers to people requiring continued care and support and who are largely unable to be educated or trained. Mental impairment-mental retardation, and reduced language, can be at issue in whether a person can waive his or her Miranda rights. See *People v Orlando LL, 188 AD2d 685, 591 NYS2d 685 (AD 3 Dept 1992).*

12.6 Language Testing

There are many tests of language acquisition and performance, and they can provide general and specific information about a child's intelligence and functional language abilities. Some tests provide a sequence of language acquisition milestones where ages and expected language behaviors are listed. There are tests of expressive and receptive vocabulary development. In a language sample, the mean length of utterances is computed in words and morphemes. (A morpheme is the smallest meaningful unit of language.) There are tests for phonological, grammar, syntax, and social-communication development. Tests of motor development are used to relate gross and fine motor development to language acquisition. Tests also address a variety of specific processing and psycholinguistic skills, such as auditory memory, attention, short-term memory, etc.

Teachers are valuable in determining whether children are delayed in their speech and language abilities. Tanner, Goedde, and Broom (1979) found that properly trained Head Start teachers can identify children with fluency, voice, articulation, and language disorders. Some authorities believe that teachers are more accurate in detecting language delay and disorders, particularly mild ones, than are standardized tests. This is because teachers have frequent contact with children, in a variety of academic contexts and social environments. Figure 12.1 lists questions for teachers that can provide information about language disorders and delay.

One of the most important determinations when examining a child's performance on psychometric tests is his or her mental age. Mental age, expressed in years and months, is the child's assumed maturation or development age of some language parameter or general measure of intelligence. It is compared to chronological age to decide relative developmental delay. Chronological age is the period elapsed since the child was born. The child's chronological age is computed by subtracting his or her birth date from when the test was administered. If the child's mental age is substantially lower than his or her chronological age on a given measure of language acquisition and functioning, then he or she is diagnosed as language delayed. There are other factors to be considered in diagnosing language delay and disorders in children, including educational, psychological, and social functioning. However, discrepancies between mental and chronological ages are important factors in the diagnosis of language delay and disorder. Large dis-

In your professional opinion, do you believe that this child has a delay in speech and language development?

Is this child able to understand questions as well as other children in the classroom?

Does this child follow instructions as well as other children in the classroom?

Do you believe that this child's understanding of vocabulary is adequate for his or her age?

Is this child able to remember information presented in classroom instruction as well as most other children in the class?

Is this child able to understand new information as well as most other pupils in the class?

How well does this child get along with other children?

Does this child cooperate with the other children in games and other activities?

Does this child have difficulty asking for help when it is needed?

Does this child have "word-finding" problems? Does the child have frequent problems selecting the correct word to be spoken?

Does this child "wander" from topic to topic when talking?

Are sentences spoken by the child of the appropriate length and complexity for his or her age?

Is the child's use of grammar similar to that of other children in his or her age group?

During reading and writing, how well does this child perform compared to the other children in his or her age group?

Figure 12.1 Questions for teachers when assessing language delay and disorders (Source: Tanner, Lamb and Secord, 1997, pp. 52–56)

crepancies between mental and chronological ages are more significant for younger children. For example, a one-year delay is more significant for a young child than an older one. A three-year-old child with a mental age delay of one year is delayed by 33 percent of his or her maturation. However, if the child is ten years old, then the delay is 10 percent.

When assessing a particular aspect of language acquisition, most tests provide a mean and standard deviation. The mean score of a test is calculated by adding a set of values and dividing the sum by the number of them. It is the average of a set of values and is one measure of central tendency. Two other measures of central tendency are mode and median. The mode is the most frequently occurring value, and the median is the middle value in a set of measurements. Standard deviation is a statistical measure showing the degree of deviation from the central tendency. It is a measure of dispersion: the square root of the variance. A standard deviation is a statistical measure that expresses how far a score deviates from the mean.

The measure of central tendency, usually the mean, and the standard deviation are used to determine normalcy on a particular language assessment. A ratio where a person's mental age is divided by his or her chronological age is called intelligence quotient or I.Q. The average score is 100. On childhood intelligence tests, children whose scores are higher or lower than the mean, as measured in standard deviations, are grouped as advanced or reduced in intelligence scores. About two-thirds of the population have intelligence scores that lay one standard deviation above and below the average. This is often called the range of normal. A consideration in determining whether a person is mentally impaired-mentally retarded is whether his or her intelligence quotient is significantly below average. As reported previously, this usually means that the person's I.Q. falls two standard deviations below the mean on a valid and reliable intelligence test. In addition, to be classified as mentally impaired-mentally retarded, the reduction in intelligence should occur during the developmental period, which is considered below the age of eighteen. Besides having a sub-average score on a standard intelligence test, to be classified as mentally impaired-mentally retarded, the person must also have an impairment in adaptive behaviors. Adaptive behaviors include personal independence and awareness and the ability to engage in socially responsible behaviors.

When it comes to testing children with language delay or disorders, it is important to consider the test's validity and reliability. Because language and culture are fundamentally related, verbal intelligence tests and tests of language delay and disorders are potentially biased, invalid, and unreliable measures. This is particularly true when the language spoken in the home is different from the language used by the test. Validity refers to the purpose of a test. A valid test measures that which it purports to measure. A valid intelligence or language test measures that which the author or authors intended it to measure. There are several specific types of validity. Validity is related to the sampling, criteria, and analysis procedures in deciding the tests' purpose. Reliability is the consistency of the scores over repeated administration. Reliable tests provide consistent results when administered repeatedly to the same group. A reliable test produces the same results when given to the same person at different times or by different forms or sections. Specific types of validity and reliability are listed and defined in Figure 12.2.

Alternate forms reliability: Extent of agreement of test scores using more than one form.
Concurrent validity: Degree a test agrees with another test or measure.
Construct validity: The extent to which a test measures a construct based on the nature of that being measured.
Criterion-related validity: Extent to which items or scores on a test agree with a given criterion measure.
Face validity: Extent to which a test appears to represent that which it is intended to measure
Split-half reliability: Extent of agreement between two halves of a test.
Test-retest reliability: Extent of agreement when administering the same test on two or more separate occasions after a short interval has passed.

Figure 12.2 *Types of test validity and reliability*

Most school districts recognize the importance of testing students in the language spoken in the home. In Arizona, students whose language is other than English, PHLOTE (Primary Home Language Other Than English), are provided comprehensive testing services to consider the special needs of bilingual students. "The district will provide comprehensive assessments for referred students which are appropriate in light of the linguistic and cultural patterns of the student, using staff qualified to evaluate language minority students" (Flagstaff Unified School District No. One, 2001, p. 8-2). These are as follows in decreasing order of preference:

1. Certified bilingual evaluators (when possible);
2. Evaluators who have proficiency and training in assessing PHLOTE students;
3. Evaluators who are trained to administer nonverbal assessment and to use caution in interpreting assessment results;
4. Evaluators who are assisted by translators trained in special education assessments and proficient in the language of the student and English.

The above are accepted as best practices and are specified in the Individuals with Disabilities Education Act (IDEA) as appropriate for assessing bilingual students.

According to the Flagstaff Unified School District No. One, (2001, p. 8-1), diagnostic reports of psychoeducational evaluation must include the following:

1. An analysis of the effect of linguistic and cultural factors on educational history and learning;
2. Documentation of the use of translation or interpretation in the administration of diagnostic instruments or procedures, and the effect on the validity and reliability of the results;
3. An evaluation of the validity and reliability of test results given the student's language proficiency and culture, and an explanation of any modifications of normal testing procedures; and;
4. An analysis of the reliability of comparisons between the results of nonverbal measures and other diagnostic measures.

12.7 Language Delay and Environmental Depravation

Children who lack environmental stimulation may experience language delay or specific language disorders. Environmental conditions can deter speech and language development in children (Van Riper and Erickson, 1996). The environmental conditions that lead to language delay and disorders include isolation from parents, siblings, and peers. There are accounts in the popular literature of children being raised by animals, but these claims are unsubstantiated in the scientific literature. However, there are children who have been subjected to extreme environmental depravation, such as confined to rooms, closets, and sheds for months and even years, and consequently suffered major communication disorders. Another examples of environmental depravation includes being reared in a remote rural area where a child is left to himself or herself during the major speech and language development period. Less dramatic environmental stimulation includes children who are

reared by intellectually limited, emotionally disturbed, or depressed parents (Haynes and Shulman, 1998). There is also the role poverty plays in environmental depravation. Hart and Risley (1995) found that as a group children of parents on welfare were less stimulated than children reared in homes of parents who are professionals. The negative effects of being reared in a low socioeconomic environment were linked to lower early vocabulary growth and subsequent poor school performance.

A child's rate and extent of language development is largely dependent on stimulation from siblings and peers. For example, Tanner, Seamon, Nye, and Lamb (1988) found that children who attend preschool have more advanced language abilities than those who are reared at home. Children who play together have opportunities to learn new words, play cooperatively, follow instructions, create and plan activities, and engage in other highly stimulating activities. Some speech and hearing clinics and schools use normal or advanced children to provide peer stimulation for language-delayed and disordered children. These normal or advanced children are called facilitators. The advantage of peer stimulation involves the role of "play" in speech and language development. Play is a child's work, and it provides him or her with the opportunity to experiment with speech and language with few negative consequences. Play provides a child with trial and error in speech and language activities. Whereas in school and other formal activities there is often adult monitoring and negativity associated with improper speech and language, during play with peers, the negativity is minimal. Play provides the child with speech and language trial and error free from negative consequences.

12.8 Language and Idioglossia

Idioglossia, sometimes called twin speech, is a unique language, one that is not identifiable with an existing one. Idioglossia can occur with a singleton where he or she produces sounds, words, and sentence-like utterances that are not identified with an existing language. Because of environmental depravation, the child is not consistently exposed to an existing language and thus speaks a unique one. True singleton idioglossia is rare because most children not exposed to language are essentially nonverbal. It can also occur when a child has a speech-impaired parent or sibling.

Most cases of idioglossia occur with twins or in children very close in age. Twins develop idioglossia when they interact primarily with each other and have very little, if any, contact with other children. Often, there is little verbal interaction with their parents. Consequently, they have no language model and develop one of their own. Idioglossia is proof that normal children will naturally learn any language to which they are exposed and in the absence of a true language will develop a unique one.

A case of idioglossia occurred with Navajo brothers reared in a remote region of northern Arizona (Tanner, 2006). They were not twins but were only a few months apart in age. They were reared by their maternal grandmother who was extremely quiet and reserved. Much of their early years were spent together tending sheep. They had little interaction with other children or adults. When the children moved to a town to live with their mother, they were enrolled in a Head Start program. During a routine speech and language screening, the idioglossia was detected. The idioglossia was highly developed, and the children would verbally communicate with each other in long utterances.

12.9 Late Talkers

A recent and evolving clinical concept is the "late talker," a toddler who is delayed in his or her language development, also called a "late bloomer" (Haynes and Pindzola, 2004). "In the research literature, late talkers are typically defined as young children (between approximately 16 and 30 months) whose language skills fall below 90 percent of their age peers" (Plant and Beeson, 2004, p. 177). Plant and Beeson's (2004) review of current research on late talkers suggests that these children tend to be at risk for continued language problems. In addition, the earlier the diagnosis of delayed language development is made, the better the outcome. Many but not all children identified as late talkers tend to remain behind their peers over time in language development. Plant and Beeson (2004) observe that there is no consensus of the types of early language deficits, e.g., poor comprehension, initial severity of the deficits, limited use of gestures and vocabulary, that predict whether late talkers will catch up with their peers. Early detection, monitoring, treatment, and follow up of late talkers likely prevents language-based educational, psychological, and social complications later in their lives. Conceivably, the failure to diagnose a late talker could be reasonable grounds for a lawsuit involving damages, compensation, and the provision of special education services.

12.10 Language Disorders and Learning Disabilities

Learning disabilities are a group of impairments that include the language disorder syndrome, attentional deficit disorders, dyslexia, and dysgraphia. Sometimes these disorders are called minimal brain dysfunctions, developmental aphasia, and deficits related to soft neurological damage.

Wiig and Secord (1998) note that the language disorder syndrome is the most common type of learning disability. Language disorder syndrome refers to children without mental impairment-mental retardation, or vision or hearing defects, who have problems learning and using symbols, particularly language.

Attention is the process of focusing on and selecting certain aspects of the environment to the exclusion of ambient stimuli. There are two types of attention deficit disorders. There are children with attention deficits who are hyperactive and those who are not. These disorders are called attention deficit hyperactive disorder (ADHD) and attention deficit disorder (ADD), respectively. According to Nicolosi, Harryman, and Kresheck (2004), children with ADHD will not give close attention to details or will make careless mistakes in schoolwork, have difficulty sustaining attention, be easily distracted, and have other behaviors showing inattention and distraction. They have difficulty following through on instructions, maintaining attention during work and play, and they shift from one uncompleted activity to another. Talking excessively, interrupting, and being impulsive, especially with dangerous activities, are also part of the attention deficit hyperactivity disorders. Generally, these children have trouble with metacognition or "thinking about thinking." Nicolosi, Harryman, and Kresheck (2004) note that for formal diagnosis of this disorder, it must have been consistently present before the age of seven and impair social, academic, or vocational functioning. Unfortunately, the general public has adopted ADHD as an all-encompassing label for children with high energy levels. Many children labeled ADHD are simply active, curious children and do not meet the clinical criteria for the disorder.

Dyslexia and dysgraphia are common learning disabilities, especially in males. These are reading and writing disorders associated with language learning deficits. Letter reversals are common symptoms of dyslexia and agraphia. A child with dyslexia may confuse "b" for "d" or "p" for "b" or be unable to recognize the significance of a letter. The child with dysgraphia may write the wrong letters or be unable graphically to put his or her thoughts on paper. The reading and writing problems seen in adult aphasia are substantially different from the dyslexia and dysgraphia seen in learning disabilities, although they are referred to by the same diagnostic labels. The alexia and agraphia seen in aphasia are the result of neurological damage and are often part of a multimodality language disorder. School districts and parents are often at odds about the type, frequency, and nature of the treatment of dyslexia. See *Livingston v. DeSoto Country School District,* 782 FSupp 1173 (ND Miss 1992).

12.11 Multiple Disabilities and Pervasive Developmental Disorders

Multiple disabilities are learning and developmental problems resulting from multiple causes. Although states define multiple disabilities differently, they usually include vision, hearing, and orthopedic impairments and moderate mental impairment-mental retardation (Arizona Department of Education, 2000). Children with syndromes, including fetal alcohol syndrome, often have multiple disabilities. Fetal alcohol syndrome (FAS) is caused by excessive alcohol consumption by the mother during pregnancy. Children with FAS often have orofacial anomalies, ADHD, and mental impairment-mental retardation. Children with multiple disabilities require ongoing support in more than one major life skill area, and the special education team works closely with the family in planning the individualized educational program (IEP). According to the Arizona Department of Education (2000), an important part of the evaluation process is assistive technology (AT) services that include a wide range of communication boards and computers.

Pervasive developmental disorders (PDD) are characterized by impairments in the development of social interaction and verbal and nonverbal communication skills. There are usually marked restrictions in activities and interests and abnormalities in cognition, posture, sensory input, motor behaviors, sleeping, eating, and mood (Nicolosi, Harryman, and Kresheck, 2004). These disorders occur as often as fifteen per 10,000 live births and are four times more common in boys than girls (Hirsch, 1998).

Autism is a pervasive developmental disorder. In the past, this disorder was thought to be a result of poor parent-child interaction. Today it is accepted that this disorder is caused by neurological impairments possibly resulting from prenatal infections and deficits with the immune system (van Gent, Heijnen, and Treffers, 1997). A current theory about autism is that sensory stimuli are not filtered by the thalamus. This disorder is caused in part by too much sensory information reaching consciousness. Autistic children are overstimulated and bombarded by sensory stimuli. Their distancing of themselves from their parents and others is an attempt to reduce sensory stimulation.

Wetherby (2000) reports that children with autism and pervasive developmental disorders have limited comprehension of verbal and gestural communication and tend to be on a concrete level mentally. They also have limited or complete lack of speech development, and there are inconsistent or hypersensitive responses to auditory stimuli. Some children are oblivious to speech and environmental sounds. These children may engage in self-stimulating behaviors that can include self-destructive actions where they strike themselves repeatedly. They can also strike and injure others.

12.12 Language Disorders, Behavioral Difficulties, and School Violence

It has long been known that many incarcerated individuals have learning disabilities, particularly dyslexia and dysgraphia. For example, studies have shown that up to 19 percent of incarcerated female juvenile delinquents have language disorders (Sanger, Moore-Brown, Magnuson, and Svoboda, 2001). Although there are many facets to behavioral problems and violence in adolescents, school failure and frustration play important roles. Not only can at-risk children reveal their frustration and violent tendencies in speech and language diagnostic and therapeutic activities, treatment for these disabilities can provide socially acceptable means of venting frustration and reducing the risk of behavioral problems and violence.

Schools are permitted to remove a child from special education placement under certain circumstances. According to the Arizona Department of Education, Exceptional Student Services Division (1999), children can be placed in an Interim Alternative Educational Setting (IAES) for up to forty-five calendar days for knowingly possessing illegal drugs, selling, or soliciting the sale of a controlled substance at school or at a school function. If the behavior of the child that led to the disciplinary action is a result of the child's disability, the Individualized Education Program (IEP) must be adjusted to remedy the deficiencies. If the child's behavior is found not to be a manifestation of his or her disability, the same procedures used with children without disabilities are used. However, if the child is suspended from school for more that ten school days or expelled, the schools must continue to provide him or her with free and appropriate public education (FAPE).

12.13 Articulation and Phonological Disorders

Speech articulation is an overlaid function. Biologically, the articulator primarily serves the function for tearing, chewing, and swallowing food. Over millions of years of evolution, the muscles and structures of the face, neck, and head adapted to make speech sounds. The ability to produce speech is secondary to that of tearing, chewing, and swallowing food; it is an overlaid function.

Articulation is the process of shaping the compressed air coming from the lungs into speech sounds. It is a highly sophisticated motor process involving hundreds of muscle and thousands of neurological impulses per second during connected speech. Humans can produce intelligible sounds in excess of 500 words per minute. Speech intelligibility is the ability to create understandable speech and is usually measured in percentages. In connected speech, the articulators move so rapidly, that speech becomes a stream of acoustic energy. Points of articulatory contact are made so rapidly that the tongue and other articulators overlap their movements. The overlapping of motor commands and movements is called coarticulation, which leads to assimilation, the effect one sound has on another when uttered in connected speech. The sounds preceding and following the target sound have an effect on its production. Rarely in connected speech are sounds produced by their ideal points of contact; they are approximated. Yet, humans can create meaningful speech very rapidly through this process of approximation.

The articulators are called the organs of speech, and there are several ways of classifying them. They can be divided into fixed and mobile, and hard and soft articulatory structures. As Figure 12.3 shows, the primary fixed articulators are the hard palate, upper incisors, and alveolar ridge (the tissue just behind the upper incisors). The mobile articulators are the tongue, velum (soft palate), mandible, and lips. The main soft articulators are the lips, tongue, and velum, and the primary hard articulators are the teeth, mandible, hard palate, and alveolar ridge.

The sounds of a language are called phonemes. They can be divided into two general categories: vowels and consonants. Vowels are dependent on the height and front-to-back position of the tongue in the oral cavity. All vowels are voiced and can be classified as low-back, high-front, high-back, etc., depending on the tongue's prominence in the oral cavity. Lip rounding also plays a role in vowel production. Consonants are produced by modification of the air stream in the oral and nasal tracts. They can be classified by the place or points in the oral cavity where they are made (place of articulation) and by the type of speech sound production (manner of articulation).

When classifying consonants in the place of articulation system, there are several points of contact. Bilabials are sounds produced by both lips; labio-dentals by the lips and teeth; lingua-dentals by the tongue and teeth; lingua-alveolars by the tongue and alveolar ridge; and lingua-palatal by the tongue and hard palate.

When classifying consonants in the manner of an articulation system there are two general categories: stops and continuants. Stops are phonemes made by ceasing completely the air stream. Continuants have a continuous flow of air rather than an abrupt release. Plosives result from an explosion of air, and affricates are explosions of air shaped into continents. Fricatives are sounds produced by constriction of the air stream, and glides are produced by a gliding action of the articulators from one position to another. Nasals involve coupling the oral and nasal cavities.

Soft	Hard	
Tongue Lips Velum	Mandible	**Movable**
	Teeth Hard Palate Alveolar Ridge	**Fixed**

Figure 12.3 Major soft, hard, movable, and fixed articulators

A. The International Phonetic Alphabet

In English there are forty-four speech sounds and there are only twenty-six letters in the alphabet. As a result, there are not enough letters to represent the speech sounds. Consequently, two phonemes may be listed by one grapheme such as happens with "th." The "th" letters represent both the voiced and voiceless "th" sounds: "th" as in "think" (voiceless), and "th" as in "that" (voiced). (Two phonemes differing only by voicing are called cognates.) Because of the confusion in representing phonemes with graphemes, the International Phonetic Alphabet (IPA) was developed. In the International Phonetic Alphabet one phoneme is represented by one grapheme and vice versa. Speech-language pathologists use the IPA both in diagnostic and therapeutic activities. Lawyers, judges, and court reporters may need to refer to Figure 12.4 and Figure 12.5 for the IPA symbols and the sounds to which they refer. (See Chapter 15 for a detailed discussion of phonetics.)

B. Etiology of Articulation Disorders

There are a myriad of diseases, injuries, birth defects, syndromes, and learning problems that can cause articulation disorders. Improper learning causes some articulation disorders, while others occur because of progressive degenerative diseases or birth defects. Some children outgrow their speech disorders, while others require intensive therapy throughout their lives to obtain and maintain intelligible speech. The primary articulation disorders etiological factors are (1) motor speech disorders, (2) structural defects, (3) hearing loss and deafness, and (4) regression in speech behaviors due to emotional shock or trauma. All articulation disorders can be evaluated and treated within the phonological or sensory-motor theories.

n	as pronounced in the word now
t	as pronounced in the word tag
d	as pronounced in the word dog
s	as pronounced in the word soap
w	as pronounced in the word water
r	as pronounced in the word rabbit
m	as pronounced in the word milk
ð	as pronounced in the word that
k	as pronounced in the word comb
l	as pronounced in the word lamb
g	as pronounced in the word go
z	as pronounced in the word zipper
ŋ	as pronounced in the word sing
b	as pronounced in the word button
p	as pronounced in the word pig
h	as pronounced in the word hurt
v	as pronounced in the word very
f	as pronounced in the word fine
θ	as pronounced in the word think
ʃ	as pronounced in the word shoot
dʒ	as pronounced in the word jump
j	as pronounced in the word yellow
tʃ	as pronounced in the word chicken
ʒ	as pronounced in the word beige

Figure 12.4 *IPA symbols and the sounds to which they refer (consonants)*

ɪ	as pronounced in the word his
a	as pronounced in the word mop
æ	as pronounced in the word cat
i	as pronounced in the word see
ɛ	as pronounced in the word head
o	as pronounced in the word over
√	as pronounced in the word mother
ɔ	as pronounced in the word all
u	as pronounced in the word you
u	as pronounced in the word cook
ɜ	as pronounced in the word bird
e	as pronounced in the word ache

Figure 12.5 *IPA symbols and the sounds to which they refer (vowels)*

Motor speech disorders are discussed in Chapter 9. Articulation is one of the five basic motor speech processes, and it is particularly vulnerable in apraxia of speech and the dysarthrias. The articulation disorders seen in apraxia of speech are the result of damage to the areas of the brain responsible for programming and sequencing speech acts. In apraxia of speech, the child knows the word or words he or she wants to say but is impaired for programming and sequencing them. Apraxia of speech in children is called developmental apraxia because it occurs during the speech and language developmental period. The patterns of speech seen in developmental apraxia are often different from what are observed in the adult with motor speech programming deficits. This is because the adult has already learned speech and is accustomed to its proper production. The young child with apraxia of speech is still developing speech and language and tends to have less groping, struggle, and compensatory activities. For the child with apraxia of speech, deficient motor speech programming and sequencing are integrated into his or her speech, and self-correction is not as extensive as is seen in the adult. Apraxia of speech is likely a predisposing factor for stuttering.

The dysarthrias are a group of motor speech disorders resulting from neuromuscular impairments. The type of articulatory impairment seen in children with dysarthria depends on the type of muscular paralysis or paresis. Flaccid speech muscles produce symptoms that are different from what is seen in spasticity. Ataxia produces articulation that is ill coordinated; and in extrapyramidal disorders, hypokinetic and hyperkinetic dysarthrias, there are unwanted speech movements that occur slowly or quickly. Several dysarthria-producing birth defects and syndromes, such as cerebral palsy and muscular dystrophy, are commonly seen in children. Flaccid, spastic, and ataxic dysarthrias are the result of various degrees of paralysis; and Parkinsonian dysarthria (hypokinetic) and the quick and slow hyperkinetic dysarthrias are considered movement disorders.

Structural defects of the articulators include cleft lip and palate, malocclusion, tongue size irregularities, glossectomy, and being "tongue-tied." They cause speech disorders because the articulators are insufficient, malformed, or damaged. Cleft lip and palate, discussed in Chapter 11, cause articulation disorders because the malformations can interfere with the child's ability to make articulatory contact and properly valve the compressed air coming from the lungs. When there is a cleft of the lip, palate, and dental arches, speech sound production can be impaired. Reconstructive surgeons are often successful in repairing these malformations, and with speech therapy the patient's articulation can become normal. Jumbled, misaligned, or missing teeth are structural defects causing articulation disorders because they cause disruptions in important points of articulatory contact, and the result is distorted speech sounds. Children can lose their temporary, deciduous teeth too early because of trauma or disease. Some children lose teeth because a milk bottle, rather than a pacifier, is used to calm them. Excessive dental exposure to milk and other liquids that damage the teeth is called early childhood caries (ECC). An insufficient palatal vault can also cause dental malocclusion because it cannot accommodate the resting tongue, thus causing it to place pressure behind the teeth. Because of the pressure, the teeth protrude. Microglossia and macroglossia refer to a tongue that is either too small or too large. Microglossia occurs when the tongue is too small relative to the oral cavity; macroglossia is a tongue that is too large compared with the oral cavity. It is common in people with Down syndrome. Besides several speech and language characteristics of this syndrome, many individuals also have macroglossia. Recently some people with Down syndrome have undergone surgery to reduce the tongue size, i.e., a partial glossectomy. Glossectomy is the surgical removal of all or part of the tongue. Although this surgery can be required because of head trauma, the leading cause of glossectomy is cancer from tobacco products. To stop the spread of cancer, it is often necessary for surgeons to remove all or part of the tongue. The articulation impairment depends on the amount of the tongue that is surgically removed. The lingual frenulum is a short cord of tissue running from the bottom of the tongue to the middle of the floor of the mouth. A person with a shortened lingual frenulum is sometimes called "tongue-tied." When the lingual frenulum is sufficiently short to reduce tongue mobility and limit articulatory contact, speech can be impaired. "Clipping" the lingual frenulum is sometimes necessary, and post-surgical articulation therapy is required. Unfortunately, some surgeons have the erroneous belief that by clipping the lingual frenulum they can cure several speech disorders, including stuttering.

Children who are born hard of hearing or deaf do not learn to articulate sounds correctly or are completely without intelligible speech. Although hearing is often called the second sense, it is the primary sense for the normal acquisition of speech sounds. Three factors are important in determining the role deafness and hearing loss play in a child's ability to articulate. First, the age at which the child acquires the deafness or hearing loss determines the severity of his or her articulation impairment. If the deafness or hearing loss occurs before or during the primary speech and language acquisition period (prelingual), i.e., before six or seven years of age, then it will significantly impair his or her acquisition of sounds. However, if the deafness or hearing loss occurs after the primary speech and language acquisition period (postlingual), it will play a less important role in speech articulation acquisition because the child will have already learned speech sounds. The second factor in determining the effects of hearing loss on speech articulation development involves the frequencies of the hearing disorder. Children learn to produce sounds properly when they hear them clearly. Consequently, when a child has a hearing loss involving the high frequencies in the speech range, he or she does not hear those sounds. Therefore, it is likely that he or she will not properly learn to produce speech sounds with a high degree of energy in the higher frequencies such as /s/, "sh," and "th." Conversely, a low frequency hearing loss will cause lower frequency speech sounds to be misarticulated. The third factor in determining the effects of hearing loss on speech articulation is the level of the hearing loss. Obviously, more severe hearing losses will result in more significant speech articulation impairments. Chapter 14 addresses audiological testing, hearing loss, deafness, and communication.

Regression is a psychological defense mechanism where an individual returns to a more secure psychological state. It occurs when the person is subjected to extreme stress. In children the stress can be related to abuse, neglect, and separation from loved ones. Usually, an aspect of the regression is the across-the-board reduction in speech and language abilities including articulation. The child returns to infantile speech, "baby talk," which is reflective of his or her regressed psychological state. When investigating whether a child's return to infantile speech is a result of emotional distress, three factors must be considered. First, the change in speech must be associated with an extreme psychological event. A psychologically devastating event prompts the regression. Second, the child must have previously been producing speech at a significantly more mature level or have had normal articulation. The regression in speech and/or language must not be the result of a neurological event. Third, mutism is often associated with the regression. Many children stop talking altogether before regressing to the infantile speech. Child abuse can result in mutism and a refusal to talk. See *People v Mills,* 1CalApp 4th 898, 2 CalRptr 614 (CalApp 1 Dist 1991). Because of a communication disorder, the child's veracity of statements can be called into question. Regression to infantile speech patterns in a child who was previously talking at a significantly more mature level requires psychiatric or psychological intervention. The child's infantile speech is one symptom of a deeper, underlying psychological disturbance. Articulation therapy is provided in conjunction with the total psychological and social management of the child.

Today, there are two general schools of thought with regard to the evaluation and treatment of articulation disorders: sensory-motor and phonology learning theories. The sensory-motor approach views articulation disorders primarily as perceptual and motor development delay. In the phonological approach, articulation disorders are viewed as a failure to learn adult rules of language phonology. "Both the traditional sensory-motor approach and the phonologic method of improving articulation have solid research and clinical history to support them. A client with an articulation disorder can benefit from the traditional sensory motor approach where the clinician works on auditory perception, production, and carryover of correct speech sound production. Similarly, treating the articulation disorders as a language-based phonology disorder and teaching the appropriate phonologic rule, rather than the speech sound error, also produces positive results" (Tanner, 2006, p. 76). Table 12.1 shows the major articulation etiological factors.

C. The Sensory-Motor Learning Theory of Articulation Disorders

There is a generally predictable order of speech sound acquisition. Speech sounds are acquired at predictable ages due to several maturational factors. For example, most children learn /m/, /b/, and /p/ sounds early, while acquiring sounds such as /r/ and /s/ later on. The sequence speech sounds are acquired is relatively invariant, while the rate of acquisition is highly variable. Some children produce speech sounds normally by the time they are three or four years of age. Other children misarticulate sounds when they are in the second and third grades. And, of course, some children never learn to produce speech sounds correctly without articulation therapy. Age normative data are contained in charts and tables listing the phonemes and corresponding developmental ages. There is a high degree of variability among these charts and tables. Two factors are important in addressing these normative charts and tables. First, the positions of the words must be considered. Do the charts and tables show when a particular sound is mastered in only the initial position of words, or do they show when a child has acquired a sound in all three positions: initially, medially, and finally? Second, what is the criterion of mastery? Do the charts and tables say when 51 percent of the children have mastered a sound or when 60 percent or 90 percent have acquired it? For meaningful interpretation,

Table 12.1
Etiology of Articulation and Phonology Disorders

Motor Speech Disorders	Apraxia of Speech
	Dysarthria: Flaccid, Spastic, Ataxic,
	  Hypokinetic, Hyperkinetic
	  (Quick-Slow), Mixed-Multiple

Structural Defects	Cleft Lip and Palate, Malocclusion, Tongue Size Irregularities, Glossectomy, Short Lingual Frenulum (Tongue-Tied)

Hearing Loss-Deafness	Variables Affecting Articulation:
	  Age (Prelingual-Postlingual)
	  Frequencies of Hearing Loss
	  Level of Hearing Loss: Mild-Moderate-Severe

Psychological-Emotional	Associated with Extreme Psychological Event Articulation Regression Mutism
Sensory-Motor Theory (Traditional)	Articulation Disorders Primarily as Perceptual and Motor Developmental Delay
Phonological Theory (Language-Based)	Failure to Learn Adult Rules of Language Phonology

both the number of positions and the criterion of mastery must be considered when deciding if a child is normally developing speech articulation. Figure 12.6 shows the consonants of English and several criteria of mastery (Tanner, Culbertson, and Secord, 1997). Figure 12.7 shows English vowels (Tanner, Culbertson, and Secord, 1997).

Auditory perception and fine motor skills are important proficiencies linked to normal articulation acquisition. Auditory perception is the ability to detect salient aspects of sensory information coming from the ears. It is the act of attending to the important stimuli, the signal, and ignoring the ambient stimuli, the noise. Children with impaired auditory perception have trouble with figure-ground perceptions. The more similar two auditory signals are, the more difficult it is to perceive their differences. Consequently, children with auditory perception difficulties often do not perceive the differences between similar speech sounds. They may engage in substitutions of similarly sounding sounds: wabbit for rabbit, ramp for lamp, thee for see. Because the child perceives little or no differences in these sounds, articulation is done incorrectly. Fine motor skills are closely associated with auditory perceptual development. Viewing and treating articulation development and disorders in this manner is called the sensory-motor approach. Usually therapy is provided for one sound, and after it is mastered the clinician addresses another defective sound.

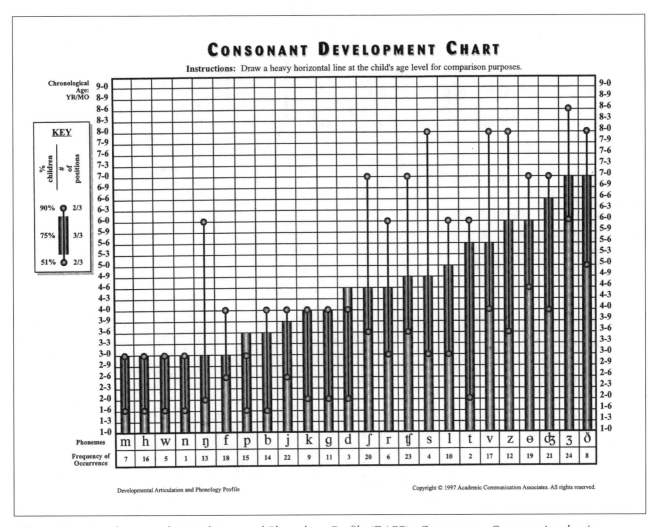

Figure 12.6 Developmental Articulation and Phonology Profile (DAPP): Consonants. Courtesy Academic Communication Associates (Source: Tanner, D., Culbertson, W., and Secord, W, 1997)

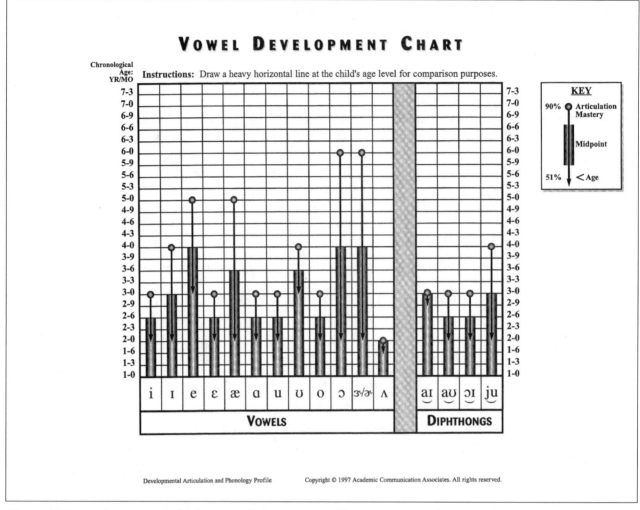

Figure 12.7 Developmental Articulation and Phonology Profile (DAPP): Vowels. Courtesy Academic Communication Associates (Source: Tanner, D., Culbertson, W., and Secord, W, 1997)

D. The Phonological Learning Theory of Articulation Disorders

The phonological approach to viewing articulation development and disorders regards speech sound development as the discovery and fusion of syllable formation principles. Rather than to consider speech sound acquisition as a product of auditory perception and fine motor skills development (sensory-motor approach), the phonological approach involves language. Phonology is the rule-governed way humans produce the sounds of language. In the phonological approach articulation disorders are thought to result from delayed acquisition of the phonological rules of the language. To treat the communication disorder the clinician helps the child discover adult phonology. In this approach more than one sound is used to teach these phonological rules. Phonological rules and their approximate ages of extinction are provided in Figure 12.8 (Tanner, Culbertson,

and Secord, 1997). This approach is particularly useful for children who have more than one articulation disorder and those who have impaired intelligibility.

E. Dialect and Accent

Accent and dialect are often used interchangeably, but technically they differ. Accent is the carryover of a native language into a second one. The phonetic traits of the first learned, native language are seen in the speech sound production of the second one. Dialect refers to a specific form of pronunciation and vocabulary spoken in a particular geographical area or social class. Many accents and dialects suggest social-economic class and status.

Technically, the speech articulation patterns of accent or dialect are not articulation disorders. However, some parents want schools to reduce or eliminate them to improve their children's social status, but school districts are usually reluctant to provide accent and dialect reduction therapies. Parents are often required to seek private services to reduce or eliminate their child's accent or dialect. Additionally, some child actors may seek articulation therapy to address accent and dialect.

F. Evaluating and Treating Articulation and Phonology Disorders

There are several clinical and forensic reasons for evaluating articulation disorders. Clinically, an articulation evaluation is conducted to decide whether a problem exists, determine its etiology, and analyze and describe the disorder. The clinical articulation evaluation is also conducted to figure out long-term and short-term goals and the methods to be used to meet them. Forensically, an articulation evalua-

tion may be required to substantiate the appropriateness of special education placement and evaluate the effectiveness of treatment. It also may be required to quantify chronic articulation problems and for vocational rehabilitation purposes.

Articulation disorders are listed by the types of impairments and their positions in words. There are three typical types of articulation errors: distortions, omissions, and substitutions. A distorted speech sound is one that can be recognized but is not made clearly or succinctly. For example, a child may produce a lateral /s/. In a lateral /s/, the airstream is diverted to the sides of the tongue and there is a lisping quality. The sound can be recognized as an /s/, but it is distorted. An omission is the child saying a word but omitting a sound: "chur_" for church. A substitution is the switching of a recognizable sound for another one: "wamp" for "lamp."

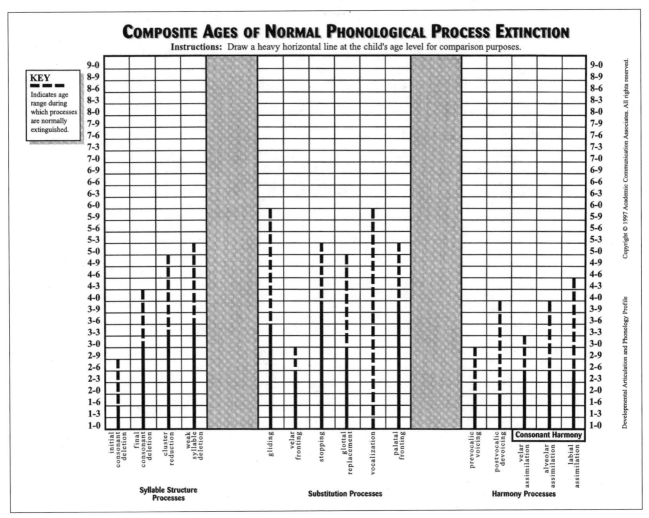

Figure 12.8 *Developmental Articulation and Phonology Profile (DAPP): Phonological rules and their approximate ages of extinction. Courtesy of Academic Communication Associates (Source: Tanner, D., Culbertson, W., and Secord, W, 1997)*

Distortions, omissions, and substitutions can occur in the initial, medial, and final (IMF) positions of words. On the report, the clinician notes "dist (IMF)" for a distortion that occurs in the initial, medial, and final positions of words. Omissions are shown by "om," and their positions in words are noted. A substitution is shown by listing the speech sound that is substituted for the appropriate phoneme, and the position in the words in which it occurs. For example, a child who produces the word "wabbit" for "rabbit" has substituted the /w/ for the /r/ sound in the initial position of a word. On the report, the clinician indicates: w/r substitution (initially). A lisp is a substitution of the voiceless "th" for an /s/ sound and would be shown on a report as a " θ/s substitution (IMF)" if the child produced the substitution in all three positions of words. A fourth type of error is the addition. In an addition, a child produces all of the sounds in the word, and adds an additional one. Additions suggest stuttering and apraxia of speech. Figure 12.9 shows several typical articulation errors and their clinical descriptions.

A phonological analysis is usually conducted on a child with multiple articulation errors. In a phonological analysis, the child's speech sample is examined in several contexts to derive the rule-governed structures in his or her speech. Usually, a determination is made about the child's intelligibility. In addition, the child's oral diadochokinesis is assessed by seeing how rapidly he or she can move the articulators. This is typically done by having the pupil say "pa," "da," and "ka" in rapid succession. Oral diadochokinesis provides general information about the strength, speed, and mobility of the articulators. With some children a determination is made whether they are stimulable.

Stimulable means the child can produce the sound when provided cues and prompts from the clinician. A child that is stimulable has the neurological and muscular integrity for making the sound; the error is likely a result of improper learning. The oral-facial examination looks at the structural or functional status of the articulators. Finally, no comprehensive articulation evaluation would be complete without a hearing screening to rule out hearing loss as a factor of the speech disorder.

The treatment of articulation disorders depends on their severity and etiology. Improving speech articulation in children with hearing loss and deafness is part of aural rehabilitation. Aural rehabilitation uses the existing communication abilities of the child to improve functional communication. Visual, tactile, and residual auditory feedback is used to improve speech sound production. Teaching speech to deaf children is part of the Total Communication Approach which combines sign language, speech reading, writing, and oral methods of communication. If the articulation errors are a result of structural or motor defects, specific therapies are provided to compensate for the impairments. For children with one or two articulation disorders such as problems with the /r/ or /s/ sounds (these are the most common articulation errors seen in school-aged children), the sensory-motor approach may be used. The goal is to improve auditory perception and fine oral motor skills. For children whose articulation disorders are phonologically based, the linguistic rules by which sounds are combined and fused are taught, often using more than one sound. For children with emotional disturbances, autism, schizophrenia, head trauma, syndromes, and so on, variations of traditional articulation therapies are incorporated into the total

"tar" for "car"	/t/ for /k/ substitution initially
"thee" for "see"	/θ/ for /s/ substitution initially
"wun" for "run"	/w/ for /r/ substitution initially
"ar" for "car"	/k/ omission initially
"bacuum" for "vacuum"	/b/ for /v/ substitution initially
"chur" for "church"	omission of the /tʃ/ finally
"bnook" for "book"	distortion of the /b/ initially
"re" for "red"	omission of the /d/ finally
"tum" for "thumb"	/t/ for /θ/ substitution initially
"dun" for "gun"	/d/ for /g/ substitution initially
"cawot" for "carrot"	/w/ for /r/ substitution medially
"buthes" for "brushes"	/θ/ for /ʃ/ substitution medially
"dod" for "dog"	/d/ for /g/ substitution finally
"nipe" for "knife"	/p/ for /f/ substitution finally
"shlaken" for "shaken"	distortion of /ʃ/ initially (lateral /s/)

Figure 12.9 Examples of clinical reporting of articulation errors

cognitive, linguistic, social, and psychological management of the child. These children often require multiple approaches to the treatment of their disorders.

12.14 Stuttering

Stuttering is a fluency disorder. Fluency is the act of speaking effortlessly, smoothly and easily, without hesitations, interjections, fillers, or blocks. Although several communication disorders can affect speech fluency, stuttering is the primary fluency-disrupting impediment. Stuttering has been around presumably since humans began to talk and it occurs in all cultures and languages. Although stuttering can begin in adults, it usually starts in childhood. Adult onset stuttering is sometimes called hysterical stuttering because it usually results from psychological trauma or shock. The definition of stuttering is important, particularly when comparing research. Some clinicians and researchers define stuttering narrowly only including obvious stuttering behaviors. Others define stuttering in a broad sense that can include mild and sometimes temporary disruptions in speech fluency and the thoughts, feelings, and attitudes associated with it. Van Riper's (1973, 1992) definition of stuttering is well-accepted among clinicians and researchers: *A word improperly patterned in time and the speaker's reaction thereto.* Stuttering is a speech planning, pattering, and coordination problem, and the speaker's reaction to the speech impediment is an important aspect to it.

Cluttering is a verbal thought-organization disorder and it is sometimes confused with stuttering. The child who clutters seems unable to organize his or her thoughts so that they can be fluently spoken. The clutterer's speech is rapid, fragmented, and contains many revisions. Whereas the stuttering child has an awareness on some level of the disorder, the clutterer appears oblivious to his or her dysfluent speech. Additionally, in cluttering, struggle on specific sounds, words, and phrases is usually absent. Research has shown that people who clutter also may have poor concentration and a reduced attention span. People who clutter are typically thought of as excited, anxious, scatterbrained, disorganized, and flighty. Cluttering is rarely treated as a clinical entity in the schools, although reduction of it may be a concurrent objective in stuttering therapy.

According to Van Riper's definition of stuttering, words are improperly patterned in time. Actually, sounds, syllables, words, and phrases are improperly patterned in time. These dysfluencies are often called the core aspect of stuttering, or the primary features. There are three ways sounds, syllables, words, and phrases may be improperly patterned in time: repetitions, prolongations, and blocks.

Repetitions are the most common types of dysfluencies, and they can occur at the sound, syllable, word, or phrase level. Prolongations usually occur on continuant sounds, although they can also involve stops. Blocks are cessations of ongoing speech and the inability to get speech started. They can occur between and within words. Some individuals who stutter typically engage in repetitions, while others may only block or prolong speech sounds. Most severe stuttering involves combinations of repetitions, prolongations, and blocks. According to Van Riper's definition of stuttering, the speaker's reactions thereto are escape and avoidance behaviors performed by the stutterer to rid himself or herself of the stuttering. Clinicians sometimes call these feelings and behaviors accessory features. They can include eye-blinks, hand slaps, head jerks and nods, and lack of eye contact. The feelings associated with stuttering can include anxiety, fear, dread, shame, and embarrassment. The primary and accessory features of stuttering are discussed later.

The following builds on Van Riper's stuttering definition and combines the primary and secondary features of stuttering into a definition of a person who stutters:

An individual who improperly patterns phonemes, syllables, words and/or phrases in time; who experiences classically-conditioned negative emotional reactions to disfluent speech and associated stimuli and who may engage in visible avoidance and escape behaviors when confronted with disfluent speech or associated stimuli (Tanner, Belliveau and Siebert, 1995, p. 6).

Diagnosing stuttering in children is a demanding clinical determination. This is because all individuals are disfluent. (In this text, "disfluency" refers to the normal breakdown in the smooth, effortless production of speech while "dysfluency" refers to a pathological breakdown in speech fluency.) No one talks completely fluently all of the time, and children often go through a normal stage where they are excessively disfluent. They hesitate, prolong, and repeat sounds, syllables, words, and phrases, particularly when they are hurried or anxious. Separating normal nonfluencies from stuttering behaviors is an exacting clinical process and can result in false positive and false negative results. As discussed below, it is difficult to know if a child is simply going through a stage of excessive normal nonfluencies or whether he or she is becoming a true stutterer.

Bloodstein (1995) reports that the incidence of stuttering, i.e., how many people have it at some time in their lives, is about 5 percent. About 1 percent of the population of the United States currently stutters. Obviously, many people only temporarily stutter, and the disorder goes away with or without treatment. It is also possible that the 5 percent figure includes children who are only going through a period of excessive disfluencies and never truly had the self-perpetuating disorder of stuttering. Nevertheless, it is safe to assume that 1 percent of the United States currently stutters and about 5 percent of school-age children are at risk for developing the disorder.

A. Theories of Stuttering

What causes some children to stutter while others are spared a life time of frustrating broken words? After nearly a century of scientific study the etiology of stuttering remains elusive. The cause or causes of stuttering have been studied by several professionals, including speech and hearing scientists, psychologists, physicians, educators, geneticists, and linguists. Over the years three general theories about the etiology of stuttering have emerged: psychogenic, learned, and organic.

The psychogenic theories of stuttering postulate that a person stutters because of psychological factors. The psychological factors usually involve anxiety, which is generated from some type of psychological conflict. The anxiety directly or indirectly results in disrupted speech. According to the psychogenic theories, stuttering can be seen as an expectancy neurosis, the result of repressed needs, a conflict between the id and the superego, or repressed anger and hostility.

Stuttering as an expectancy neurosis suggests that people who stutter are verbally impotent. They stutter because they have developed an unrealistic fear of speaking: logophobia. Other types of expectancy neuroses include nonorganic sexual impotence, writer's cramp, and stage fright. According to this theory, stutterers have experienced failure with speech in the past and as a result of that failure, they expect to fail in the future. Speech fluency failure becomes a self-fulfilling prophecy.

The theory that stuttering is a result of repressed needs postulates that the disorder results from maladaptive child-rearing practices where the infant was unable to satisfy normal psychological desires and needs. Consequently, as the child matures, he or she acts out those needs in a socially acceptable manner through stuttering. The repressed needs theories have provided some of the most bizarre explanations for this speech disorder. In the early and mid-1900s, some theorists proposed that stuttering was an oral fixation where a person symbolically obtained oral gratification through sucking on an illusionary nipple. There was even an anal fixation theory where the stutterer supposedly displaced his or her anal fixation orally and was symbolically smearing the listener with feces. Although these theories received some attention from scholars, there is no empirical support for them, and they have been rejected.

The idea that stuttering results from a conflict between the id and the superego gained some support from psychogenic theorists. The conflict between the id and the superego generates anxiety that results in speech disruptions. Central to this theory is the hypothesis that people who stutter have deficient egos. There have been empirical studies supporting the belief that stutterers have reduced self-esteem and a general reduction of the ego. The repressed anger and hostility theory suggests that people who stutter do so because they have "unspeakable feelings." The anger and hostility are just below the surface and cause stuttering. There is a logical basis to this theory, because anger and hostility do cause some people to be disfluent.

In the past, some professors cautioned their students not to "cure" stuttering without finding a substitute for their client's repressed needs, anger, and hostility. Stuttering therapy needed to be provided with psychoanalysis. According to these professors, stuttering was a safe manifestation of the patient's psychological turmoil, and to remove it without the benefit of psychotherapy could result in the patient engaging in destructive outlets. Again, although this belief was held by some experts on the disorder, there have been no reports in the scientific literature where a person was cured of stuttering and engaged in violence or other destructive acts as a result of the cure. Some people who stutter engage in socially unusual patterns of behavior such as repetitively protruding their tongues and snorting. Clinically, these are avoidance and escape behaviors developed over the years in an attempt to stop stuttering. These accessory behaviors can be confusing and distressing to listeners. In one case, they resulted in an accusation of sexual harassment (A Case Study of Alleged Sexual Harassment and Stuttering).

The above psychogenic theories on stuttering are not widely accepted as identifying the primary cause of stuttering by current speech and hearing scientists and clinicians. However, it is likely that stuttering is caused, in part, by psychological factors, especially the disruptive effects of anxiety and excessive speech muscular tension. It is also apparent that stuttering causes anxiety and other negative emotions in the speaker. Most people who stutter feel negativity during the moment of stuttering. Psychologically, stuttering is a doubled-edged sword. It is caused in part by psychological factors, and the disorder itself results in anxiety and other negative emotions.

In basic terms, the learning theories propose that stuttering is a bad habit, and variations of these theories have been around since the late 1700s. In the learning theory framework, stuttering begins and is maintained by rewards and reductions of anxiety and can be stopped through behavior modification. Most current theories of the nature and treatment of stuttering recognize the role learning plays in this speech disorder. In stuttering, there are two major variations of current learning models: operant and classical conditioning.

In the operant conditioning framework, stuttering is a product of rewards. The child's normal nonfluencies are rewarded, and because of the rewards, the nonfluencies increase in frequency and magnitude until they constitute stuttering. The providers of the rewards are the child's family, peers, and teachers, and stuttering can be self-reinforcing. There are several types of rewards provided for dysfluent speech. Sometimes family, peers, and teachers will not interrupt the stuttering child, thus providing the reward of noninterruption for stuttered speech. All children want to be special, and by stuttering a child can achieve special status. Other types of rewards are specific to each individual child.

In the classical conditioning (Pavlovian) framework, stuttering is a result of the disruptive influence of anxiety. It has long been known that anxiety disrupts fine motor movements, and speech production is no exception. As anxiety increases, so do dysfluencies. According to this theory, stuttering is the result of classically conditioned negative emotions (Brutten and Shoemaker, 1967). In this type of learning paradigm, stuttering is the result of negative emotional learning where the child reacts to dysfluent speech with anxiety. The anxiety is paired with sounds, words, situations, and certain people. Soon, the child expects to stutter on those stimuli, creating more anxiety, which further disrupts speech fluency. A vicious spiral of anxiety, stuttering, more anxiety, and increased stuttering results from this type of emotional learning. There is one important difference in the operant and classical learning paradigms. In the operant model, stuttering begins as too many normal nonfluencies, whereas in the classical model, the dysfluencies are unique and different from normal hesitations, prolongations, and repetitions. All speech is learned, and consequently, learning must play a role in its disorders. Modern learning principles play an important role in the treatment of stuttering. They are the foundation of the drills, exercises, and counseling approaches. Through learning models, people who stutter are taught to talk differently and to speak more normally.

The organic theories of stuttering postulate that stuttering is caused by a neurological or physical irregularity or defect. One of the most popular myths about stuttering is that a child is thinking faster than his or her mouth can utter the words. Some parents believe that their stuttering child has normal or above-average intelligence but the organs of speech are clumsy or slow. Studies have shown that as a group, stutterers have normal or even above-average intelligence. This is particularly true of research that factors out from the sample Down syndrome people who have a higher occurrence of stuttering and are also mentally impaired-mentally retarded. However, the research has not shown that stutterers as a group have slow or sluggish speech musculature and impaired fine motor control. And, in fact, all normal people think faster than they can talk. Humans can produce intelligible speech rapidly, but the words in internal monologues occur much faster. If a disparity between thought and the speed of speech muscular movements caused stuttering, everyone would stutter.

In looking for a cause of stuttering, scientists have examined the biochemistry of stutterers and compared them to normal speakers. To date, there have been no conclusive studies showing that stutterers have significant biochemical differences. People who stutter and those who speak normally have remarkably similar biochemistry. In the majority of individuals, stuttering is not related to seizures, abnormal blood sugar levels, calcium levels, and so forth.

Researchers have also tested whether stuttering is an abnormality in auditory feedback. It has long been known that delayed auditory feedback (DAF) causes normal speakers to be temporarily dysfluent. If a person hears his or her own speech through air conduction a fraction of a second later than through bone conduction, disfluencies result. (Bone conduction is the perception of sound through the vibration of the skull, bypassing the middle ear. It is the reason a person sounds different to himself or herself on a tape recorder.) The effects of DAF can be observed when a public address system delays a speaker's feedback. The public speaker talks with a stutter because of the auditory feedback disruption. This organic theory of stuttering proposes that stutterers have a delay in air and bone conduction or that one ear delays the feedback. Although this theory is plausible, studies have yet to confirm it.

One of the areas people who stutter may differ from normal speakers is in the functional areas of the brain activated during speaking. New generations of brain imaging techniques have provided evidence that people who stutter are atypical in the areas of the brain used during speech.

However, this research is not conclusive, and studies occasionally report contradictory results.

A promising organic theory to explain stuttering involves genetics. Several studies have shown that people who stutter may be genetically predisposed to the disorder. There may be a sex-linked gene for stuttering accounting for the fact that the disorder runs in families. "Fifty percent of people who stutter report that they have a relative who stuttered at some time in his or her life" (Owens, Metz, and Haas, 2000, p. 252). Few theorists believe that a gene for stuttering directly causes the disorder. It is generally accepted that if there is a gene for stuttering, it predisposes the person to the disorder. People with a gene for stuttering are more likely to stutter given precipitating and perpetuating environmental conditions.

The above stuttering etiology theories revolve around the age-old question, "Do people who stutter do so because of nature or nurturing," which is asked about many human maladies. Is the disorder a result of organic factors and/or genes, or does it occur because of learning, psychology, and social factors? Given the complexities of this communication disorder, and the fact that no single cause of the disorder has been discovered during nearly a century of research, it is probable that people stutter for multiple reasons. It is likely that the majority of stuttering is the result of learning and psychology, although some youngsters may be at risk for the disorder because of genes and other organic factors. People who develop stuttering later in life probably have it occur because of psychological factors such as shock and trauma. In most cases of the disorder, speech anxiety and fear complicate and perpetuate the disorder.

B. The Typical Course of Stuttering Development in Children

Most stuttering begins between the ages of three and seven. Typically, the stutterer is a male who may have additional communication disorders. The incidence of stuttering in males is three to four times greater than in females. The at-risk child goes through a stage where his or her speech is very nonfluent, possibly as a result of organic predisposing factors. These repetitions, prolongations, and hesitations occur in all people and are normal speech behaviors throughout life. Children who are at risk for stuttering, however, may have a greater frequency of them.

In the typical course of stuttering development, a parent, teacher, sibling, or peer brings those normal nonfluencies to the child's attention as being abnormal; normal nonfluencies are labeled as stuttering by a lay person. (The child may also independently and erroneously reach the conclusion that they are abnormal.) The role of misdiag-

nosis of normal nonfluencies as stuttering which eventually contributes to the onset of the disorder is called the Semantic or Diagnosogenic Theory of Stuttering and was first postulated in the 1940s by Dr. Wendell Johnson. It is a well-accepted clinical concept. Because of the reactions of others, the child begins to believe normal nonfluencies are abnormal and attempts to produce perfectly fluent speech, of which most humans are incapable. He or she tries harder to make the sounds of speech perfectly fluent, an act that actually increases self-consciousness and causes more disruptions in fluency. This increase in the number and type of the dysfluencies causes increased negative reactions by listeners, and a sense of verbal impotence is created in the child. A negative spiral is set into motion: stuttered speech, increased negativity, more stuttered speech, etc. Rewards for stuttered speech may also be causal agents. Over time the child's speech fluency deteriorates, and he or she acquires the secondary features of eye squints, hand slaps, head jerks, nasal snorts, and the like as an attempt to avoid or escape the moment of stuttering.

C. Diagnosing Stuttering in Children

There are three diagnostic categories of stuttering in children: normally nonfluent, developmental stuttering, and confirmed stuttering. All verbal children can be placed in one of these three categories. Children who are diagnosed as normally nonfluent may have excessive dysfluencies, but they are not symptomatic of stuttering. These children are not enrolled in therapy, and parents are counseled about the nature of speech fluency. Children in the developmental stuttering category have more disfluencies than are normal, or the ones they have are abnormal, but these children are not clearly stuttering. There are several indicators that these children are at risk for stuttering (see Figure 12.10). Developmental stuttering is sometimes called incipient stuttering. Children in the developmental stuttering category may be seen for direct therapy, and their parents and teachers counseled to eliminate the precipitating factors for stuttering. The confirmed stuttering category includes those children who have shown a sufficient number and type of dysfluencies to require direct therapy and the stuttering has been confirmed by a speech-language pathologist. Parent and teacher counseling is also a part of the treatment of the young confirmed stutterer.

The proper diagnosis of stuttering in children is important for several reasons and there are legal ramifications to improper placement. First, the earlier stuttering is detected and the therapies provided, the more successful the treatment. A child who is just beginning to stutter has not developed the response strength or experienced the psychological and social negativity that perpetuate the disorder. Second, improperly diagnosing a child as a stutterer when in fact, he or she is only normally nonfluent can cause the disorder. Because of the risk of causing stuttering in a child who is only normally nonfluent, clinicians are conservative when placing a child in the confirmed stuttering category. Third, stuttering can be prevented. For children in the developmental stuttering category, counseling and instruction of parents and teachers and therapies for the child have proven successful in preventing the disorder.

Struggled attempts to produce speech
Presence of the schwa vowel "uh" during dysfluencies
Tongue, lip, and/or jaw tremor
Excessive repetitions, prolongations, and blocks
Circumlocutions
Lack of eye contact
Pitch rise during struggled speech
Airflow interruptions-gasping
Pauses within word boundaries
Fear of speech
Speech frustration

Figure 12.10 *Indicators of stuttering in children (Source: Tanner, 1990)*

D. Stuttering Variability in Children

Stuttering is a highly variable disorder, especially during early stages of onset. Some children who stutter may only struggle on a few sounds or words or in specific situations, while others may stutter on most of their words and in many situations. Stuttering may come on rapidly in some children, and in others it may take months and years to develop fully. In some cases, the disorder may be obvious during the school year yet apparently disappear during the summer months. Some stutterers report that their stuttering began because of a shift of handedness and that when they returned to their natural handedness, the stuttering disappeared. Most people stutter more when under stress, while some others stutter when they are relaxed. Stuttering may be an inconvenience for one child and devastating for another. The factors discussed below that usually affect the frequency and severity of stuttering in children include singing, audience threat, fatigue, masking noise, and the general propositionality of speech. (Alcohol consumption affects speech fluency in adults.)

Most people who stutter can sing normally and without stuttering. There are several reasons why most stutterers can sing and not stutter. First, singing uses additional areas of the brain that are not typically used during speech. The rhythmic patterns of speech and singing are controlled differently. Second, singing without stuttering may also result from the rhythm of the tune. The imposed rhythm of the song causes the words to be timed easier and more smoothly. Third, when a person sings, he or she may adopt a different role, the role of entertainer which diminishes the insecurity and speaking fear. Finally, most songs are rehearsed, and the frequent practice may also contribute to the normal fluency during singing.

Stutterers usually do not stutter when talking to animals or children, aloud to themselves, or through a hand puppet. Conversely, most stutterers stutter more when talking to lawyers, judges, doctors, teachers, the police, and potential mates. The degree to which an audience is threatening affects most stutterers, and the more threatening the audience, the more stuttering there is. In most people who stutter, the extent of stuttering is a barometer of how threatening they perceive the audience.

People who stutter can speak normally when repeating what has been spoken by someone else. They can also talk fluently when doing so in unison with other speakers. For most stutterers, loud background sound or masking noise provided through earphones improves their speech fluency. Fatigue causes some people to stutter more severely, while others report that being tired improves fluency. Alcohol consumption causes improved fluency in most people who stutter, and some stutterers report that even the weather can affect their speech fluency. As a rule in stuttering, as the propositionality of an utterance increases, so does the likelihood of stuttering. Propositionality is the importance and significance of an utterance.

E. Essentials of Stuttering Treatment

The comprehensive treatment of stuttering involves addressing four factors: audible symptoms, visible features, anxiety and associated negative emotions, and personality factors (Tanner, 2006; Tanner, 2003; Tanner, 1999; Tanner, 1994; Tanner, Belliveau, and Siebert, 1995). Regardless of whether the client is a child or an adult, the four factors are addressed in any comprehensive treatment regime. Not all factors need to receive extensive focus, but because of the complexities, of stuttering each is addressed more or less.

Early in the treatment of stuttering it was discovered that if a stutterer is told, "Do not stutter" the result was actually an increase in stuttering. Telling a person who stutters to stop the act actually increases the behavior because of increased self-consciousness, anxiety, and tension. However, if the stutterer is taught to stutter unobtrusively, e.g., lightly, gently, and easily, the audible features can be reduced to the point where most people do not detect the disorder. The stutterer has permission to stutter but minimizes the behavior. This approach to therapy was developed by Dr. Charles Van Riper and is the therapy of choice for this aspect of the disorder. It is called by several names including fluent stuttering, the Van Riper Approach, and symptom modification. There are other approaches to removing or reducing the audible symptoms, including behavior modification and systematic desensitization. However, the fluent stuttering approach is time tested and has a high success rate in treating both children and adults who stutter.

The visible features of stuttering include eye squints, hand slaps, head nods, lack of eye contact, etc. They are the result of avoidance and escape behaviors where the stutterer attempts to avoid or stop the moment of stuttering. They tend to be superstitious in that the stutterer believes they help, but the results are only temporary improvements in speech fluency. Over time, the person who stutters acquires several visible features which are activated immediately before and during the moment of stuttering. Behavior modification is successful in eliminating these accessory or secondary features of stuttering. Operant conditioning is used to reward normal visible features during speech and discourage abnormal ones.

Not all people who stutter experience anxiety and negative emotions before, during, or after the moment of stuttering. Stutterers also have anxiety-free normal nonfluencies like everyone else. However, in the majority of the cases stuttering is anxiety and tension based. The more the anxiety and tension, the more the stuttering. In addressing the anxiety and associated negative emotions of stuttering, systematic desensitization is used (Brutten and Shoemaker, 1967). The person who stutters becomes relaxed and calm, and the stuttering stimuli are gradually and systematically presented to him or her. The stuttering stimuli are sounds, words, situations, and people. As a result, there is an elimination of the anxiety and associated negative emotions that have been paired with the stuttering stimuli. In this aspect of therapy, stuttering is treated in the same way as other phobias.

The effects of stuttering on personality depend on the duration and severity of the disorder and the age of the stut-terer. Studies have shown that, as a group, people who stutter are disturbed by the disorder, but not psychologically devastated; it affects their personality but not profoundly. As expected, their speech-related self-esteem suffers, and there is evidence of general self-concept disturbances. Children are understandably concerned about peer rejection, and their academic performance may suffer. Comprehensive stuttering therapy involves improving general and speech-related self-esteem and, for those who do not eliminate the disorder, strategies for dealing with rejection.

In adults who have stuttered for years, the psychological, cognitive, and behavior patterns of stuttering are so ingrained that completely eliminating the disorder may be an unrealistic goal. The response strength of stuttering for many years may be resistance to elimination. For some adults who have stuttered for many years, the idea of curing stuttering is unrealistic, and the clinical objective is to control the disorder. Some experts on stuttering liken this approach to the treatment of alcoholism. The stutterer always has the propensity to stutter, but by attending to certain attitudes, thoughts, and behaviors, the disorder can be controlled. However, in children and adolescents, it is realistic to seek a cure for the disorder. Although the person cured of stuttering may always remember being a young stutterer, the disorder can be effectively eliminated. Uncontrolled stuttering in adults can be a source of litigation such as the case of a person denied candidacy for firefighter training. See, for example, *Columbus v Liebhart,* 86 Ohio App3d 469, 621 NE2d 554 (Ohio App 10 Dist 1993).

The treatment of stuttering in the schools is controversial. Many clinicians complain that they do not have the expertise or the time to treat properly young confirmed stutterers (Tanner and Derrick, 1981). Goldberg (2002, p. 1) notes that in the best of situations in many public schools, a stutterer may receive no more than forty minutes of therapy per week, and most of that in group sessions: "In group settings, your child may have individual attention for as little as 10 minutes per session. Both of these limited time treatment approaches are inefficient and ineffective." For a true cure of the young stutterer, therapy must be provided intensively, include family and teachers, and involve individual and group sessions. Individual therapy should be provided for a minimum of three hourly sessions per week with additional group therapy. Time should also be provided for counseling teachers, parents, and other relatives. In school-aged children, the therapy may continue for several school years. The minimum duration of time necessary to know whether the disorder is controlled or eliminated is two years. However, even after two years some children require booster sessions to maintain normal levels of fluency.

12.15 The Individuals with Disabilities Education Act (IDEA)

Federal law guarantees all children the right to a free and appropriate education program, and the IEP details the services provided to children in special education. The Individuals with Disabilities Education Act of 1997 (IDEA) requires that eligible children with disabilities receive free and appropriate public education (FAPE) and related services in the least restrictive environment (LRE). The Individualized Education Plan, sometimes called the Individualized Education Program, describes the services provided to the child, and failure to provide one can be a source of litigation. Because of no or an unacceptable IEP, parents sometimes enroll their children in private schools and sue to have the public schools pay for the services.

All IEPs must include the following:

1. Projected dates for initiation of services.
2. Anticipated duration of services.
3. The extent to which the child will be able to participate in regular classroom activities.
4. A statement of the child's present level of educational performance.
5. List of short-term and long-term objectives.
6. A statement of annual goals.
7. Appropriate objective criteria and evaluation procedures to determine whether the objectives are being met.

Most students in special education should have a completed IEP before the delivery of services. However, a relatively new federal program, "Response to Intervention," allows the provision of some speech and hearing services without entering the realm of special education to determine if short-term therapy would alleviate the problem.

Special education departments are required to review annually each child's IEP. An annual IEP meeting is held with the child's parents (or surrogate parents) and the special education team, the composition of which is established by law for each type of disability. During the meeting, there is a review of the evaluation results for new enrollees or a progress report made on the current IEP. If changes are made to the IEP, written notices are given and the appropriate signatures obtained. During the IEP meeting, parents are expected to advocate for their children, be participants in goal setting, and be critical of progress. Sometimes the children are also invited to attend the IEP meeting. A source of litigation can involve the type and nature of the services to speech-impaired children. See *Matter of Anthony E., 159*

Misc2d 508, 605 NYS2d 645 (Fam Ct 1993). In a preliminary study, Tanner and Guzzino (2002) found that issues related to IDEA were the most frequent sources of litigation for speech-language pathologists and audiologists over a ten-year period.

Federal and state laws protect the rights of parents and children with disabilities. The Arizona Department of Education, Exceptional Student Services Division (1999), has detailed the special education rights of parents and children under federal and state laws. Below is a summary of those rights, especially as they pertain to children with communication disorders.

1. Children suspected of having communication disorders are to be evaluated at no charge, and the results supplied to the parents within 60 calendar days of receipt of written parental consent. A reevaluation can be conducted without parental consent if reasonable measures were taken to obtain parental consent and there was no response from the parents. Parents have the right and the responsibly to be a part of all aspects of their children's free and appropriate public education.

2. There are three written notices supplied to parents: Procedural Safeguards Notice, Prior Written Notice, and Meeting Notice. The Procedural Safeguards Notice explains the rights of parents and the child throughout the special education process. The Prior Written Notice details what the school proposes or refuses to do, states how the decision was reached, and provides a description of test and evaluation results. The Prior Written Notice must contain a statement that the parent and child have protection under the Procedural Safeguards Notice. The Meeting Notice informs the parents of the purpose, time, and location of any meeting concerning the identification, evaluation, educational placement of the child, or provision of special education. These written notices must be in the language spoken by parent or interpreted and adapted to any communication limitations.

3. In providing FAPE, there are provisions for surrogate parents, transfer of rights, and parental access to educational records.

4. Schools are required to permit and fund an Independent Educational Evaluation (IEE) if parents disagree with the results of the school's evaluation.

According to the Arizona Department of Education, Exceptional Student Services Division (1999, p. 6), schools may be required to reimburse a parent for the cost of private school placement under certain circumstances:

These reimbursement provisions apply only if your child previously received special education and related services under the authority of a public agency, and you enrolled your child in a private elementary or secondary school or facility without our consent or referral. Under these circumstances, reimbursement can be ordered if a court or hearing officer finds that we did not make a free appropriate public education available to your child in a timely manner before you enrolled your child in the private school or facility.

Unilateral placement of children with communication disorders by parents, and their subsequent request for reimbursement, is a common source of litigation See for example, *Livingston v DeSoto Country School District,* 782 FSupp 1173 (ND Miss 1992). Placement issues also involve enrollment in extended school year services for children with communication disorders. See *Myles v Montgomery Country Board of Education,* 824 FSupp 1549 (MD Ala 1993).

12.16 Disputes, Mediation, and Due Process

When parents of children with communication disorders disagree with the identification, evaluation, educational placement, or provision of FAPE, mediation and complaints through the State are available, and the resolution process is specified for both parties (Arizona Department of Education, Exceptional Student Services Division, 1999). The school district also may request mediation, but both parties must agree to the process. If parents choose not to participate in mediation, they may be required to meet with a disinterested party from one of the parent information centers or another appropriate dispute resolution group, and have the benefits of mediation explained. Discussions that occur during the process may not be used as evidence in any subsequent proceeding, and the parties may be required to sign a confidentiality document before beginning mediation.

Parents have the right to file a written complaint with the state alleging that a school is not complying with federal or state special education laws and regulations. Complaints need to be filed within one calendar year of the alleged violation, although longer periods are considered if the viola-

tion or violations are ongoing. The state investigates the complaint and may conduct an on-site investigation if deemed necessary. The results of the investigation are reported within sixty calendar days. A corrective plan is initiated if warranted by the investigation.

An Impartial Due Process Hearing (IDPH) is used to resolve disputes between schools and parents. This involves an impartial and trained third party familiar with state laws, the Individuals with Disabilities Education Act Amendments of 1997 (IDEA), and other relevant laws and regulations. The due process hearing results must be delivered to both parties forty-five calendar days after the written request was submitted. The decision can also be appealed through administrative review. Unless both parties agree, there will be no change in the child's placement during the dispute resolution procedures.

12.17 Stuttering Misdiagnosis

As reported previously, diagnosing stuttering in children requires knowledge of both normal and abnormal speech nonfluencies. Some children are simply going though a temporary stage of excessive normal nonfluencies, while others are showing signs that they are in the first stages of what may be a lifetime of stuttering. The diagnosis of stuttering is a complex and detailed process, and false positive and false negative diagnoses may result in litigation.

A false positive diagnosis is where a child is diagnosed as a stutterer or likely to become one, when in fact he or she is normally nonfluent. Normal nonfluencies are diagnosed as stuttering, and the child is placed in stuttering therapy. Because of this misdiagnosis, the child's normal nonfluencies are brought to his or her attention, and he or she can be made to feel self-conscious, anxious, and tense during speech. As a result, anxiety and negative emotions are paired with the dysfluencies, and the child may begin to stutter. The child may have been predisposed to the stuttering, and the wrongful placement in therapy precipitated and perpetuated the disorder. Had a proper evaluation and counseling been conducted, the child would have been spared a possible lifetime of stuttering. Understandably, when parents and the stutterer are provided the facts regarding the self-fulfilling prophecy of stuttering diagnosis, they may seek damages from the school and/or the clinician responsible for the misdiagnosis.

A false negative diagnosis occurs when a child is in the early stages of stuttering but the school and the clinician do not detect it. The child is a true stutterer but because of the misdiagnosis of stuttering symptoms as normal nonfluencies, he or she is not placed in therapy in a timely manner. Valuable therapies are delayed because of the misdiagnosis. Stuttering therapy is most effective when provided as soon as possible after the onset of the disorder. The stuttering thoughts, feelings, attitudes, and behaviors are not as ingrained and habitual during the initial course of the disorder and consequently are more easily changed or eliminated.

Misdiagnosis of stuttering can also involve ineffectual preventative measures. Stuttering is preventable even in those children predisposed to it when environmental precipitating factors are eliminated. There are several stuttering prevention strategies and programs available; they involve removing stress, self-consciousness, and fear from the child's speech. They also involve improving the child's speech-related self-esteem. Usually parents and teachers are counseled, and often the child is not seen for direct therapy. The success rate in preventing stuttering is far greater than in curing it.

Stuttering can occur as an unwanted consequence of articulation or language therapy. Several studies have shown that children who stutter also have a higher occurrence of other communication disorders. Articulation and language therapies involve bringing speech errors to the attention of the child and encouraging him or her to correct them. In most cases, this is done in an accepting, tolerant manner, and negativity over speech imperfections is minimized. However, in rare instances too much pressure may be placed on the child for speech improvement, and he or she may begin to stutter. The child is required to produce a sound or sound combinations that are beyond his or her physical capabilities, and he or she forces speech musculature, becoming anxious and tense. There is verbal impotence, a feeling of being out of control. The negative spiral of stuttered speech and speech negativity is set in motion. If the clinician recognizes the problem, stuttering preventative measures can be taken and the disorder rapidly eliminated. It may be prudent to discharge the child from articulation or language therapy at this time. However, the clinician can miss the signs of incipient stuttering, or the child may be resistant to the preventative measures, and consequently permanent stuttering may result. The parents and the stutterer may not be aware of the cause of stuttering for months, or even years, after the onset.

12.18 A Case Study of Alleged Sexual Harassment and Stuttering

An adolescent with severe stuttering made very few gains in eliminating or controlling the disorder even though he received therapy for most of his life. He displayed several accessory features during the moment of stuttering because of avoidance and escape behaviors. One of the accessory features was rapidly protruding his tongue. During a stuttering moment, he would protrude and retract his tongue several times, especially during blocks. The behavior was so extensive that he damaged and scarred the surface of his tongue. Several behavior management techniques were used to modify or eliminate the tongue protrusions. The most successful procedure was to reward the incompatible behavior of talking with clenched teeth. Protruding the tongue and having clenched teeth are incompatible behaviors. The long-term goal of therapy was to eliminate both the tongue protrusions and clenched teeth. Unfortunately, the tongue protrusions had occurred for many years, and the behavior was resistant to elimination. The stutterer also engaged in nasal snorting during attempts to speak. Because this person had been in stuttering therapy for many years with poor results, he was finally encouraged to accept the disorder as a permanent part of his life. Long-term goals of therapy were changed from attempting to overcome the disorder, to accepting it. He was discharged from stuttering therapy with continued severe symptoms involving tongue protrusion and nasal snorting behaviors.

Several years after being discharged from therapy, he was accused of sexually harassing a woman in a laundromat. She complained to the police that he engaged in nonverbal sexually suggestive acts to her. The woman said he approached her and made sexually obscene tongue and lip movements, and when she turned away he grasped her arm. She reported the events to the police, and he was arrested. The stutterer told the court of his stuttering problem, and stated that he was simply requesting change for a washing machine. He explained that when she turned away, grasping her arm was an attempt to delay her for more time to clarify the request.

The stutterer did approach the woman in the laundromat and in his typical stuttering manner attempted to ask her for change. The woman was understandably startled by his manner, and her fearful reactions caused him to be even more verbally impotent, thus producing more bizarre accessory symptoms. Here, the stutterer's actions were misinterpreted by the woman. He was not sexually harassing her. The court was told of his longstanding stuttering accessory features and the likelihood that his actions were innocent and merely typical symptoms of his communication disorder.

12.19 Case Study in Childhood Language Disorders Litigation

The parents of a four-year-old male brought a medical malpractice suit against an obstetrician alleging that preventable complications occurred during pregnancy and delivery. Consequently, the child allegedly suffered several birth abnormalities and defects including spastic hemiplegia and suspected language delay and dysarthria. There were two normal older children in the family, and the eldest brother and father had a history of communication disorders and special education placement. The eldest brother had subsequently been discharged from special education and the father was a practicing attorney. Central to the issues involved in the medical malpractice suit were the definitions and clinical manifestations of spastic dysarthria versus apraxia of speech, and, if the child suffered from the latter, whether or not it was an inherited disorder. If spastic dysarthria is determined to be inherited and typical of the brother and father's disabilities, then the communication disorder might not be a result of the preventable complications. The following are the opinions of the merits of the case supplied by the plaintiff's expert witness. (Identifying information has been changed for privacy purposes.)

You have requested my opinion regarding the nature, etiology, symptoms, and prognosis for (Child)'s motor speech disorder. Having reviewed pertinent medical records and psycho educational reports, and conducting interviews with his mother and father, I believe I have sufficient information to provide the following opinions:

1. (Child) suffers from severe spastic dysarthria consistent with spastic cerebral palsy and resulting hemiparesis. Of the five basic motor speech processes (respiration, phonation, articulation, resonance, prosody) that can be compromised in spastic dysarthria, his speech symptoms are primarily limited to the articulatory mechanism.

2. (Child)'s spastic dysarthria is typical and characteristic of upper motor neuron damage resulting from cerebral anoxia. I believe that his motor speech symptoms, as present thus far, are probably a result of the spastic hemiparesis. Based on the evaluation conducted on him, I do not believe his primary symptoms are a result of apraxia of speech, also a motor speech disorder. Apraxia of speech is a speech conceptualizing, programming, and planning disorder for volitional movements. (Child)'s speech is typical of many adult and pediatric spastic dysarthria patients I have evaluated, and consistent with research showing the damage to be of the upper motor neurons. I find

nothing unusual about his cerebral palsy speech symptoms or the likely cause of them.

3. For (Child) to make maximal gains in motor speech habilitation and to maintain them, he will probably need speech pathology services throughout his lifetime. With regular therapy, it is likely that his speech will be 75% intelligible for two and three word utterances.

3. You have asked my opinion about whether his motor speech disorder is of genetic origin because his brother has experienced a communication disorder. Having reviewed (Brother)'s evaluation, it is my opinion that he does have apraxia of speech as a component of his communication disorder. I am certain, however, that (Child)'s motor speech disorder, and (Brother)'s communication disorders are fundamentally different, caused by different conditions, and not genetically related or inherited. There are no relevant histories in paternal or maternal pedigrees for motor speech disorders or phonological disorders. Having reviewed the literature on the subject of genetics and communication disorders, (especially Lewis, B. A., 1990, Familial phonological disorders: Four pedigrees, *Journal of Speech and hearing Disorders*, Vol. 55, 160-170, and others), I find it improbable that (Child)'s motor speech disorder, in part or whole, is an inherited malady.

This case was settled out of court with the child receiving an undisclosed amount for special education, medical, and other related services.

12.20 Chapter Summary

The primary childhood communication disorders are language, articulation disorders, and fluency. Because of federal laws such as the Individuals with Disabilities Education Act (IDEA), the schools are responsible for providing communication-disordered children with a free and appropriate public education (FAPE). Issues related to IDEA and FAPE are common sources of litigation in childhood communication disorders. Pivotal to these issues are the accuracy of diagnoses and the appropriateness of Individual Education Plans (IEPs) where the long-term and short-term goals of articulation, language, and fluency disorders are detailed and the methods by which they are to be achieved are detailed.

Suggested Readings and Resources

Ruben, R.J. (2000). Redefining the survival of the fittest: Communication disorders in the 21ˢᵗ century. *Laryngoscope, 110*: 241-245. This article provides data about the effects of communication disorders on vocational opportunities in the 21st century.

Tanner, D. (1999). *Understanding Stuttering: A Guide for Parents.* Oceanside, CA.: Academic Communication Associates. This pamphlet explains childhood stuttering in easy to understand terminology.

Tanner, D. (2003). *Exploring Communication Disorders: A 21st Century Introduction Through Literature and Media.* Boston: Allyn & Bacon. This book has several chapters addressing childhood communication disorders and uses references to literature and media to introduce and explain them.

Tanner, D. (2006). *Case Studies in Communication Sciences and Disorders.* Upper Saddle River, NJ: Pearson Merrill Prentice Hall. Several chapters of this book address communication disorders in children including case studies illustrating litigation issues.

Tanner, D. (2006). *An Advanced Course in Communication Sciences and Disorders.* San Diego: Plural Publishing. This book addresses scientific and philosophical issues in childhood communication disorders and describes the Unified Model of Communication Sciences and Disorders.

Van Riper, C. (1992). *The Nature of Stuttering* (2nd ed.). Englewood Cliffs, NJ: Prentice-Hall. (Reissued by Waveland Press, Prospect Heights, Illinois). This is the classic text on the nature of stuttering.

Wiig, E. and Secord, W. (1998). Language disabilities and school-age children and youth. In G. Shames, E. Wiig, and W. Secord (Eds), *Human Communication Disorders: An Introduction* (5ᵗʰ ed.) Boston: Allyn & Bacon. This chapter provides detailed information about language delay and disorders in children.

References

American Association on Mental Retardation (2006). Retrieved May 15, 2006 from the World Wide Web: http://www.aamr.org/.

Arizona Department of Education, Exceptional Student Services Division (1999). Special education rights of parents and children under federal and state requirements. Revised by ADE/ESS 10/14/99. Phoenix: Arizona Department of Education.

Arizona Department of Education. (2000). ADE School Support Programs. Retrieved September 13, 2000, from the World Wide Web: //www.ade.az.gov/ess.

Bloodstein, O. (1995). *A handbook on stuttering* (5th ed.). San Diego: Singular.

Brutten, G.J., and Shoemaker, D. (1967). *The modification of stuttering.* Englewood Cliffs, NJ:Prentice-Hall.

Flagstaff Unified School District No. One (2001). *Special education manual.* Flagstaff, Arizona.

Goldberg, S. (2002). Reaching out. *The Association of Young People Who Stutter.* Pacifica, CA:

Grossman, H. (1983). *Classification in mental retardation.* Washington, DC: American Association on Mental Deficiency.

Hart, B., and Risley, T. (1995). *Meaningful differences in the everyday experience of young American children.* Baltimore: Paul H. Brookes.

Haynes, W.O., and Shulman, B. (1998). *Communication development.* Baltimore: Williams & Wilkins.

Haynes, W.O., and Pindzola, R. (2004). *Diagnosis and evaluation in speech pathology.* Boston: Allyn & Bacon.

Hirsch, D. (1998). Ask the doctor: Pervasive developmental disorders. *Exceptional parent.* Oradell, NJ.

Moore-Brown, B., Sanger, D., Montgomery, J. and Mishida, B., (2002). Communication and violence: New roles for speech-language pathologists. *The ASHA Leader*, Vol. 6, No. 6. April 30

National Institute of Neurological and Communicative Disorders and Stroke. (1988). *Developmental speech and language disorders: Hope through research.* Bethesda, MD: National Institutes of Health.

Nicolosi, L, Harryman, E., and Kresheck, J. (2004). *Terminology of communication disorders (5ᵗʰ ed).* Baltimore: Lippincott Williams & Wilkins.

Norris, J.A. (1998). Psycholinguistic foundations of communication development. In W. Haynes and B. Shulman (Eds), *Communication development: Foundations, processes, and clinical applications.* Baltimore: Williams & Wilkins.

Owens, R. (1998). Development of communication, language, and speech. In G. Shames, E. Wiig, and W. Secord (Eds), *Human communication disorders: An introduction* (5th ed.). Boston: Allyn & Bacon.

Owens, R., Metz, D.E., and Haas, A. (2000). *Communication disorders: A life span perspective.* Boston: Allyn & Bacon.

Plante, E. and Beeson, P. (2004). *Communication and communication disorders: A clinical introduction.* (2nd ed.). Boston: Allyn & Bacon.

Ruben, R.J. (2000). Redefining the survival of the fittest: Communication disorders in the 21st century. *Laryngoscope, 110*: 241-245.

Sanger, D., Moore-Brown, B., Magnuson, G. and Svoboda, N. (2001). Prevalence of language problems among adolescent delinquents: A closer look. *Communication Disorders Quarterly*, 23(1), 17-25.

Tanner, D. (1990). *Assessment of stuttering behaviors.* Oceanside, CA: Academic Communication Associates.

Tanner, D. (1994). *Pragmatic stuttering intervention for children* (2nd ed.). Oceanside, CA.: Academic Communication Associates.

Tanner, D. (1997). *Handbook for the speech-language pathology assistant.* Oceanside, CA: Academic Communication Associates.

Tanner, D. (1999). *Understanding stuttering: A guide for parents.* Oceanside, CA.: Academic Communication Associates.

Tanner, D. (2003). *Exploring neurogenic communication disorders: A 21st century approach through literature and media.* Boston: Allyn & Bacon.

Tanner, D. (2006). *Case studies in communication sciences and disorders.* Upper Saddle River, N.J.: Pearson Merrill Prentice Hall.

Tanner, D., Goedde, K. and Broom, C. (1979). An examination of communication disorders in Head Start children. A paper presented to the Annual Convention of the American Speech-Language-Hearing Association, Atlanta.

Tanner, D. and Derrick, G. (1981). The treatment of stuttering in Arizona public schools. *Journal of the Arizona Communication and Theatre Association*, Volume XII, No. 2.

Tanner, D., and Lamb, W. (1984). *The cognitive, linguistic, and social-communicative scales.* Tulsa: Modern Education Corporation.

Tanner, D., Seamon, M., Nye, C. and Lamb, W. (1988). Direct and indirect measurements of preschool versus non-preschool language enhancement. A paper presented at the Annual Convention of the American Speech-Language-Hearing Association, Boston.

Tanner, D., Belliveau, W. and Siebert, G. (1995). *Pragmatic stuttering intervention for adolescents and adults.* Oceanside, CA: Academic Communication Associates.

Tanner, D., Culbertson, W., and Secord, W. (1997). *Developmental articulation and phonology profile (DAPP).* Oceanside, CA: Academic Communication Associates.

Tanner, D., Lamb, W., and Secord, W. (1997). *The cognitive, linguistic and social-communicative scales* (2nd ed.). Oceanside, CA: Academic Communication Associates.

Tanner, D. and Guzzino, A. (2002, April). Westlaw search of litigation areas in communication sciences and disorders: A paper presented at the 2001-2002 Honors Day Program. Northern Arizona University, Flagstaff, Arizona.

Van Gent, T., Heijnen, C., and Treffers, P. (1997). Autism and the immune system. *Journal of Child Psychology and Psychiatry.* 38(3): 337-349.

Van Riper, C. (1973). *The treatment of stuttering.* Englewood Cliffs, NJ: Prentice-Hall.

Van Riper, C. (1992). *The nature of stuttering* (2nd ed.). Englewood Cliffs, NJ: Prentice-Hall. (Reissued by Waveland Press, Prospect Heights, Illinois).

Van Riper, C., and Erickson, R. (1996). *Speech correction* (9th ed.). Boston: Allyn & Bacon.

Wetherby, A. (2000). *Understanding and enhancing communication and language for young children with autism spectrum disorders.* Flagstaff, AZ: Northern Arizona University.

Wiig, E. and Secord, W. (1998). Language disabilities and school-age children and youth. In G. Shames, E. Wiig, and W. Secord (Eds), *Human communication disorders: An introduction* (5th ed.). Boston: Allyn & Bacon.

Chapter 13

Medical-Legal and Forensic Aspects of Communication Disorders Resulting from Dementia

13.1 Chapter Preview

In this chapter, reversible and irreversible dementias are discussed including their causes and treatments. There is a review of Alzheimer's disease, dementia resulting from multiple infarcts and other neurological diseases and deficits. The communication disorders seen in dementia are discussed including pragmatic deficits, circumlocutions, confabulation, perseveration-echolalia, logorrhea, and tangential speech. Although dementia patients, as a group, cannot benefit from speech and language rehabilitation, individuals may benefit from direct and indirect intervention and patient management procedures. There is also an analysis of the role dementia-related communication disorders play in determining mental competence and other medical-legal and forensic issues.

13.2 Reversible and Irreversible Dementia

Dementia is the progressive loss of previously acquired mental functioning. Davis (2007) observes that dementia is a general category of cognitive deficits with many causes. Deterioration of the personality and communicative functions are considered to be part of dementia (Bayles, 1994). Other terms and conditions associated with progressive general mental deterioration include senility, mental and cognitive deterioration, organic brain disease (OBD), and generalized intellectual impairment (GII). Delirium is a state of disordered thinking where the patient is confused and disoriented. However, in delirium, the patient also is hyperactive, agitated, and distracted. Dementia is a frightening condition because many early symptoms of the disorder can resemble normal forgetfulness, and as it progresses, the person may become completely mentally impaired and dependent on others. Dementia jeopardizes the basic integrity of the self and is the ultimate psychological threat. Many diseases and disorders causing dementia are fatal.

One of the most common misconceptions about dementia is that it is a natural and normal part of the aging process. Dementia is a product of pathological aging. Although many people in their later decades of life lose mental acuity, the clinical symptoms of dementia are a result of pathological aging. Certainly, dementia is a frequent occurrence in the elderly, but it is not a necessary aspect of a lengthy life. With the dramatic increase in the life span of Americans, more people are living into their seventh, eighth, ninth decades, and beyond. And with the aging of the baby-boom generation, the number of demented patient in the United States has increased and will continue to do so. It is estimated that by 2050, 14.4 million Americans could have dementia (Ripich and Ziol, 1998). Ripich and Ziol go on to note that as many as 50 percent of people by the age of eighty-five have some of the symptoms of dementia and that currently it touches one in three families.

With regard to rehabilitation, there are two types of dementia: reversible and irreversible. Reversible dementia, sometimes called pseudo-dementia, is the type of generalized intellectual impairment that can be successfully treated or that resolves on its own, and several medical conditions can cause it. A frequent cause of reversible dementia is abuse of prescription medications. When most patients stop the abuse of the medication or cease taking a combination of drugs, the cognitive and intellectual impairments are reversed. Transient ischemic attacks (TIAs) also cause reversible dementia. A TIA is a temporary interruption of the blood flow to the brain due to partial occlusion of one or more arteries. TIAs are similar to strokes, but the blood flow to the brain is interrupted for fewer than twenty-four hours and the symptoms are temporary. Transient ischemic attacks can cause the cognitive and intellectual changes seen in dementia, and some people may have multiple episodes. Other causes of reversible dementia include tumors and biochemical deficiencies that when removed or corrected improve the patient's cognitive functioning. Severe organic depression can cause some people to appear demented. In reversible dementia, when the underlying cause of the disorder is successfully treated, all or part of the cognitive and intellectual deterioration resolves. Unfortunately, only a small percentage of dementias are completely reversible or can be arrested. Davis (2007) reports that the most common types of reversible dementia are depression, alcohol abuse, and drug toxicity. Most dementias are not responsive to treatments and do not resolve on their own.

The early symptoms of irreversible dementia are often minor memory deficits or temporary bouts of confusion. As irreversible dementia progresses, there may be severe disorientation, amnesia, and speech and language pathologies. Most types of dementia are variable and progressive; however, some types are relatively unchanging.

Alzheimer's disease and multiple infarct vascular disturbances are the most common causes of dementia. Toxins, heavy metal poisoning, fever, genes, a history of head trauma, and Parkinson's, Pick's, and other neurological diseases are also linked to dementia. The areas of the brain damaged in dementia depend on the type of dementia-causing disease or disorder. The hippocampus, located in the temporal lobe of the brain, is important for memory, orientation, and learning, and is considered a likely site of the lesion in many dementia-causing diseases and disorders. Diseases of other organs of the body, such as the kidneys, pancreas, and liver can also cause dementia. Toxin-induced dementia include those resulting from exposure to poisons. Heavy metals that build up in the body can cause dementia. Extremely high fevers can damage brain cells and result in cognitive and intellectual impairments. One occurrence of a head trauma, or repeated head traumas such as are often experienced by professional boxers, is associated with dementia. There is some evidence that early onset dementia (progressive cognitive and intellectual deterioration at a relatively young age) is related to an occurrence of childhood traumatic brain injury. Parkinson's disease, a result of damage to the basal ganglia and a deficiency of the neurotransmitter dopamine can cause dementia, particularly during its late stages. Pick's disease causes a deterioration of the tem-

poral and frontal lobes of the brain (Ripich and Ziol, 1998), leading to dementia. Acquired Immune Deficiency Syndrome (AIDS) and late-stage syphilis can also result in dementia. The dementia seen in AIDS patients is called AIDS Dementia Complex.

Alzheimer's disease accounts for about one-half of the cases of irreversible dementia (Hooper and Bayles, 2001). It is the fourth leading cause of death in the United States (Kennedy, 1999). Alzheimer's disease is difficult to diagnose as the cause of irreversible dementia, and until recently, the only way to confirm it was by autopsy. However, today there are neuropsychological tests, biochemical analyses, and brain scanning technologies that are useful in confirming the disease. Divergent diagnostic criteria for Alzheimer's disease also affect the accuracy of diagnosis. Research has shown that women tend to have a higher risk for Alzheimer's disease (Ripich and Ziol, 1998).

Vascular dementia is caused by cortical and/or subcortical infarcts. An infarct is the death of tissue due to an interruption of blood flow. Vascular dementia is usually a result of multiple strokes. Vascular dementia may have a more rapid onset of symptoms than what is observed in Alzheimer's disease. In vascular dementia, the number, site, and size of the lesions to the brain cause the patient's symptoms. However, because the brain operates as whole, other factors such as the patient's education, premorbid personality, intelligence, and social support influence the symptoms in vascular dementia. In brain damage, simply projecting the patient's symptoms from the site and size of the lesions is fraught with error. A strict localization approach to brain functioning is insufficient in explaining behavior, particularly language and other aspects of communication (Tanner, 2006; Tanner, 2003b).

Dementia is not synonymous with aphasia. Although aphasia is a multimodality reduction in language usually cutting across all modalities of communication, the aphasic person is not demented. The Linguistic Regression Theory of Aphasia, which postulated that the disorder returns the person to the mentality of a child, has been disproved and discounted. Although these patients tend to be on a concrete level and have disrupted language, other forms and aspects of cognition are available to the patient. Aphasia does not return a person to the intellect of a child (see Chapter 2). Dementia and mental impairment-mental retardation are not one in the same because the cognitive and intellectual impairments seen in dementia are a decline in previously acquired cognitive abilities. Dementia and psychosis are not interchangeable diagnoses. A patient who has lost contact with reality is not necessarily demented. However, aphasic, mentally impaired-mentally retarded, and psychotic people may also have dementia, and vice versa.

Patients with dementia often become disruptive. They will not take instruction, follow requests, or cooperate with caregivers. With some demented patients, there is social disinhibition, impulsiveness, and aggressiveness. They can strike out and injure family and staff. There are four major sources of disruptive behavior occurring in dementia: organic or physically related causes, environmental precipitants, cognitive origins, and emotional factors (Hartke, 1991).

Organic and physically related causes of disruptive behavior include pain, sensory losses, medication reactions, illness, fatigue, and acute confusional states. Environmental precipitants include changes in caregivers or routine, noise, lack of privacy, and unfamiliar people. Cognitive origins include impairments of memory, communication, insight, judgment, and problem solving. Emotional factors include anxiety, depression, lowered self-esteem, attention seeking, fear, and suspicion.

13.3 Communication Disorders in Multiple-Infarct-Induced Dementia

The neurogenic communication disorders seen in multiple infarct dementia depend on the type of brain damage and/or the nature of the neurological impairments. Although most dementias present with learning, memory, behavioral, and orientation impairments, those caused by toxins, heavy metal poisoning, traumatic brain injuries, fever, and certain neurological diseases may also cause varying degrees of aphasia, apraxia of speech, and the dysarthrias. For patients suffering from vascular dementia, the size of the infarcts is important in deciding the severity of the neurogenic communication disorders. The site of the brain damage also influences the nature of the neurogenic communication disorders because some vascular dementias include damage to the speech and language centers of the brain and the tracts leading to and from them. Besides the dementia, these patients also present with unusual symptoms of aphasia, apraxia of speech, and/or the dysarthrias. However, through careful testing, the expressive language, auditory comprehension, and motor speech deficits can be detected through the cloud of dementia.

Aphasia is divided into predominantly expressive and predominately receptive categories. The disorder, to various degrees, impairs reading, writing, speaking, and understanding the speech of others. (See Chapter 9 for a comprehensive discussion of aphasia.) Indications that Broca's and Wernicke's areas of the brain and the tracts leading to and from them have been damaged can be observed by whether the patient has nonfluent or fluent speech output. Demented patients who speak haltingly with hesitations and reduced cadence and melody of speech and with word-finding problems often also have symptoms of expressive aphasia. The nonfluent word-finding problems can occur on confrontation naming tasks and during spontaneous speech. The patient with dementia may also be disorientated, impaired with regard to memory, have deficiencies in judgment and intellect, and have symptoms of nonfluent aphasia. The symptoms of nonfluent aphasia will be present and detectible during conversations with the patient. Typically, patients with dementia-related aphasia will have association and approximation naming errors. They will substitute a word that is semantically related or rhymes with the word they have trouble remembering or uttering. Many demented patients with aphasia word-finding problems will also have random naming errors, where the substituted word has no apparent relationship to the desired one. Patients with damage to Wernicke's area of the brain usually present with fluent output. In dementia-related aphasia, fluent jargon is clinically indistinguishable from many other dementia-related symptoms. If they can write, patients with dementia-related aphasias typically write like they speak, and their abilities to read parallel their verbal abilities.

Acalculia is the inability to perform and understand simple mathematics, and dyscalculia is a less severe form of the disorder. There are two aspects of dyscalculia seen in dementia patients and reflect varying degrees of the disorder. In the first aspect of acalculia, the patient is unable to do simple arithmetic or understand monetary values. This is the type of problem typically seen in aphasia where the patient has lost the language of mathematics. Patients cannot make change, answer simple arithmetic questions, or understand mathematical symbols. In the second aspect of acalculia, the demented patient may have lost the language of mathematics and also the ability to appreciate problems related to financial expenditures and mathematical reasoning. Higher level mathematical problem solving and abstraction are lost, especially as they pertain to money. Patients will pay exorbitant amounts of money for insignificant items, although they may be able to write checks or give correct change; the sense of financial responsibility is lost.

Many symptoms discussed above are seen in dementia-related apraxia of speech. This is because apraxia of speech is often a part of expressive aphasia. When the demented patient's motor speech planning and sequencing are disrupted by the brain damage, speech struggle, substitutions, and additions of sounds are apparent in purposeful speech. In nonpurposeful speech, these symptoms are usually absent, and many patients with apraxia of speech can say off-the-cuff statements fluently. This volitional-nonvolitional dichotomy is called an automatic speech phenomenon. Because dementia often affects the patient's awareness of speech errors, self-corrective behaviors will be highly variable. Additionally, in some patients with dementia the motor speech planning and sequencing areas of the brain will be severely damaged, eliminating purposeful speech.

As discussed in Chapter 9, the dysarthrias are a group of communication disorders classified by the site of the neuromuscular damage and the subsequent type of weakness, paralysis, or movement disorders that disrupt motor speech. The dysarthrias affect, to various degrees, respiration, phonation, articulation, resonance, and prosody. When dysarthria occurs in addition to dementia, patients may have slurred, hypernasal, and/or generally indistinct speech. If the patient's respiratory-laryngeal functioning is impaired, he or she also may have a breathy or harsh voice quality. Patients with extrapyramidal disorders, as is sometimes seen in heavy metal poisoning or head traumas, may produce speech slowly and with reduced volume and have the speech characteristics of Parkinsonian dysarthria. Other patients with extrapyramidal disorders may have unwanted movements that disrupt speech production. These unwanted movements can occur slowly, as is seen in athetoid cerebral palsy, or rapidly, as happens with myoclonic jerks and tics. Usually, the dysarthric speech in patients with dementia is easily identified because it is not significantly affected by mental and intellectual deterioration. However, when the dysarthria is severe, the patient may be rendered mute.

Because of the dementia, most patients cannot benefit from aphasia and apraxia of speech therapies. Improving speech programming and sequencing, auditory comprehension, reading, writing, expressive language, etc., in these patients is futile because of the global memory deficits and inability to learn. To profit from these therapies, patients must be able to learn and retain new information in the short and long term. Consequently, most patients with significant dementia are unable to benefit from aphasia and apraxia of speech therapies. As a rule, patients with dysarthria are more likely to benefit from therapy in the early stages of the dementia because the emphasis is on muscular control and functioning. However, because of the progressive nature of dementia and poor prognosis, lengthy treatment of the dysarthria is contraindicated.

13.4 Communication Disorders in Alzheimer's-Disease-Induced Dementia

Most texts on Alzheimer's disease simply chronicle its progression into early, middle, and late stages. However, *Lippincott's Textbook for Clinical Medical Assisting* (1999)

lists seven levels of Alzheimer's disease, providing a more detailed description of the course of the memory deficits, confusion, behavioral problems, and ability to perform activities of daily living (ADLs). At Levels I and II, the brain changes are not significant, and the only remarkable symptom may be forgetfulness. At these two stages the presenile dementia may end with no further progression. At Level III, there are more problems remembering facts, faces, and names, and the person will recognize the problem by becoming increasingly frustrated and angry.

At Level IV, the first problems with ADLs are noted as the patient begins to neglect them. Here the individual is aware of the problems but denies them. This level is considered mild Alzheimer's disease or a late confusional state. Custodial care is required for the patient in Level V because of the severe lapses in memory and disorientation compounded by frustration and anger.

Level VI is moderately severe Alzheimer's disease, and the patient has immense anger, hostility, and combativeness, suffers severe memory loss, and is disoriented most of the time. Interestingly, at Level VI, many patients have fear of water. Patients in late dementia, Level VII, require full-time care and may need tube feeding. Patients in this, the final stage of the progression of the disease, rarely speak and are incontinent.

Bayles (1994) observes that the speech symptoms of Alzheimer's disease are unlikely to be confused with nonfluent aphasia because the motor strip is not affected throughout most of the course of the disease. In the progression of Alzheimer's disease, there is a fundamental deterioration of the semantics, syntactical, and/or phonological aspects of language. Semantics refers to the meanings of words. Syntax is an aspect of the grammatical structure of an utterance: the linguistic rules for arranging words into connected utterances. The phonological aspects of language are the rules governing the way sounds are combined. Beyond the above semantic, syntactic, and phonological aspects of language affected by Alzheimer's diseases the context and intent in which language is used are often impaired. This is the social-communicative function of language, or pragmatics.

Ripich and Ziol (1998) have identified the communication changes seen in early stage Alzheimer's disease. They and others report that syntax and phonology errors are absent during the initial course of the disease. Problems with word order, and the breakdown of the rules by which sounds are combined, are usually not present in patients with early stage Alzheimer's disease. Word fluency may be compromised but, as Bayles (1994) notes, not because of motor speech difficulties. Word fluency is disrupted because of semantic difficulties. In the initial stages of Alzheimer's disease, patients are generally aware of their deficits and may request clarification and confirmation of what has been spoken.

It is in the pragmatic aspects of communication that patients with early stage Alzheimer's disease usually show the most problems. They have difficulty storytelling and giving instructions. During storytelling they may drift and wander from the topic, forget the intent of the story, and go on and on without ever completing it. They may be vague in giving instructions leaving the listener without an understanding of the intent or the actions required. According to Ripich and Ziol (1998), there may be specific difficulties understanding humor, analogies, sarcasm, and abstract expressions. These patients are similar to many aphasic patients concerning higher level language. They are concrete and tend to be literal in dealing with language concepts.

In the middle stage of Alzheimer's disease, there is less self-awareness of communication problems. According to Ripich and Ziol (1998), comprehension of complex grammatical structures is impaired. Studies have shown that as elderly people age there may be an overall impairment in comprehending grammatical and syntactical structures, but what is observed in middle stage Alzheimer's disease is more significant and debilitating. Word fluency continues to suffer because of increased word-finding problems.

The pragmatics of language continues to be the most obvious problem area in communication. Patients jump from topic to topic, and there are fewer ideas to be expressed. There are frequent requests to repeat statements, and they utter automatic and stereotypical statements such as "It's OK," "Uh huh, yes," and "That's all right." In the middle stage of Alzheimer's disease, there is poor self-correction of communication mistakes. Conversations with middle stage patients lack substance and may be limited to discussions of past events.

Ripich and Ziol (1998) report that in the late stage of the progression of Alzheimer's disease patients are unaware of their communication disorders. There is poor comprehension of others' speech, and some patients are mute. For many patients with late-stage Alzheimer's disease, their verbal communication consists of jargon speech and denial of the communication problems. Essentially, there are two types of jargon. First, there are words used improperly, i.e., a string of words that makes no sense. The patient may say, "Just butterfly crib." Second, some patients make up words. A made-up word is called a neologism. The patient may say, "Cala, tulu, des tula." Neologisms may be related to phonological disorders and/or apraxia of speech. Most patients with jargon speech use a combination of words strung together incorrectly and made-up words. For verbal patients without jargon there is a general impoverishment of vocabulary, although grammar may be preserved. Phonological errors may be present. In the pragmatic category of language functioning, there may also be a lack of coherence and poor eye contact. Verbal patients with late-stage Alzheimer's disease have poor conversational turn taking, and utterances may appear to be monologues.

13.5 Verbal Manifestations of Dementia

Many patients with dementia have one or more of the following verbal manifestations of the disorder: circumlocution, confabulation, perseveration, echolalia, logorrhea, tangential speech, and cluttering. They may occur at any stage or level and are usually chronic verbal aspects of the generalized intellectual deterioration and motor-sensory impairments.

Circumlocution is the saying of an alternate sound, word, or phrase for one that is feared, difficult to produce, or unavailable for recall. Although circumlocution is a frequent pattern of speech in people who stutter, demented patients also circumlocute; they substitute an easily produced word for another. In demented patients, the circumlocution may also be related to the difficulty producing a word, but it can also be used during word-finding behaviors. When the desired word cannot be recalled, they will use an alternate one. Sometimes the alternate word is distant from the meaning of the desired one, causing disrupted communication. This behavior can also occur on the phrase level.

Confabulation is remarking about something without regard to the truthfulness of the statements. Some authorities equate confabulation with lying, but it is more than knowingly making false statements. Confabulating patients disregard truth, accuracy, and facts, and appear to be cognitively oblivious and morally detached from the deception. They make up events and distort real ones. They appear to say what comes to mind, trying to satisfy some psychological need or for no reason whatsoever. Sometimes patients with right hemisphere damage who are disoriented to place engage in confabulated journeys (Pimental and Kingsbury, 1989). They talk on and on about some made-up event. These confabulated journeys are tied to delusions and disorientation. One patient with organic brain syndrome engaged in morbid confabulation. She continuously talked about how some animals eat other animals, and the train of thought got progressively more morbid until she began talking about cannibalism. When she realized where her story had taken her, it appeared to frighten her, and she stopped talking altogether (Tanner, 1977). As discussed below, the tendency to confabulate has implications for knowing the veracity of any statements made by the patient during legal proceedings.

Perseveration is the tendency to continue an activity for a longer period than is appropriate, a speech or motor act that lasts longer than the significance of the stimuli warrants. When verbally perseverating, a patient will repeat the sound, word, or phrase over and over, and when writing, he or she will repeatedly produce the same letter or word. A good way of understanding perseveration is to compare it with a song or melody that gets stuck in a normal person's mind. The song or melody continues for a longer period than is appropriate or warranted by the significance of the stimulus. With brain-injury-induced perseveration, this type of phenomenon occurs more frequently and intensely. In severe cases, most or all thoughts and behavior patterns may be perseverated. Perseveration is particularly disruptive to communication because the patient will only be able to respond to questions with the same answer once the perseveration has begun. The patient with severe perseveration is obviously stuck in a train of thought and/or motor act and cannot shift to another.

Related to perseveration, echolalia is the tendency to repeat the last sound, word, or phrase spoken by someone else. According to Benson and Ardila (1996), echolalia is a feature of many degenerative brain diseases. The echolalia seen in demented patients is different from what normal people do when they repeat the last statement made by someone. Usually, normal individuals are simply repeating what the speaker said to bid for more time to process the information or to obtain a clarification, and this behavior is called "mitigated echolalia." The echolalia seen in demented patients also differs from normal childhood echolalia. Most children go through a stage where they repeat what others have spoken, and it is a natural and expected part of childhood acquisition. Dementia-induced echolalia is related to the patient's need to communicate, but because of the impoverished vocabulary, he or she is limited only to repeating the sounds, word, and phrases of others. There is little cognitive processing involved in simply echoing what someone else has said.

Logorrhea is the continuous incoherent talking resulting from a cognitive disorder or psychological aberration. The garrulousness and unrestrained talking are incoherent because the strings of words are not connected semantically or because the speech act has no point or conclusion. It is rambling incoherently. Logorrhea differs from confabulation in that the latter is coherent, albeit untruthful and factless. Patients with logorrhea may also say untruthful and factless statements, but knowing the veracity of their statements is difficult because they are often incomprehensible.

Tangential speech lacks continuity and consistency. The train of thought of the speaker wanders, and his or her speech reflects a lack of disciplined concentration. Often in dementia the last words spoken stimulate a tangential thought, and the patient begins a new topic as if prompted by them. During the new topic another word or other words sparks a tangential thought, and the patient embarks on that monologue. Tangential speech shows a lack of concentration and a poor attention span but also may be founded in a reduced memory span. The patient cannot keep the integrity and continuity of a thought because he or she cannot store it in memory long enough to maintain the intent of the speech act.

Cluttering is a verbal thought-organization fluency disorder characterized by short attention span, an excessive rate of speech, and omissions and substitutions of sounds and words. The cluttering person often speaks rapidly, with sentence fragments, word repetitions, and many revisions. He or she appears to be unable to organize thoughts clearly and is persistently unsatisfied with the output. The following is an example of cluttering (Tanner, 2003a):

> I would like to go. What I want to do after class is to go to the, go to the, uh. Hey, why don't you and I go to the student union. The thing is that a cup of coffee would taste good at the student…Would you like to go to the student union and have a cup …Espresso coffee is good at the student union. Hey, let's go to the student union and have a cup of espresso.

Table 13.1 provides communication patterns seen in some patients and categorized by the stage or level of dementia.

13.6 Evaluating and Treating Communication and Swallowing Disorders in Dementia Patients

There are four reasons to evaluate the communication disorders in patients with dementia. First, an evaluation is conducted to determine the presence of dementia-related communication disorders. The goal is to assess the patient's communication strengths and weaknesses. Second, an evaluation is used to separate the symptoms of dementia from the typical and usual manifestations of neurogenic communication disorders. The characteristics of dementia such as disorientation and impaired global memory, judgment, and intellect are separated from the speech and language disorders of aphasia, apraxia of speech, and the dysarthrias. Third, some dementia-related communication disorders are reversible and can be treated. Evaluation is conducted to figure out treatment goals and objectives and prognoses in these patients. In addition, some patients with irreversible dementia may be able to profit from experiences and thus are candidates for therapy. Training and counseling of medical staff and the patient's family may be necessary, and the evaluation results can serve as a foundation for these endeavors. The fourth reason for evaluating communication disorders in patients with dementia is for forensic purposes. Assessing the communication abilities and disabilities in patients with dementia may be necessary when litigating issues related to mental competence, standards of practice for medical professionals, and abuse and neglect.

The diagnostic procedures used to assess the communication disorders in patients with dementia depend on the level of cognitive and intellectual deterioration. Many assessments are done in conjunction with neuropsychological testing. For patients in early-stage dementia, the goals of assessment are to find out the degree of awareness, and to quantify and qualify the word finding, tangential speech, concretism, and pragmatic communication disorders that may be present. Early signs of dysphagia are also examined, including impulsiveness and motor and sensory deficits. Important in evaluating patients with dementia is a hearing screening or comprehensive audiological assessment to rule out hearing deficits. Some patients have apparent symptoms of mild dementia, such as frequently requesting clarification, failure to follow commands, and auditory comprehension problems, because of an undiagnosed hearing disorder. Comprehensive audiological assessment and treatment are necessary for most patients with apparent early stage dementia (see Chapter 14).

In middle-stage dementia, an assessment of the patient's degree of awareness of the communication disorder is made. There is often only partial awareness of the communication disorders. Awareness can be estimated as a percentage. For example, a patient who knows he or she has erred in counting change or remembering names can be assigned a percent awareness score of 50 percent if awareness of the mistakes occurs about one half of the time. Related to a patient's awareness of communication disorders is his or her ability to self-correct. Obviously, patients who are not aware of mistakes do not try to correct them. For aware patients who attempt self-correction, a determination is made about the success rate, and this too is recorded in percentages. Patients who are aware of communication errors and yet are unsuccessful in correcting them often have increased frustration and anger.

Specific speech and language testing often depends on the severity of the middle stage/level dementia. Tests of auditory comprehension are particularly valuable in finding out how well the patient understands the speech of others. Token testing is an appropriate assessment tool for auditory comprehension in demented patients. There are several varieties of token tests and different methods of scoring them. Token tests involve having the patient place differently shaped, colored, and sized objects or pictures on, above, or below other tokens based on verbal requests from the examiner. This type of language testing is relatively free of cultural complications because of the simple, basic nature of the tests. The words used are culturally neutral, such as large, red, triangle, etc. The testing of pragmatic communication disorders involves observing the patient during communication for impairments in the context and intent in

Table 13.1
Communication Patterns and Disorders in Some Patients with Dementia

Early Stage/Level	Middle Stage/Level	Late Stage/Level
Awareness of communication errors	Partial awareness of communication errors	Lack of awareness of communication errors
Occasional word finding deficits, pragmatic deficiencies	Increased word finding deficits, pragmatic deficiencies	Mutism, perseveration-echolalia, monologues, pragmatic deficiencies
Concrete language	Stereotypical utterances, confabulation	Phonological errors
Occasional tangential speech	Increased tangential speech and impaired comprehension	Jargon, logorrhea
Occasional frustration and anger	Increased frustration and anger	Denial of disability Extreme anger/hostility

which language is used. Storytelling, giving instructions, and tangential speech are noted, as is higher level language such as understanding humor, analogies, sarcasm, and abstract expressions.

In some medical settings, a dysphagia screening may be an aspect of all the evaluations conducted by a speech-language pathologist. As reported below, dysphagia assessment is particularly important in middle stage/level dementia. Whereas patients in early stages of the disorder may only be impulsive and have minor sensory or motor swallowing deficits affecting swallowing, dysphagia in middle stage/level dementia may be mild or severe. Patients in the middle stage/level of dementia pose the most challenge in assessing swallowing and abilities to meet their hydration and nutritional needs orally. Comprehensive swallowing assessment is often required for them.

Dysphagia evaluation and treatment may be clinically irrelevant in late-stage dementia because the patient may have an IV, NG, or PEG tube. An IV, or intravenous line, is a needle inserted into a blood vessel. An NG is a nasogastric tube that goes through the patient's nose to his or her stomach. A PEG tube is like a nasogastric tube, but it goes directly into the patient's stomach. The above are used to supply the patient with needed fluids and nutrients. IV and NG tubes are usually temporary ways of providing fluids and nutrients to the patient. The PEG tube is usually permanent. It is used for patients who are never able to meet their nutritional needs orally. Of the patients who are still capable of meeting their hydration and nutritional needs orally, most require comprehensive swallowing assessment and monitoring. Because of the severity of the cognitive and intellectual deterioration, dysphagia therapy is often unsuccessful and patients must be carefully fed by nurses or aides. The testing of communication functioning in patients with late stage/level dementia is dependent on the degree of cognitive and intellectual deterioration. Because some patients are mute and unable to comprehend the speech of others, detailed and in-depth testing for communication disorders is contraindicated. Speech, voice, and language functioning can be described, but most late-stage patients are unable to participate meaningfully in formal diagnostic testing.

There are three areas of clinical management for the communication disorders seen in patients with dementia. First, ongoing comprehensive speech, language, and hearing evaluations are necessary to gain an understanding of the patient's changes in functioning over time. Evaluation is particularly important in early stages/levels of the disorders. "Early identification is extremely valuable for patients with reversible dementia, and also for those with irreversible dementia. Patients with reversible dementia need treat-ment, and patients with irreversible dementia and their families need information about how to maximize communicative performance" (Bayles, 1994, p. 541). As noted previously, a comprehensive hearing assessment is necessary to rule out hearing loss and/or deafness as a cause or contributor to problems in following commands, understanding information, and being detached from conversations. Hearing aids and other treatments are appropriate and available for many patients. Second, evaluation of communication functioning is also important for identifying deficiencies and designing appropriate therapies for neurogenic communication disorders.

Clinical management of communication disorders includes providing direct therapy to those patients who can benefit from it. There are individual and group therapies that can improve orientation and memory and therapies for aphasia, apraxia of speech, and the dysarthrias. Although the research has shown that, as a group, patients with dementia are unable to benefit from direct treatment of communication disorders per se, some individuals with irreversible dementia can profit from experience. The treatment approaches for patients with dementia are similar to the ones used for patients with traumatic brain injuries. They include orientation drills, memory enhancement exercises, and reality orientation, as well as the standard therapies for aphasia and motor speech disorders. Ongoing evaluation is necessary for determining whether the patient can continue to benefit from the therapies.

The third area of clinical management for the communication disorders seen in patients with dementia is the counseling of family and training of medical staff. Family members are told of the typical communication symptoms seen in dementia and ways of dealing with them. What is most important, they are helped in preparing for the eventualities that the impaired communication may bring to relationships, quality of life, and home care. Medical staff, including physicians, nurses, therapists, aides, orderlies, and food service personnel, are provided information about the nature and course of communication and swallowing deterioration in dementia. They are trained in how to reduce problems with communication and how to use the patient's remaining communication abilities maximally. Training can be informal discussions about these disorders during conferences or provided during formal inservice training programs. Communication problems in dementia can also interfere with medical management of nondementia illnesses in patients (Brauner, Muir, and Sachs, 2000). Medical management relies, in part, on optimal communication between the patient and physician. The information provided by speech-language pathologists and audiologists about communication disorders in dementia can be helpful to physicians when addressing nondementia illnesses. Ongoing training and counseling of medical staff and family are important aspects of the management of communication disorders in dementia patients. Care should be taken to address caregivers' stress when dealing with demented patients (Dean, 2004). Table 13.2 describes the treatment considerations in dementia patients.

13.7 Dementia and Dysphagia

Dysphagia is a swallowing disorder that when broadly defined can include impairment of the emotional, cognitive, sensory, and/or motor acts involved with transferring a substance from the mouth to stomach, resulting in a failure to maintain hydration and nutrition, and posing a risk of choking and aspiration. Dysphagia is common in elderly nursing home residents and is associated with aspiration pneumonia and death (Cowen, Simpson, and Vettese, 1997). As reported in Chapter 8, approximately one-third of hospitalized patients have dysphagia, and approximately two-thirds

of nursing home residents may be compromised concerning eating and swallowing. According to Cefalu (1999), high-risk patients with dementia who are suspected of having dysphagia include those with feeding difficulties, those requiring assistance with feeding, and those with concurrent depression or a history of cerebrovascular accidents. Patients with a 5 percent weight loss in six months or a 10 percent loss in twelve months are also high-risk patients.

The dysphagia can result from the psychological and emotional aspects of the generalized cognitive and intellectual deterioration. Patients may lose the desire to eat, refuse food and liquids, and begin to "waste away." This failure to thrive is a result of malnutrition and dehydration and recent studies have shown that significant loss of weight often precedes acute onset of Alzheimer's disease symptoms. Sensory and motor deficits associated with Alzheimer's disease, and more commonly vascular dementia, can result in chewing, sucking, and swallowing disorders at the oral, pharyngeal, and laryngeal-esophageal stages. With dysphagia patients there is the risk of aspiration and choking. The occurrence of pneumonia is 7.5 times greater in stroke pa-

Table 13.2
Communication Disorders Treatment Considerations in Dementia Patients

Ongoing Speech, Language, and Hearing Evaluation	- Audiological assessment to rule out hearing deficits and to provide treatment as appropriate. - Motor speech assessment to identify speech pathologies and appropriate therapies. - Language and cognitive assessment to determine deficiencies and whether or not patient can benefit from therapy.
Designing Therapies for Appropriate Patients	- For patients who can benefit form speech language, and dysphagia therapies, individual and group therapy. - Group therapies to improve orientation and memory. - Continuous monitoring of treatment objectives and outcomes to determine whether patient can continue to profit from experience.
Inservice Training of Medical Staff and Family Counseling	- Inservice training for hospital, nursing home, home health care agencies' medical staff including physicians, nurses, nursing aides, and food service staff. - Therapy, training, and counseling to address dysphagia. - Ongoing training and counseling of family members and friends. Goals and objective adjusted to the changing conditions of the patient. - Ongoing training and counseling of medical staff, family and friends to address safety issues - Address stress levels of caregivers

tients who aspirate than in those who do not (Schmidt, Holas, Halvorson, and Reding, 1994). Pneumonia has a mortality rate of 43 percent in hospitalized elderly patients who develop it (Gonzalez and Calia, 1975).

Traditional dysphagia management is complicated and often compromised by dementia. Especially in middle and late stages/levels of the disorder, patients may be careless and impulsive about eating. Because of their cognitive and intellectual impairments, they may talk with food in their mouths and pose choking risks. They also can perseveratively put food in their mouths until it cannot be contained, and then try to swallow, talk, or spit it out. Many patients refuse to eat and turn their heads and clench their teeth when spoonfuls of food are presented to them. Patients with dementia also can have sensory and motor deficits of varying severity affecting the ability to chew, suck, and swallow.

At the oral stage, patients may not have the neuromuscular ability to chew sufficiently and create a bolus. Consequently, particles of food are distributed throughout the oral cavity and are unmanageable for swallowing. Food pocketing is common, i.e., patients put food in a cheek and cannot or will not clear it. Pocketing can be related to sensory deficits where the patient is unaware of the food mass or is simply unconcerned about the pocketed bolus and not inclined to clear it. The laryngeal-esophageal stage of the swallow involves the protective action of being able to clear particles of food and liquid from the airways. Many demented patients with dysphagia can clear the airways but are not inclined to do so or are perplexed at the task. They simply allow the food to compromise the airway, increasing the choking and aspiration risks.

In patients with middle and late stage/level dementia, assessing the pharyngeal stage of swallowing requires a video swallow study (VSS). Bedside dysphagia assessment of this stage of the swallow is fraught with error even in patients who can cooperate and are cognitively intact. Even the VSS procedures must be adjusted to the patient's cognitive and intellectual status; the results can be highly variable, and some patients are untestable. It may take several video swallowing studies to achieve a level of confidence about the patient's risk for choking and aspiration. And, of course, many dementias are progressive, requiring ongoing evaluation.

Dysphagia management in late stage/level dementia requires video swallowing studies. Reliance on bedside assessment results is contraindicated. In some patients with early stage/level dysphagia, a bedside assessment may provide valid and reliable clinical information about the oral stage of swallowing, but even in these cases, because of the cognitive, intellectual, and communication disorders, the veracity of the patient's reports is suspect. In many demented patients with dysphagia, IV lines or the placement of NG or PEG tubes eventually are necessary to meet their hydration and nutritional needs and eliminate the risk of aspiration pneumonia. Brush, Slominski, and Boezko (2006, p. 9) observe: "Many clients with AD require a thorough dysphagia evaluation. Preserved abilities should be identified and a treatment plan that builds on preserved abilities and past and current meal preferences should be developed, with an eye to the possible facilitators and barriers in the environment." Sometimes, a continued oral intake of food and liquid can lead to the death of the patient, and healthcare professionals and family members may be aware of the risks, but they are accepting of them given a poor prognosis for a meaningful future quality of life for the patient.

There are incidental and anecdotal reports, but no empirical studies, showing that in some cases, patients with dementia are permitted to take in foods and liquids orally, and the medical professionals know there is a likelihood that they will aspirate and suffer aspiration pneumonia, probably leading to death. Swallowing therapy or an IV, NG, or PEG tube placement does not occur, though it is generally known that the patient is at risk for aspiration pneumonia. These patients may be confronted with major surgeries from which they are not likely to survive or are in late stages/levels of dementia with few prospects for a reasonable quality of life. These instances also occur when the oral intake of foods and liquids is left to the discretion of the family and there is ambiguity or no wording about tube feeding in living wills or medical power of attorney. In some cases, the ethics and legality of knowingly permitting a demented and dysphagic patient to ingest food and liquids, rather than to be NPO, may be at issue.

13.8 Dementia and Determining Veracity of Statements

Confabulation is making incorrect statements and giving tangential answers to questions. It is remarking about something without regard to the truthfulness, facts, or accuracy of the statements. As noted previously, confabulation is more than lying. The confabulating patient disregards truth, accuracy, and facts and is morally detached from the deception. Confabulation has been linked to right hemisphere damage (Pimental and Kingsbury, 1989). The tendency to confabulate brings into question the veracity of all statements made by the patient during legal proceedings. Sometimes confabulating patients produce answers to questions and stories that are bizarre, but confabulations can also be plausible deceptions and inaccuracies. Separating fact from fiction in demented patients who confabulate requires careful analysis.

Statements made by confabulating patients can be confirmed or rejected by questioning accessible family, friends, and medical staff. They can provide information about the veracity of the patient's statements. For example, a patient with dementia reported a fall in a bathtub, casting doubt on her ability to live independently. Confabulation was suspected because of the absence of bruising and other injuries. Her husband confirmed that the event occurred several years in the past, not recently, and that the patient was confabulating. The patient, however, was very convincing about the recency of the accident. For patients without accessible family or friends, the accuracy and truthfulness of reports of past events are difficult to confirm. Unfortunately, looking at the consistency of the reports is not appropriate because many confabulating patients are consistent in their inaccuracies and deceptions. They will be steadfast in the confabulations over time. Polygraph results are also questionable because many patients are not knowingly making false statements. Many patients, on some level, believe them and consequently will not have psychophysiological reactions to deceptions that can be measured by the polygraph.

13.9 Dementia, Communication Disorders, and Mental Competence

By definition patients with dementia have suspect mental competence. They have a loss of cognitive and intellectual functions with accompanying disorientation and impaired memory and judgment. Demented patients are more or less incompetent with regard to understanding, creating, modifying, and changing wills and trusts, the ability to distinguish right from wrong, manage affairs, and assist counsel in legal proceedings. The medical diagnosis of dementia calls into question all aspects of the patient's mental competence. However, as reported previously, some dementias are reversible, and there are degrees of irreversible dementia. The patient's communication abilities are important in knowing the stages of mental competence at any given time. In mental competency hearings, a comprehensive communication evaluation can provide valuable information about current intellectual and cognitive functioning, and a review of reports can suggest the patient's retrospective competence.

In vascular dementia, the presence of cooccurring motor speech disorders, i.e., apraxia of speech and the dysarthrias, does not contribute to the patient's impaired mental competence. Because pure motor speech disorders do not impair the fabric of language, or necessarily impair cognitive and intellectual functioning, these neurogenic communication disorders do not contribute to mental incompetence. However, because patients may have apraxia of speech to the extent they cannot program and sequence speech or may have neuromuscular impairments to the degree they are anarthric, they may appear less competent because of the communication disorders. (Anarthria is the inability to speak due to lesions of the peripheral nerves and/or the muscles they enervate, a severe form of dysarthria.) In motor speech disorders, if patients are provided with alternative communication devices such as communication boards or speech synthesizers, their communication abilities will be more reflective of their levels of cognitive and intellectual functioning. The competence of patients with aphasia depends on the severity and type of language impairment. Benson and Ardila (1996) note that aphasia does not necessarily impair the patient's ability to manage his or her affairs although it can impair the ability to make important decisions and thus require that the patient have the protection of a conservator or guardian. Benson and Ardila go on to note that aphasia can make patients appear less intelligent than they are in reality. In this sense, aphasia is similar to motor speech disorders.

When deciding the mental competence of patients with dementia, the same procedure discussed in Chapter 9 should be followed, but with variations to address the progressive nature of the disorder. Test stimuli should be provided gradually and on a segmented basis. Most patients with dementia will have difficulty understanding long verbal or written requests and statements. Care should be taken that when the testing on an item is completed, it should be completely removed from the visual field of the patient to reduce sources of distraction. The testing rooms should be free of distractions such as open windows, overhead paging, posters, painting, and clutter.

When testing patients with dementia, it is also important to schedule the time for the evaluation to consider the effects of medication. Some anti-dementia medications cause drowsiness, and others may cause the patient to be optimally alert and responsive within two or three hours of administration. The goal is to review the medication regime and to test the patient during periods of optimal alertness. When testing communication abilities in patients with dementia, it is particularly important to videotape the sessions, carefully noting the dates and times to document the processes followed and the patient's responses to them over the course of the illness.

Pivotal to determining a patient's mental competence are his or her receptive language impairments. As noted above, token testing is a desirable way of assessing the patient's auditory comprehension, because the test is relatively free of cultural and linguistic bias. Questionnaires provided to family and friends of the patient can also provide accurate measures of how well he or she understands directions, follows instruction, and comprehends the speech of others. In vascular dementias, brain scans can also provide information about the patient's auditory comprehension. Patients with damage to the left temporal, parietal, and temporal-parietal lobes are likely to be compromised with regard to auditory comprehension and reading. However, it is not prudent to assume the nature and degree of the deficits from the site and size of lesions based solely on brain scan data, for there is much individual variation in speech and language cortical representation. Many subtests of aphasia batteries are available to assess graphic involvement, visual processing, auditory comprehension, and expressive speech and language. No single test of aphasia is appropriate for assessing the communication abilities of patients with dementia. However, the *Porch Index of Communicative Abilities* (PICA) has an elaborate numerical scoring system and can provide objective data about dementia patients' overt communication strengths and weakness. Unfortunately, the test is weak concerning the quality of communication, higher level language, high-level auditory comprehension, and abstraction.

The accuracy of a patient's yes-no responses is fundamental to assessing mental competence. When a patient responds in the affirmative or negative, has he or she completely understood the question and its legal implications? Deciding the accuracy of yes-no responses requires repeated trials with gradually more difficult questions. Patients with vascular dementia may produce paraphasias similar to those seen in aphasic patients. Verbal paraphasias compromise the patient's yes-no accuracy because they can cause the patient to answer incorrectly, not because he or she did not understand the question, but because of word-retrieval behaviors associated with damage to the speech and language centers of the brain. Verbal paraphasias are common word-retrieval behaviors in aphasic patients; a patient will produce a word that has a semantic relationship to the desired word. Both "yes" and "no" are one-word, closed-end responses, and they are associated. Consequently, for demented patients with this type of word-retrieval error, accuracy when answering these types of questions is suspect. This is particularly true of patients who are unaware of their errors and unable to self-correct. The tendencies for perseveration and echolalia also compromise the accuracy of patients' yes-no responses.

Cognitive and intelligence testing conducted by neuropsychologists can be used in conjunction with testing done by speech-language pathologists. Together the results can provide a basis by which judgments can be made about the communication abilities in patients with dementia. Unfortunately, no single psychometric test or brain scan can provide reliable and valid measures of a patient's mental competence. Often, informal information from nurses can provide a better picture of the patient's real-life performance than can brain scans or psychometric tests.

Retrospective competency testing involves determining whether a person was competent to read, understand, and sign a legal document. The goal is to know whether the patient was in early-stage dementia when the legal document was signed, and if he or she was competent to understand it. In retrospective competency determinations, the patient's communication status at the time of the document signing cannot be accurately determined unless the examiner has the benefit of videotape or witnesses who have complete recall of the conditions surrounding the test. A review of the medical reports about the patient at the time of the signing can provide general information about the patient's status.

13.10 Case Study in Dementia-Induced Dyscalculia

This case illustrates how early signs of dementia can be difficult to diagnose. It involves dyscalculia and the appreciation of monetary values. A wealthy seventy-nine-year-old woman first started showing indications of dementia when she provided her children an ordinary kitchen object, a butter dish, and demanded that they sell it for an exorbitant amount of money. On one occasion she asserted that the butter dish was worth "a hundred thousand dollars." She demanded that they "put the butter dish in the Internet" and provide her with a check within a week. Because some elderly people have incomplete understanding of the Internet, it was difficult to know whether her request reflected this ignorance of the workings of the World Wide Web or was a delusion. And although unlikely, there was the possibility that the butter dish was a rare and valuable antique. For several weeks her children were confused about the butter dish, yet she persisted in her demands. A few weeks later, the woman paid $500.00 to an acquaintance for an amateurish, self-made cassette tape of songs. Unfortunately, her ability to write checks was unimpaired during the early stage of the disorder. Although she was a generous woman by nature, she became excessive with tipping. Several times she would leave tips totaling ten times the amount of the meal. It gradually became clear to her children that the woman was having increasing difficulty appreciating monetary concepts and understanding the value of goods and services. They also feared that she was being taken advantage of by strangers. The episode that clearly showed her progressive dementia was when she entered a car dealership and attempted to purchase several luxury cars for herself, members of her family, and total strangers.

13.11 Chapter Summary

Dementia is the loss of previously acquired cognitive and intellectual functions and is usually progressive. Reversible and irreversible dementias are not natural occurrences of the aging process; they can be caused by several diseases and disorders. Vascular dementia and Alzheimer's disease are the most common causes of the disorientation, impaired memory, judgment, and disruptive behaviors. Patients with dementia are usually diagnosed as being in early, middle, or late stages of the disorder. Patients with dementia can have motor speech disorders and aphasia as well as other verbal symptoms of the disorder. Dysphagia is common in dementia. As a group, demented patients have a poor prognosis and are not candidates for speech and language rehabilitation because they cannot profit from experience. Quantifying and qualifying current and retrospective mental competence in dementia patients involves a comprehensive and ongoing evaluation of their speech and language symptoms.

Suggested Readings and Resources

Cefalu, C. (1999). Appropriate dysphagia evaluation and management of the nursing home patient with dementia. *Annals of Long-Term Care*, 7(12):447-451. This article provides guidelines for the management of dementia-related dysphagia.

Davis, G. A. (2007). *Aphasiology: Disorders and Clinical Practice* (2nd ed.). Boston: Allyn & Bacon. Chapter 13 addresses diagnosis and assessment of dementia, medical treatments, and cognitive intervention.

Hooper, T. and Bayles, K. (2001). Management of neurogenic communication disorders associated with dementia. In R. Chapey (Ed), *Language Intervention Strategies in Aphasia and Related Neurogenic Communication Disorders* (4th ed.). Philadelphia: Lippincott, Williams, & Wilkins.

Ripich, D., and Ziol, E. (1998). Dementia: A review for the speech-language pathologist. In A. Johnson and B. Jacobson (Eds), *Medical Speech-Language Pathology: A Practitioner's Guide.* New York: Thieme. These chapters, in edited books, review the management of dementia-related communication disorders.

References

Bayles, K. (1994). Management of neurogenic communication disorders associated with dementia. In R. Chapey (Ed), *Language intervention strategies in adult aphasia* (3rd ed.). Baltimore: Williams & Wilkins.

Benson, D. and Ardila, A. (1996). *Aphasia.* New York: Oxford University Press.

Brauner, D.J., Muir, C.J., and Sachs, G.A. (2000, June). Treating nondementia illnesses in patients with dementia. *JAMA*, 283(24): 3230-3235.

Brush, J., Slominski, T., and Boczko, F. (2006, May). Nutritional and dysphagia services for individuals with Alzheimer's disease. *ASHA Leader, May 23, 2006, Vol 11. No. 7.*

Cefalu, C. (1999). Appropriate dysphagia evaluation and management of the nursing home patient with dementia. *Annals of Long-Term Care*, 7(12):447-451.

Cowen, M., Simpson, S., and Vettese, T. (1997). Survival estimates for patients with abnormal swallowing studies. *J. Gen. Intern. Med.*, 12:99-94.

Davis, G. A. (2007). *Aphasiology: Disorders and clinical practice* (2nd ed.). Boston: Allyn & Bacon.

Dean, C. (2004). *The everything Alzheimer's book.* Avon, M.A.: Adams Media.

Dirckx, J. H. (2001). *Stedman's concise medical dictionary for the health professions* (4th ed.). Philadelphia: Lippincott Williams & Wilkins.

Gonzalez, C., and Calia, F. (1975). Bacteriologic flora of aspiration-induced pulmonary infection. *Archives of Internal Medicine*, *135*: 711-714.

Hartke, R.J. (1991). *Psychological aspects of geriatric rehabilitation.* Gaithersburg, MD: Aspen.

Hooper, T. and Bayles, K. (2001). Management of neurogenic communication disorders associated with dementia. In R. Chapey (Ed) *Language intervention strategies in aphasia and related neurogenic communication disorders (4th ed.).* Philadelphia: Lippincott, Williams, & Wilkins.

Hosley, J.B. and Molle-Matthews, E.A. (Eds.) (1999). Lippincott's textbook for clinical medical assisting. Baltimore: Lippincott Williams & Wilkins. Cited in Dirckx, J. H. (2001).

Kennedy, W.Z. (1999). Delirium, dementia, amnesia, and other cognitive disorders. In P.G. O'Brien, W.Z. Kennedy, and K.A. Ballard (Eds). *Psychiatric nursing: An integration of theory and practice*. New York: McGraw-Hill.

Pimental, P., and Kingsbury, N. (1989). *Neuropsychological aspects of right brain injury*. Austin: ProEd.

Ripich, D., and Ziol, E. (1998). Dementia: A review for the speech-language pathologist. In A. Johnson and B. Jacobson (Eds), *Medical speech-language pathology: A practitioner's guide*. New York: Thieme.

Schmidt, D., Holas, M., Halvorson, K., and Reding, M. (1994). Videofluoroscopic evidence of aspiration predicts pneumonia and death but not dehydration following stroke. *Dysphagia, 9*: 7-11.

Tanner, D. (1977). Differential diagnosis of organic brain syndrome. A paper presented to the Annual Convention of the Arizona Speech and Hearing Association, Tucson.

Tanner, D. (2003a). *Exploring communication disorders: A 21st century introduction through literature and media*. Boston: Allyn & Bacon.

Tanner, D. (2003b). *The psychology of neurogenic communication disorders: A primer for healthcare professionals*. Boston: Allyn & Bacon.

Tanner, D. (2006). *An advanced course in communication sciences and disorders*. San Diego: Plural Publishing.

Chapter 14

Medical-Legal and Forensic Aspects of Hearing Loss and Deafness

Synopsis

14.1 Chapter Preview

In this chapter, the hearing mechanism is examined from external ear to the central auditory pathways. There is a review of professionals and their roles in the management of diseases and disorders of the hearing mechanism. This chapter contains an overview of the anatomy and physiology of the hearing mechanism and the types of disorders that occur at each stage of hearing. There is a general discussion of hearing tests, giving lawyers and judges basic information to interpret audiological reports and examine expert testimony. Several forensic issues are discussed including malingering and the accuracy of hearing testing. There is also a case study involving hysterical deafness.

14.2 Hearing, Hard-of-Hearing, Deafness, and Audiology

Hearing has been called the "second sense," with vision being the primary one. However, hearing is the primary sense when it comes to the development of speech and language. Children born deaf will not naturally learn to speak; a child must hear the sounds of a language to be able to speak them. The degree to which a child has a hearing loss will also affect his or her language development. A child with severe hearing loss will suffer more in language development than one with a mild hearing loss. The sensation of hearing also suffers because of aging and living in a noisy society; many people experience partial hearing loss as they age. There are many diseases, traumas, and defects that can cause hearing loss and deafness, but fortunately, medicine and technology are making giant leaps in treating them. From cochlear implants to digital hearing aids, people who are deaf or hard-of-hearing are provided with new and improved options for restoring hearing. As the number of people with hearing loss and deafness increases in society, so too will litigation involving compensation, medical malpractice, and eligibility for special education and other social services.

Audiology got its start as an independent clinical discipline at the close of World War II (Martin, 1997). This was a direct result of the high number of soldiers returning from the war with noise-related hearing losses. In the United States, the terminal degree for practicing audiologists is the master's, but soon audiologists will have a clinical doctorate (Au.D.) as the highest required degree. The American Speech-Language-Hearing Association (ASHA) and the American Academy of Audiology (AAA) have guidelines and requirements for educational and clinical preparation for audiologists. There are also state licensing regulations. Audiologists are responsible for assessing and managing hearing disorders including conducting comprehensive hearing screening and testing, and selecting, fitting, and dispensing hearing aids. As the audiology profession evolves, increasingly important responsibilities of audiologists are aural habilitation and rehabilitation.

In the United States, hearing loss and deafness are the most common communication disorders (Public Health Service, 1994). The American Academy of Audiology (2006) reports that more than 31 million Americans have some type of hearing problem. In the elderly population, about 33 percent of people over the age of sixty-five experience a hearing problem (National Center for Health Statistics [NCHS], 1988). Martin and Clark (2003) report that two million people are classified as deaf and 26 million people are hard-of-hearing. As many as 15 percent of school-aged children may fail school hearing screenings, often due to transient ear infections. The economics of hearing loss and deafness can be staggering. Over his or her lifetime, a child with a severe hearing impairment may have an economic cost of two million dollars (Northern and Downs, 2002).

Otologists, otolaryngologists, and otorhinolaryngologists are physicians specializing in diseases and disorders of the ear. Some physicians are known as ENTs, or ear, nose, and throat specialists. Today most medical specialists concerned with the ear, hearing loss, and deafness are otologists, but in the past, combined specialties were common. Even the eye was included in some early specialty training: EENTs- eye, ears, nose, and throat specialists. Pediatricians and general practitioners also evaluate and treat diseases and disorders of the ear.

Teachers of the hearing impaired are responsible for educating children with hearing loss and deafness. They are special education professionals with training in educating children with hearing loss, deafness, and multiple disabilities. They are employed in special schools, have self-contained classrooms, or work individually with disabled children. These teachers are proficient in sign language and educational philosophies for hard-of-hearing and deaf individuals. Speech-language pathologists also work with hard-of-hearing and deaf individuals. For children learning to speak, speech-language pathologists teach them how to make speech sounds and also learn language. In some work settings, speech-language pathologists also teach sign language and other aspects of the total communication approach. In the total communication approach, hard-of-hearing and deaf children are taught all methods of communication.

As noted above, audiologists are professionals who assess and provide nonmedical treatment of hearing disorders. In the past, the American Speech-Language-Hearing Association (ASHA) prohibited them from dispensing hearing aids, but now audiologists select, fit, and dispense hearing aids. Specialties in audiology include industrial, pediatric, and educational audiologists, depending on their employment setting. Many audiologists work in physicians' offices and in private practice.

14.3 Survival and Human Hearing

The range of human hearing is approximately between 20 Hz and 20,000 Hz and evolved from a survival imperative. As prehistoric humans evolved, the sense of hearing played an important role in their ultimate successful adaptation. Prehistoric humans evolved the 20–20,000 Hz hearing sensitivity because animals threatening to them, or serving as sources of food, typically produced sound in that frequency range. What is most important, the 20–20,000 Hz frequency range provided the hearing sensitivity for speech communication and a powerful survival advantage. Through speech communication, prehistoric humans could plan and cooperate for individual and collective survival: relative loudness, shadow effect, and the speed of sound.

An important survival benefit for humans, and many other animals, is the ability to localize sound. Knowing the directional source of a sound alerts hunters to prey, and provides combatants with warning and avenues to avoid and escape threats to safety. Even for casual conversations, directional hearing is a convenience for the communicators, and contributes to the ease of conversational turn-taking. There are three factors involved in knowing the directional source of a sound:

> The first and most important factor in sound localization is the relative loudness of the sound in each ear. Environmental sound can be localized because a person has learned the general direction of a sound source; it is perceived louder in one ear compared to the other. Certainly this loudness difference is small, but perceptible. The reason for the loudness difference is that the energy is blocked and consequently damped more in one ear than the other by the head. Second, speech and hearing scientists believe that there is a shadow effect. A shadow effect is acoustic energy casting a shadow behind the external ear (pinna). This results in a person being able to sense differences in acoustic energy as a function of the direction from the sound source. The third and possibly negligible reason for sound localization has to do with the speed of sound and differences in its arrival to each ear. Brief in duration though it is, sound reaches the ear closer to the source sooner than when it reaches the distant ear (Tanner, 2006, pp.187-188).

14.4 Anatomy and Physiology of the Hearing Mechanism

The main structures of the hearing mechanism are the external ear, ear canal, ear drum, ossicular chain, cochlea, cranial nerve VIII, and the central auditory pathways. Figure 14.1 shows the basic structures of the ear including the pinna, external auditory meatus (ear canal), tympanic membrane (ear drum), ossicles (bones of the middle ear), and cochlea (end organ of hearing).

The external ear is the least functional of all the hearing structures and is an S-shaped passageway about one-half of an inch in length. The pinna, or auricle, is the cartilaginous structure on a person's head which allows sound to be directed into the ear canal. It captures the sound energy and funnels it into the ear canal. The ear canal is also called the external auditory meatus. "The external auditory meatus, in its normal anatomic form, enhances sounds within the acoustic range of speech, and protects the sensitive deep structures of the auditory system" (Culbertson, Cotton, and Tanner, 2006, p. 227). Cerumen is a wax-like substance secreted in the lining of the external auditory meatus.

In the middle ear, the acoustic energy produced by a sound source is transformed into mechanical energy. The tympanic membrane, also called the ear drum, is a sensitive, thin membrane that vibrates at a corresponding frequency and amplitude (intensity) with the air molecules. It vibrates in response to sound waves. Attached to the tympanic membrane are the ossicles. These are the smallest bones in the human body and are known as the malleus (hammer), incus (anvil), and stapes (stirrup). Collectively, these structures are called the ossicular chain, and they too vibrate at a frequency and amplitude that corresponds to the sound source. Without the eustachian tube the middle ear would be a closed structure and be unable to equalize its pressure to that of the outside atmosphere. The eustachian tube is a duct or passage between the middle ear and the nasopharynx (back of the throat). It allows for the drainage of fluids and the equalization of pressure in the middle ear.

The inner ear is where sound is transformed from mechanical, hydraulic, and then electrochemical (neural) energy. The cochlea is the end-organ of hearing and is snail-shaped. A convenient way of knowing the function of the cochlea is to compare it to the sense of vision: "The eyes are to vision as the cochlea is to hearing." The organ of Corti is a structure in the cochlea containing hair cells that are sense receptors. They are hair cell nerve endings that move and vibrate. At the level of the cochlea, the mechanical energy is transformed into hydraulic energy when the fluid in the cochlea is set in motion, thus causing the hair cells to move and vibrate, setting off electrochemical or neural discharges. "Between the threshold of hearing and the sound of a raging rock concert, these hairs are sensitive to sounds ranging in power over 14 orders of magnitude" (Young and Geller, 2007, p. 386). The semicircular canals are also located in the inner ear and are partially responsible for the ability to maintain balance. Consequently, some diseases and disorders of the inner ear also result in balance difficulties.

Cranial nerve VIII is also known as the auditory-vestibular nerve because it carries hearing and balance information to the brain. "Although the auditory nerve is relatively thick, it contains a surprisingly small number of nerve fibers, about 50,000 in the cat and 30,000 in the human" (Zemlin, 1998, p. 499). This paired nerve (there are two of them) enters the brainstem at the pons. From the pons, the neural information is sent to other structures of the brain that permit perception of sound. An important structure in perception is the thalamus, also known as the "gatekeeper," because it regulates incoming sensory information. Martin and Clark (2003, p. 316-317) summarize central auditory pathways:

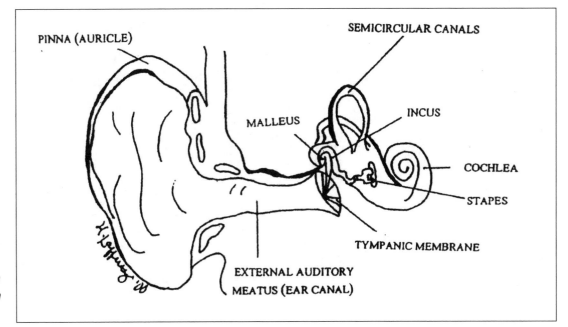

Figure 14.1
Cross section of the human ear

The medial geniculate body, located in the thalamus, is that last subcortical relay station for auditory impulses. Only one of its three main areas, the ventral division, is responsible specifically for auditory information. There is some spiral organization in this area, but tonotopicity is uncertain. Most of the fibers come from the ipsilateral inferior colliculus, and a few fibers come from the lateral lemniscus. After this point, nerve fibers fan out in the auditory radiation and then ascend to the auditory cortex. Because there are no commissural neurons at the level of the medial geniculate body, no desussations exist there.

The auditory cortex of the brain is where sound is finally decoded and associated. It is on the surface of the temporal lobe.

When speaking, humans get two types of auditory feedback. The first type of auditory feedback is through air conduction. When speaking, a person hears his or her voice through the ears. The second type of auditory feedback is through bone conduction. In bone conduction, sound is transmitted to the cochlea through the vibration of the bones of the skull. This process bypasses the outer and middle ear structures and accounts for the observation that people sound different to themselves on a recording than during speaking. When speaking, a person hears himself or herself through air and bone conduction. On a recorder a person is only hearing himself or herself through air conduction.

14.5 Categories of Hearing Loss

As Table 14.1 shows, there are three general ways of classifying hearing loss. The most common way is by the site of lesion or impairment in the process of sound transmission. Conductive hearing loss occurs when there is damage or impairment of the external or middle ear. Sensorineural hearing loss results from damage to the cochlea and/or cranial nerve VIII. Mixed hearing loss has both conductive and sensorineural components. Central hearing loss is caused by damage or impairment of the central auditory nervous system.

The hallmark of a conductive hearing loss examination is that during a bone conduction test, the person can hear tones because the outer and/or middle ear structures are bypassed in the transmission of sound. Damage to or abnormalities of the outer ear can cause conductive hearing loss. A buildup of cerumen can prevent the conduction of sound to the cochlea. Although the external ear canal is a self-cleaning structure, sometimes this wax-like substance can be impacted. There are commercial solutions that can soften and remove cerumen, but sometimes it needs to be removed by a physician or nurse. Foreign objects can also prevent conduction of sound through the external ear. Children, in particular, sometimes put objects in their ear canals, such as eraser heads, pebbles, raisins, corn, etc., thus impeding sound conduction. Some birth defects can cause narrowing or occlusion of the external ear canal. Otitis externus is the swelling of the external ear and can occur in swimmers. It is known as "swimmers' ear." The external ear is irritated by the chemicals in swimming water.

Table 14.1
Types of Hearing Loss and Site of Lesion

Type of Hearing Loss	Site of Lesion
Conductive	Damage or impairment of the external or middle ear
Sensorineural	Damage or impairment of the cochlea and/or VIIIth cranial nerve
Mixed	Damage or impairment of both conductive and sensorineural components
Auditory Processing (Central)	Damage or impairment of the central auditory nervous system

Otitis media is an infection of the middle ear. It is very common in children with about 70 percent of them having at least one episode by the time they are two years old and more than half of them having further episodes (Martin and Clark, 2003). Martin and Clark go on to note that factors predisposing an individual to otitis media include poorly functioning eustachian tubes, abnormalities in the action of the cilia of the mucous membranes, anatomical deformities of the middle ear and eustachian tube, age, race, socioeconomic factors, and the integrity of the immune system. Genes may play a role in otitis media, as does the flu. A sudden change in air pressure, a barotrauma, also has been linked to otitis media. Serous otitis media is a buildup of fluid in the middle ear. A surgical procedure known as a myringotomy, where a pressure-equalizing tube is inserted in the ear drum, is frequently used for children with otitis media. Historically, there has been disagreement between otologists and pediatricians as to the benefit of this surgery for children. Whereas otologists recommend it, some pediatricians have suggested that medication, including antihistamines, should be used as the treatment of choice for otitis media or that no treatment be provided at all. One of the problems of surgery is that myringotomy tubes sometimes become dislodged.

Otosclerosis is a progressive disorder where there is new formation of spongy bone in the ossicular chain. It causes a conductive hearing loss because the new bone growth interferes with the movement of the ossicles. Otosclerosis usually occurs in adults in their middle and later years of life. The disorder is usually surgically correctable. A stapedectomy is a surgical procedure where the stapes is replaced by a prosthesis. Other causes of conductive hearing loss include head traumas and loud noise. Sometimes people who experience severe head traumas and skull fractures have the ossicular chain damaged or the tympanic membrane punctured. Extreme noise and probes can also rupture the tympanic membrane. Polyps and tumors can also disrupt the conduction of sound in the hearing mechanism.

A sensorineural hearing loss occurs when there is damage to the inner ear and/or the auditory nerve (cranial nerve VIII). Exposure to loud noise is a common cause of sensorineural hearing loss, particularly among men. The noise exposure need not be prolonged; even brief periods of loud sounds can cause sensorineural hearing loss. Sometimes the hearing loss will be temporary, and hearing will return. Other times noise exposure can cause permanent loss of all or part of hearing. When hearing is temporarily lost, the transient disorder is called a temporary threshold shift (TTS). When there is irreversible loss of hearing sensitivity,

it is called a permanent threshold shift (PTS). These changes in hearing sensitivity cause the threshold of hearing, the point at which hearing sensation first occurs, to be increased. Loudness must be increased to permit awareness of sound. The types of noise exposure causing threshold shifts vary greatly.

Presbycusis is a general term for the loss of hearing as part of the aging process. It includes biological factors and also noise exposure. Sociocusis is a term used by some authorities to refer to threshold shifts due to aging and living in a noisy environment. Musicians and their fans exposed to loud music at concerts often have noise-induced hearing loss. Children are also subject to threshold shifts due to noise because of playground activities, toys, and musical devices. Sometimes children risk of noise-induced hearing loss is even greater than for adults because their arms are shorter, thus causing the source of loud sound to be closer to their ears (Martin and Clark, 2003).

Drugs can cause sensorineural hearing loss. Threshold shifts have been noted in people taking large doses of aspirin for long periods for arthritis, back injuries, and other sources of chronic pain. Alcohol has also been linked to sensorineural hearing loss, and it appears to exacerbate the effects of noise exposure. Antibiotic and chemotherapy regimens can also have sideeffects of hearing loss and deafness. Other causes of sensorineural hearing loss include congenial defects, tumors, head traumas, syndromes, and diseases such as Meniere's disease.

Meniere's disease causes progressive hearing loss and is associated with nausea, vomiting, vertigo, and tinnitus. Tinnitus is a buzzing, ringing, or roaring noise in the ear and vertigo is a dizziness and falling sensation. Meniere's disease is caused by a buildup of fluid, or hydrops, in the cochlea. The hearing loss in Meniere's disease is usually unilateral, although occasionally both ears may be affected. Martin (1997, p. 209) describes the typical onset of symptoms: "The difficulty may begin with a sensation of fullness in one ear, followed by a low frequency roaring tinnitus, hearing loss with great difficulty in speech recognition, the sensation of violent turning or whirling in space, and vomiting." There continues to be speculation as to the cause of Meniere's disease and authorities suggest it is related to trauma and biochemical disturbances. Treatment involves medication and surgery to relieve the pressure.

Permanent sensorineural hearing loss can be caused by relatively moderate trauma to the skull (Northern and Downs, 1991). Complications of a traumatic head injury can include meningitis which can cause complete deafness. Meningitis is an inflammation of the membranes surrounding the brain and spinal cord. Autoimmune inner ear disease

(AIED) also causes sensorineural hearing loss. In this disorder the body's own immune system attacks the normal, healthy tissue of the inner ear. There are effective treatments for this sensory-neural hearing loss, including steroid therapy and surgical implants. The auditory nerve can also be damaged during surgery and by acoustic tumors.

Recently the classification of *central auditory processing disorders* was changed to *auditory processing disorders* to provide a more clinically descriptive, rather than an anatomically referenced, category of hearing disorders. Terms used sometimes for hearing loss and processing disorders resulting from damage to the auditory cortex and the tracts leading to it include central auditory defects, cortical deafness, pure-word deafness, auditory agnosia, and acoustic agnosia. They are caused by strokes, tumors, head traumas, brainstem compressions, diseases, and birth defects. These types of hearing disorders often occur with neurogenic speech and language disorders and are difficult to isolate with traditional audiometric tests. Particularly in aphasia, they are difficult separately to diagnose and treat.

14.6 Hearing Screening and Testing

Two important aspects of a sound wave are its frequency and its amplitude. The frequency of vibration is how often the molecules of air compress and rarefact. The compression stage is where the air molecules are compressed from their resting position, thus increasing pressure in that area. Rarefaction is when the distance between the molecules increases from their neutral or resting position, thus decreasing pressure. Sound moves as a wave of progressive compressions and rarefactions of air molecules, and a visual sound wave is a graphic representation of molecular movement. They are high and low pressure changes traveling through the medium of air. Frequency of vibration is how many pressure changes occur in a period (e.g., one second). This frequency of vibration, in the past, was labeled cycles per second (CPS). Today, it is called Hertz (Hz). The "H" in Hertz is in deference to Heinrich R. Hertz, a German physicist. Frequency of vibration is perceived as pitch. Pitch is the subjective impression of how frequently molecules vibrate. As frequency of vibration increases, so does the psychological perception of pitch, although this is not a one-to-one relationship. Pitch and frequency are not linearly proportional. A unit change in frequency of vibration does not necessarily translate into an identical unit change of pitch. The frequency range of the human ear is between 20 and 20,000 Hz. Frequencies below 20 Hz are perceived as vibration, and those above 20,000 Hz are ultrasonic, above the range of human hearing. The energy for speech is primarily around 2,000 Hz, with most of it below 4,000 Hz.

The amplitude is the extent of the mass movement from its resting position to a point farthest away from the neutral position. Intensity is the energy created during this movement. The psychological perception of the force of vibration is called loudness. As the amplitude or intensity of a sound wave increases, so does loudness. Loudness is measured in decibels. A decibel, dB, is one-tenth of a unit of sound called a Bel. The "B" in decibel is capitalized in deference to Alexander Graham Bell for his contribution to the study of sound and hearing. Extremely loud sounds, about 140 dB to 160 dB, are made by chainsaws and jets during takeoff. Breathing is about 10 dB. The distance from the source of a sound affects its intensity. Loudness decreases the farther away a listener is from a sound source. As sound energy moves away from the sound source, it spreads over an increasingly larger area. The inverse-square law states that energy decreases in proportion to the square of the distance from the source. Loudness also affects the perception of pitch. Low-frequency sounds, when made louder, are perceived as lower in pitch. High-frequency sounds, when made louder, are perceived higher in pitch.

There are two related but qualitatively different types of hearing tests which are conducted by individuals with varying levels of training: hearing screening and hearing aid testing. These types of hearing testing are less complex and comprehensive than a medical site of lesion testing. Hearing screening is a longstanding and widespread practice, particularly in schools. It is also done, usually at no charge, by clinics and hearing aid dispensers for adults, particularly the elderly. In a screening hearing test, the goal is to detect a hearing loss and refer the patient for a comprehensive audiological assessment if warranted. The objective of a hearing screening is to detect a problem, not to evaluate the nature and severity of it. Many children are screened in schools and, as reported previously, as many as fifteen children in 100 fail the screening, usually because of head colds and allergies. Hearing screenings in schools are often conducted by school nurses who have been trained in screening methods using portable audiometers. Sometimes, particularly in larger school districts, they are conducted by audiometrists under the supervision of the school audiologist. Often speech-language pathologists also screen hearing as part of speech and language screenings which are conducted at the first of the academic year.

Screening for hearing loss and deafness involves the presentation of pure tones. Each ear is tested separately. The tones usually include 500 Hz, 1,000 Hz, 2,000 Hz, 4,000 Hz, and 6,000 Hz. Many clinicians consider the 6,000 Hz tone to be unnecessary, and some believe it advisable to administer the 250 Hz tone during the screening process.

Some believe 8,000 Hz should be tested. The most important frequencies tested are those in the speech range and include 500 Hz, 1,000 Hz, 2,000 Hz, and 4,000 Hz. Screenings are done in the quietest room available. Each frequency is tested at the same decibel level, such as 20 dB or 25 dB, given the ambient noise levels. If a child fails to hear two or more of the frequencies at the determined decibel level, then he or she is referred for a follow-up screening in about two weeks or for an audiological assessment.

If an individual must be tested in a room with loud ambient noise, there must be adjustments made to the testing protocol. One method of adjusting to the presence of ambient noise is a biological calibration. In biological calibration, the tester places the earphones on his or her head and learns at which loudness levels the sounds can be detected. If the noise level is such that the individual must increase the amplitude level to 30 dB, for example, then testing is conducted at that level. It is assumed that if the student can hear the test tones at the same level as the tester, then the child's hearing must be within the normal range. It is important to note in the report that biological calibration was completed because of the ambient noise levels.

Depending on state licensing requirements, hearing aid fitting and dispensing testing is conducted by ASHA-certified audiologists or hearing aid audiologists who have been specially trained. There are a wide variety of requirements in the United States for fitting and dispensing hearing aids. When fitting and dispensing hearing aids, otoscopic, middle ear, and speech audiometry examination are usually conducted, and hearing aids are selected to compensate for the hearing loss. Hearing aids are then provided by the hearing aid company (factory), and many hearing aid dispensers allow the customer a trial period, typically two weeks, to see if the aids are beneficial.

An otoscope is an instrument for examining the external ear and tympanic membrane. It has a light source and a probe that is placed in the patient's ear. It is used to look for impacted wax, foreign bodies, and other defects and deviations of the ear canal and tympanic membrane. Many audiologists now use a video otoscope rather than the handheld variety. With a video otoscope, the examiner and the patient can view the otoscopic examination on a video display. Slow-motion and still shots can be used to help evaluate the structure and function of the external ear and tympanic membrane, and also to explain the results to the patient.

A pure-tone audiometer is an instrument that measures hearing of pure-tone thresholds. A threshold is the intensity (loudness) at which the sound is first detectible. It is the decibel level at a particular frequency that is barely detectible. Patients are instructed to show when they first

"think they hear the tones." Thresholds are obtained across frequencies, and an audiogram is produced. An audiogram is a graphic chart showing these thresholds. This is done in a step-by-step manner where the patient indicates the quietest sound he or she hears. The decibel levels are increased and decreased until the threshold is found. For air conduction testing, a red O shows right ear results, and a blue X indicates the results in the left ear. Other symbols used in audiometric testing are shown on most audiograms. The typical frequencies available to be tested include 125, 250, 500, 750, 1,000, 1,500, 2,000, 3,000, 4,000, 6,000, and 8,000 Hz. The decibel range of typical audiometers is from -10 dB HL (hearing level) to 110 dB HL. Most audiometers have bone conduction vibrators which are usually placed behind the ear on the mastoid process of the skull. Used for bone conduction testing, they vibrate the skull and bypass the external and middle ear. Sometimes masking is necessary to eliminate sound from being heard in the ear opposite from the one being tested. Noise, usually white noise containing energy in all frequencies, is presented in the opposite ear from the one being tested. Patients are often told that the masking sound is like a waterfall or a rushing river. An air bone gap is usually indicative of middle ear dysfunction. Some audiometers are used in soundproof booths, of which there are several varieties. Portable audiometers are also available.

Speech audiometry is a method of testing hearing whereby the loudness of the speech signal is adjusted to provide information about the patient's understanding of speech. Speech audiometry is conducted in soundproof booths to eliminate the effects of ambient noise on the patient's responses. Speech audiometry provides information about the threshold for speech, most comfortable and uncomfortable loudness levels, and the patient's word-recognition ability (Martin and Clark, 2003). Speech-detection threshold (SDT) is the lowest decibel level at which a patient can just barely detect speech. Speech-reception information (SRT) is the lowest decibel level at which a patient can understand speech. Comfortable and uncomfortable loudness levels provide information about the patient's tolerance of overall loudness levels. Speech discrimination of words with and without hearing aids and in quite and noisy environments can be pivotal in vocational rehabilitation issues. See *Eddy v. Massanari,* 180 Fsupp2d 1255 (d Kan 2002).

There are several diagnostic tests in audiology that provide information about the site of the lesion along the auditory pathways. Otoadmittance, acoustic immittance, impedance, tympanometry, and acoustic reflex tests automatically compare the acoustic energy flowing into and reflected out of the ear. Impedance is the opposition to energy flow. Acoustic impedance audiometry measures resistance in the middle ear and is used in detecting conductive hearing disorders. A hand-held probe is held against the ear, creating a seal between it and the tympanic membrane. Sound and air pressure changes are used to measure the status of the middle ear.

The objective of acoustic impedance audiometry is to assess the energy reflected in the ear canal. If more energy is reflected, the tympanic membrane and/or the ossicular chain are less compliant than normal, suggesting a problem at the mechanical energy stage of the hearing process. Compliance is the flexibility and responsiveness of a structure. Part of impedance audiometry is assessing the acoustic reflex. This reflex action is sometimes called the stapedial reflex. It is the contraction of the stapedius and tensor tympani muscles in response to loud sounds. About 85 dB will produce the stapedial reflex in people with normal hearing. The reflex is an involuntary, protective reaction. Not only does acoustic reflex testing provide information about the middle ear, sometimes it can provide information about the higher levels of the hearing process.

Otoacoustic emission testing (OAE) helps determine the status of the cochlea, VIIIth cranial nerve and brainstem structures. Otoacoustic emissions are echoed sounds created by the expansion and contraction of a normal cochlea and are used in newborn screening programs (Yellin, Culbertson, Tanner, and Adams, 2000). This test is helpful in determining whether a person is feigning a hearing loss or whether it is caused by psychogenic factors. Evoked response audiometry (ERA) involves the placement of electrodes on the patient's head and recording the electrochemical discharges associated with hearing certain sounds. Evoked response audiometry can be helpful in assessing the hearing abilities in infants and adults who cannot respond to traditional testing.

There are other audiological tests and brain scanning devices that are helpful in finding the site of the lesion, types of hearing loss, and auditory perceptual and cortical impairments. They are useful even in patients who are unable to respond to testing. Over the past thirty years, site of lesion testing for hearing disorders has evolved into a highly sophisticated and accurate process. Although false negatives and false positives can be made, audiological testing, when done by competent audiologists and medical specialists, yields reliable and valid diagnostic information.

14.7 Aural Habilitation and Rehabilitation

Technically, aural habilitation and rehabilitation involve different goals and objectives although the therapies are similar. Aural habilitation is provided to individuals who have never developed speech and language skills because of their hearing disorders. Usually these individuals are children born deaf or hard-of-hearing. However, there are instances where older individuals are provided with aural habilitation later in their lives. In contrast, aural rehabilitation is given to individuals who have lost their hearing later in life after they have learned all or part of speech and language. The goals of both therapies are to help improve communication by developing new skills and abilities and strengthening existing ones. Amplification, auditory training, speech reading, and manual communication are procedures and techniques of aural habilitation and rehabilitation. Cochlear implants have also dramatically improved the ability for some individuals to hear.

In recent years, the quality of hearing aids has increased dramatically, largely due to the development of digital models. In the past, hearing aids operated by amplifying an electronic signal and directing it into the ear canal. They were simply small amplifiers. With digital technology, an analog-to-digital converter, a computer chip, converts sound energy into digits, thus providing more clarity when amplified. The difference between analog and digital hearing aids is analogous to the difference between a phonograph record and a musical recording played on a CD player. The quality of the music is substantially improved by digital technology.

In auditory training, the patient is trained to have improved general awareness of sound with and without hearing amplification. Emphasis is placed on auditory discrimination ability, which is the ability to perceive differences in individual sounds. Improving auditory discrimination is particularly important in similarly sounding phonemes and words. Sounds that differ only by voicing, one distinctive feature, are called cognates. Words that differ only by one sound are called minimal pairs.

Speech reading is using the lips, body, and facial gestures to comprehend speech. In the past speech reading was simply called lip reading. The accuracy of speech reading is highly variable and less than 100 percent. This is because many sounds are produced in the back of the mouth and thus do not provide visual cues. In speech reading either the sentence or phrase is broken down into isolated components or each individual sound and word is synthesized into a communication act. Some speech readers use a combination of analysis and synthesis.

Manual communication is the use and understanding of sign language and finger spelling. Sign language is using one or more gestures to express a word or phrase, and finger spelling is using gestures of the fingers to indicate individual letters. Finger spelling is also called dactology. Total communication is using any or all of the above methods to improve communication.

Cochlear implants work by sending sound directly to the auditory nerve. Electrodes are placed into the scala tympani within the cochlea, and a microphone attached to an earhook feeds electrical impulses to a speech processor housed in a behind-the-ear casing or a body-worn unit (Martin and Clark, 2003). Currently cochlear implants are appropriate only for individuals with damage to the hair cells of the cochlea and not neural defects. According to Martin and Clark (2003, p. 380): "Children selected for cochlear implantation typically have a profound bilateral hearing impairment, have reached 18 to 24 months of age, and ideally have no concomitant handicaps in addition to deafness. Active and dedicated family support is a primary key to the successful habilitation of a child with a cochlear implant." Although the quality of speech perception is improving with cochlear implants, they do not create normal hearing in children, nor do they return complete sense of hearing in adults.

14.8 Deafness, Hearing Loss, and Mental Impairment-Mental Retardation Misdiagnosis

There have been instances where children with significant hearing loss or deafness were not identified, and because of their communication disorders, were erroneously classified as mentally impaired-mentally retarded. Sometimes these children were confined to institutions for the mentally retarded, and only later in life was their hearing loss or deafness discovered. Although these tragic occurrences were rare, they can still happen today and consequently be a source of litigation. Issues surrounding litigating misdiagnosis of deafness, hearing loss, and mental impairment-mental retardation include deciding who was responsible for the misdiagnosis, the types of hearing tests administered, and their interpretation. Accuracy of hearing tests can also be called into question when the children are seeking eligibility for special education services.

The reason children with undiagnosed deafness or hearing loss can be labeled mentally impaired-mentally retarded is that a hearing impairment significantly affects speech and language development. The speech patterns and language characteristics of deaf and hard-of-hearing children can resemble mental impairment-mental retardation. Failure to make sounds and words at expected ages, lack of auditory comprehension, difficulty following directions, and poor social interaction can be symptoms of both mental impairment-mental retardation and hearing disorders. In addition, to further complicate diagnostic procedures, some birth defects and syndromes causing mental impairment-mental retardation also have hearing impairments as part of their symptoms. Finding out the degree to which the hearing loss affects the child's scores on intelligence and cognitive tests is necessary. Undiscovered or misdiagnosed hearing loss and deafness in these children compromise the determination of the type and degree of mental impairment-mental retardation.

14.9 Calibration of Audiological Instruments and Tester Competency

The validity and reliability of audiological tests are dependent on the audiometers' calibration and the testers' competency. Calibration is the standardization of an instrument. It is a test and adjustment of the instrument to insure it provides valid and reliable results. Some hearing instruments automatically calibrate themselves, but this process also needs to be periodically checked for accuracy. Public schools, in particular, may not regularly calibrate hearing instruments. Thomas, Preslar, Summers, and Stewart (1969) found poor calibration compliance. In their sample of audiometers in public schools and physicians' offices not one was in proper calibration.

Because hearing screening appears to be straightforward and simple, some schools, physicians, hearing aid dispensers, and clinics do not properly train and monitor testers. This can lead to suspect screening results. The types of testing errors made by poorly trained and insufficiently monitored personnel include failing to place the earphones on the proper ears (red earphone on right ear), making incorrect symbols on the audiogram, and not following standard screening protocols. Perhaps the most common screening error is not adjusting for ambient noise and testing in rooms where the noise levels are too great for accurate results. Speech-language pathologists are trained to screen hearing and their responsibilities include pure tone and screening tympanometry.

14.10 Hearing Aid Sales and Conflicts of Interest

As reported previously, early in the evolution of audiology as an independent discipline, the dispensing of hearing aids by certified audiologists was prohibited. The reason for this prohibition was that there may be a conflict of interest in selling hearing aids when the audiological tests were also conducted by dispenser. It was feared that the profit motive might obscure clinical judgment. Today certified audiologists and hearing aid dealers conduct hearing tests and also dispense hearing aids, and there exists the potential for the misrepresentation of test results and exaggeration of the benefit of hearing aids.

In the 1970s a public interest research group in Michigan studied the claims made by people selling hearing aids and found several misleading statements made to customers. The most misleading statement was that if the person did not purchase the hearing aid his or her hearing would continue to deteriorate. The implications were that the hearing aids would stop and even reverse progressive hearing loss. The rationale given by some in the hearing aid industry was that a person with hearing aids would not adjust for his or her hearing loss by increasing loudness, consequently decreasing overall noise exposure and the risk of noise-induced hearing loss. However, there have been no studies supporting this claim, and in fact, the case can be made that hearing aids stimulate the cochlea, thus increasing the likelihood of continued noise-induced hearing loss. Hearing aids amplify sounds and do not prevent or cure hearing loss.

14.11 Deafness and the Oralist-Manualist Controversy

The oralist-manualist controversy concerns the question of whether American Sign Language is a primary language and whether deaf children should be educated using it. Some in the deaf community are adamant that manual communication is the "natural" language of deaf individuals. They believe attempts by some deaf educators, physicians, speech-language pathologists, and audiologists to teach oral communication are repressive and professionally self-serving. The belief of some in the deaf community is that being deaf and using sign language are cultural issues. To some, deaf individuals are members of a unique culture, one that needs to be respected and preserved. Teaching speech and speech reading and providing cochlear implants are invasive to their culture, and deprives them of membership in the Deaf Community. On the other side of the controversy are those who note that few people outside the Deaf Community use or understand American Sign Language, and that oral communication is necessary to succeed in education, business, and industry. Limiting communication to American Sign Language is needlessly restrictive.

Central to the oralist-manualist controversy is whether being deaf is a disability or an example of being in a repressed linguistic minority. *Stedman's Concise Medical Dictionary for the Health Professions* (Dirckx, 2001) provides two definitions of disability both of which classify deafness as a disability. Most dictionaries define deafness as a disability and include words such as "defect," "disorder," and "inability."

On one side of the controversy, deafness is a defect in the organ of hearing and fits the disability definition. Deafness also fits the definition of disability in the sense that it restricts the ability to perform activities within the range normal for human beings. In contrast to these arguments, some in the Deaf Community note that there is a strong bond among manualists, and American Sign Language, a true language unto itself, creates a sense of linguistic community. This community is similar to one whose members prefer to speak Spanish, French, or another language. Parents and guardians are ultimately responsible for determining a minor child's options for special education. It should be noted that a child taught speech and speech reading can choose to be a manualist at a later time.

14.12 Deafness, Hearing Loss, and Malingering

Malingering is where an individual willfully and deliberately feigns or exaggerates a hearing loss for exemption, attention, sympathy, academic, and/or employment rewards or, more commonly, for financial gain. A true malingerer consciously feigns hearing loss for a self-serving end. Malingering is included in the broad category of "functional" hearing loss. Functional hearing loss is nonorganic in nature; that is, there is no physical basis to the disorder.

When discussing cases of suspected malingering, it is necessary to address psychogenic factors. In some cases where a broad definition of malingering is used, it may be postulated that psychogenic hearing loss, particularly hysterical deafness, is a type of malingering. Hysterical deafness is the complete loss of hearing due to psychological factors. It is thought to result from a conversion reaction. According to Aronson (1990), a conversion reaction can include the loss of a sense (hearing) from interpersonal conflicts or environmental stress. Some persons lose their hearing because of anxiety and interpersonal distress. Often the loss of hearing symbolizes psychic trauma associated with negative relationships. The psychological mechanism underlying the conversion reaction provides the patient with relief from distress, and thus many patients appear relieved at having the hearing loss. They may present with "la belle indifference." In these cases, the hearing loss may be an attention-getting device and an attempt to repair the relationship; the motives may be only partially conscious. The case can be made that some people with psychogenic hearing loss are simply malingerers who at some conscious level receive rewards for feigning the disorder. The issue becomes at what level is the patient conscious of the cause and rewards associated with the hearing loss.

The most common causes of hearing-loss-related malingering are for financial gain and exemption. Financial gain can be associated with automobile or industrial accidents or prolonged noise exposure, and the individual feigns loss of hearing to seek compensation. Malingerers may exaggerate the existing hearing loss. It is likely that exaggerating a hearing loss is more common than feigning one where there is no actual hearing pathology. Parents may exaggerate a child's communication impairment resulting from a hearing loss to increase the amount of compensation in medical malpractice and accident disability cases.

Feigning hearing loss to be exempt from the military draft or assignment is the most common form of malingering for exemption purposes. Obviously a person with a significant hearing loss is unfit for many military assignments. During periods of military drafting, draftees may feign hearing loss or deafness to be designated 4-F, unfit for military service. Also, concerning military service, some individuals may feign or exaggerate a hearing loss to obtain military disability compensation.

Other situations where an individual may feign or exaggerate a hearing loss include issues related to Miranda rights and participation with legal counsel. A person with a hearing loss may indicate that he or she did not understand his or her Miranda rights, when in fact, they were understood. Feigning or exaggerating a hearing loss can bring into question whether a client can meaningfully participate with legal counsel. Hearing loss and malingering may also be an issue under the Americans with Disabilites Act and other disability legislation.

Currently there is no single audiological test that can prove malingering. No test, or series of tests, can conclusively prove that a person is malingering. However, there is a battery of audiological tests and brain scans that can provide credible evidence that a person is "probably" malingering. Through a process of elimination, audiological tests, particularly automatic ones, can shed light on the function of the external, middle, and inner ear. Tests can be performed that can show lesions on cranial nerve VIII, and scans can indicate deficits at higher auditory perceptual, and association areas of the brain. Consequently, expert testimony can be used in cases of suspected malingering.

14.13 A Case Study Hysterical Deafness

A young woman was seen by a university speech and hearing clinic for apparently hysterical deafness allegedly resulting from parental abuse when she was a child. This was before the development and refinement of present-day audiological tests, such as evoked response and acoustic impedance audiometry, and current brain scanning devices.

Although the woman's history of the onset of hearing loss was difficult to confirm, it was thought that her deafness originated when she was a preschooler. Medical reports showed no organic cause of her deafness, and the audiological site of lesion testing also suggested that it was functional.

It was hypothesized that the hysterical deafness was the result of a conversion reaction. The conversion reaction caused her deafness and stemmed from the environmental stress and parental abuse. Reportedly, she was also subjected to extreme verbal abuse, and the deafness symbolized the psychic trauma. She also presented with "la belle indifference," appearing unconcerned about the deafness.

Central to whether the deafness was indeed a result of a conversion reaction was the woman's speech. She spoke with "deaf speech" typical of an individual who has lost hearing before or during the speech and language development period. Prelingual deafness is the loss of hearing before or during the speech and language development period. Deaf speech is often abnormally nasal, produced with imprecise articulation, and an "open mouth" feature. There is also a "singsong" trait to ongoing utterances. Deaf speech results from the person's lack of auditory feedback with regard to speech sounds. The question arose about why she would present with deaf speech if there was no organic reason for the deafness.

The argument for an organic pathology causing her deafness was supported by the observation that a hysterical conversion reaction would not completely block auditory feedback for several years. Given that the woman had left home and the abusive environment several years previously, the auditory feedback might have returned, thus eliminating or reducing the deaf speech characteristics. On the other hand, some specialists opined that a conversion reaction can completely block auditory feedback over long periods. The sensory block occurs at the perceptual level and eliminates auditory feedback in a manner similar to bilateral hearing deficits and perceptual disorders. As noted above, this case occurred before current sophisticated audiological tests and brain scanning devices. It is likely that today an organic pathology, if present, would be identified, thus eliminating the speculation about the functional nature of her deafness and deaf speech.

14.14 Chapter Summary

In the past three decades, the diagnosis and treatment of hearing loss and deafness have dramatically improved. Advances in audiological assessment procedures, especially those that automatically perform site of lesion tests, combined with current brain scanning devices, permit the comprehensive evaluation of the hearing mechanism from external ear to the auditory cortex. Many of these tests can be conducted without patient participation. Cochlear implants and digital hearing aids can restore a degree of hearing in deaf individuals and provide improved clarity of amplification for hard-of-hearing people. These advances in the diagnosis and treatment of hearing disorders have also influenced medical malpractice litigation, eligibility for special education services, malingering, and other legal issues.

Suggested Readings and Resources

Martin, F. and Clark, J. (2003). *Introduction to Audiology* (8th ed.). Boston: Allyn & Bacon. This book provides a comprehensive overview of audiology and a CD-ROM is included for illustration purposes.

Tanner, D. (2003). *Exploring Neurogenic Communication Disorders: A 21st Century Introduction Through Literature and Media*. Boston: Allyn & Bacon. Chapter 6 addresses hearing loss and deafness and uses references to literature and media to introduce and explain them.

Tanner, D. (2006). *An Advanced Course in Communication Sciences and Disorders*. San Diego: Plural Publishing. This book explores the hearing mechanism, auditory perception, and verbal association from a scientific and philosophical perspective.

References

American Academy of Audiology (2006). About Audiology. Retrieved September 22, 2006 from the World Wide Web: http://www.audiology.org/aboutaudiology/ (Author)

Aronson, A. (1990). *Clinical voice disorders: An interdisciplinary approach* (3rd ed). New York: Thieme.

Culbertson, W., Cotton, S., and Tanner, D. (2006). *Anatomy and physiology study guide for speech and hearing*. San Diego: Plural Publishing.

Dirckx, J. H. (2001). *Stedman's concise medical dictionary for the health professions* (4th ed). Philadelphia: Lippincott Williams & Wilkins.

Martin, F. (1997). *Introduction to audiology* (6th ed.). Boston: Allyn & Bacon.

Martin, F. and Clark, J. (2003). *Introduction to audiology* (8th ed.). Boston: Allyn & Bacon.

National Center for Health Statistics. (1988). Current estimates from the National Health Interview Survey, United States, 1988. *Vital and Health Statistics*, Series 10, No. 173 DHHS Publication No. (PHS) 89-1501.

Northern, J., and Downs, M. (1991). *Hearing in children* (4th ed.). Philadelphia: Lippincott Williams & Wilkins.

Northern, J. L. and Downs, M.P. (2002). *Hearing in children* (5th ed.). Baltimore: Lippincott Williams and Wilkins.

Public Health Service. (1994). Vital and health statistics: Prevalence and characteristics of persons with hearing trouble: United States 1990-91. Series 10: Data from the National Health Survey No. 188. DHHS Publication No. 94:1516.

Tanner, D. (2006). *An advanced course in communication sciences and disorders*. San Diego: Plural.

Thomas, W., Preslar, M., Summers, R. and Stewart, J. (1969). Calibration and working conditions of 100 audiometers. *Public Health Report*, 84, 311-327.

Yellin, M., Culbertson, W., Tanner, D., and Adams, T. (2000). Gender differences in transient evoked otoacoustic emissions (TEOAEs) of newborns. *Infant-Toddler Intervention*, 10(3): 177-200.

Young, H. and Geller, R. (2007). *Sears & Zemansky's college physics* (8th ed.). San Francisco: Pearson, Addison Wesley

Zemlin, W. (1998). *Speech and hearing science* (4th ed.). Boston: Allyn & Bacon

Part III
The Forensic Aspects of Voice Prints

Chapter 15

Speech Production and Phonetics

15.1 Chapter Preview

This chapter provides an overview of the various aspects of speech production and serves as a basis to understanding voice prints. The distinction between speech and language is made and there is a review of relevant terminology. Discussed in this chapter are the five basic motor speech processes: respiration, voice, articulation, resonance, and prosody as they relate to speech acoustics. This chapter also examines phonetics, the science concerned with the perception, classification, description, acoustics, and production of speech sounds. There are several figures showing the International Phonetic Alphabet and the symbols used to represent speech sounds.

15.2 Speech Communication

Speech communication is a process, a series of events allowing the speaker to express thoughts and emotions and the listener to understand them. Speech communication begins as thought which is transformed into language for expression, and the brain programs and activates the body movements necessary to produce speech sounds. Respiration provides the compressed air for the production of speech sounds, and the vocal cords vibrate, providing voiced energy for loudness and resonance. The articulators, primarily the tongue, lips, teeth, and soft palate, valve the air stream and shape it into speech sounds. Energy is transmitted through the medium of air as sound waves, and the structures of the ear detect that energy. From the ear, the speech signal goes to the brain, where sound is perceived, decoded, and understood by the listener.

Speech and language are often used interchangeably, but they are different aspects of communication. Language is the use of symbols for thinking, and expressing and understanding ideas and information. Language is multimodality; there are several avenues or ways of communicating. Expressively, one sends ideas and information through writing, speaking, and gesturing, and receptively, the listener understands what has been spoken, written, and gestured. The primary expressive avenues of communication are speaking, writing, and using expressive gestures. The primary receptive avenues of communication are reading, auditory comprehension, and understanding the gestures used by others. Mathematics is also a language; people express and receive ideas and information using mathematical symbols.

There are three primary aspects to any language: phonology, syntax, and semantics. Language is rule governed and grammar is a general term for the rules of a language. Phonology is the set of rules by which speech sounds are combined into words and is indirectly depicted on voice prints. Syntax addresses word order and semantics deals with word meanings. Semantics is the relationship between the word and what it means.

Speech is one aspect of language. Speech is the use of the muscles and structures of the body to shape compressed air into sound. Speech patterns are commonalities among speech sounds, similarities and differences in the way people speak. Speech patterns can be detected on acoustic levels with minor changes in air pressures, vibratory modes, and resonance characteristics. Speech and language are interconnecting aspects of communication.

15.3 Motor Speech Production

Speech programs, i.e., neurological impulses and muscular movements necessary to produce voluntary speech sounds, are planned in the cortex of the brain. The cortex (Latin for "bark") of the brain is a thin surface layer of cells. It is dark in appearance and sometimes called the gray matter. In most people, purposeful and voluntary speech is planned, at least partially, in Broca's area of the frontal lobe of the left hemisphere. Broca's area is named after the 18th century French neurologist, Paul Broca, who discovered that speech and language occur in the left hemisphere of the brain in most people. However, it should be remembered that the brain operates as a whole, and no single part of it works independent of other areas especially when it comes to communication. In addition, the areas of the brain responsible for speech and language differ among individuals. For example, some left-handed individuals have aspects of speech and language located in the right hemisphere of the brain. Therefore, it is difficult to say with precision where in the brain the speech act is programmed in all people. (See Chapter 2 for a detailed discussion of brain localization issues.)

The speech program includes the neurological commands to produce sounds, syllables, words, and phrases. Speaking is a very complex neurological and muscular event. It involves hundreds of muscles and thousands of neurological impulses per second. The program includes every muscle movement to be used in the production of speech. For example, to produce a word, the breathing muscles must take air into the lungs, compress it, and allow it to be released slowly. The vocal cords must vibrate on some sounds, and not on others, and with proper loudness and pitch. The tongue, lips, lower jaw, and soft palate must move rapidly and smoothly from one articulatory point to another when forming speech sounds. Besides the motor, or movement commands, sensory feedback occurs. The sensory feedback allows the speaker to know whether the sounds are being produced correctly, and to make corrections if necessary. Motor speech occurs very rapidly. A speaker can talk intelligibly at more than 500 words per minute, and he or she can do so for several hours. There are five physical processes to motor speech production: respiration, phonation, articulation, resonance, and prosody.

15.4 Respiration for Speech Purposes

The primary function of respiration is to sustain life by providing the cells of the body with oxygen and removing carbon dioxide. The secondary function of respiration is speech production. Respiration for speech involves expanding the chest cavity, allowing air to enter the lungs, and then gradually decreasing the size of the cavity to expel it. Boyle's law and the Kinetic Theory of Gases account for this process; a given quantity of gas varies inversely with its pressure, and gas flows from a region of high to low pressure and vice versa. Inspiration is the taking of air into the lungs. During inspiration, the diaphragm, a dome-shaped muscle separating the thorax (chest) from the abdomen (stomach or belly), contracts and compresses the lower abdominal tissue. Also during inspiration, the chest wall muscles expand the chest cavity. This creates a condition where the pressure in the lungs is lower than the outside atmospheric pressure. When the speaker's mouth and nose are opened, air rushes from the higher atmospheric pressure to the lower pressure in the lungs. During expiration, or expelling air from the lungs, the opposite pressure change occurs. During expiration, the pressure in the lungs is greater than the atmospheric pressure, and air flows outward through the speaker's mouth and nose. Speech sounds are made on this outwardly flowing air.

15.5 Phonation

Phonation is the act of vibrating the vocal cords to produce sound. Not all speech sounds are voiced, and cognates are two sounds differing only by voicing. For example, the cognates /s/ and /z/ differ only by one feature: voicing. Voicing occurs in the larynx (lair-rinks), a structure made up of cartilage, muscles, and soft tissue, and suspended by muscles in the center of the neck. The thyroid cartilage is shaped differently in males and the notch or prominence is called the "Adam's Apple." Another cartilage, the epiglottis, snaps down over the vocal cords to protect the airway during swallowing. The vocal cords (folds) are inside the larynx and they are capable of vibrating very rapidly due to the myoelastic-aerodynamic principle of voice production. This principle states that the rapid vibrations of the vocal folds are due to their muscular elasticity and a suction effect related to the velocity of air flowing through a constriction. The vocal cords are tightened and loosened by the sliding, rocking, and rotating action of the arytenoid cartilages. The frequency of vocal cord vibration creates the perception of pitch. In men, the vocal cords vibrate, on average, 130 times per second. In women, the average rate of vocal cord vibration is about 250 cycles-per-second giving the perception of a higher pitch. The frequency of vocal cord vibration primarily depends on how tightly the vocal cords are stretched and their thickness. The amplitude or force of vocal cord vibration creates the perception of loudness. The amplitude of vocal fold vibration primarily depends on air pressure and how forcefully they close. The quality of a person's voice, e.g., whether it is harsh, hoarse, or breathy is a result of the efficiency of vocal cord vibration and the resonance characteristics of the system. As discussed below, the voicing mechanism can be viewed as a resonating system. It is similar to musical instruments where the source vibrations are transformed into distinctive musical qualities. The vibrations occurring in the larynx are resonated in a person's neck and head giving him or her a distinctive voice quality. Figure 15.1 shows the human larynx.

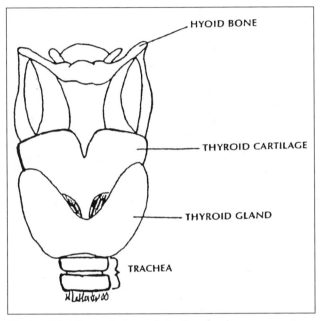

Figure 15.1 *Frontal view of the human larynx*

15.6 Articulation

Articulation is the shaping of the oral cavity into distinctive speech sounds. The primary articulators are the lips, tongue, teeth, lower jaw (mandible), and palates (hard and soft). The alveolar ridge, the tissue just behind the upper incisors (front teeth), is also an important articulatory site. For example, /d/ and /l/ are produced when the tongue contacts the alveolar ridge. The primary articulators are divided into those fixed, e.g., alveolar ridge, teeth, and hard palate, and the movable ones, e.g., lips, tongue, mandible, and soft palate (velum). The articulators are also divided into those that are hard and soft. The primary hard articulators are the teeth, mandible, alveolar ridge, and hard palate, and the soft articulators are the lips, tongue, and soft palate. Figure 15.2 shows the primary articulators.

Static articulation is producing of speech sounds in isolation. In static articulation, there are no sounds produced before or after the one being made. Dynamic articulation is producing speech sounds in connected utterances. Connected speech is usually done so rapidly that the articulators do not make their ideal points of contact; they only approximate them. This is the concept of serially ordered speech events; dynamic speech is a stream of articulatory gestures. In dynamic speech, the sounds preceding and following the target one affect the points of contact. Coarticulation is the overlapping of movements during dynamic speech. Coarticulation leads to assimilation; the effect one sound has on another. In rapid speech, sounds become more like each other and their differences diminish.

15.7 Speech Resonance

The vibrations of vocal cords in the larynx serve as the source of sound for the resonating chamber. In adults, the speech resonating chamber, a double Helmholtz system, is approximately 17 cm in length. The length, size, texture, and configuration of the oral tract affect the resonance characteristics, and give speech sounds their acoustic qualities. As noted above, the comparison of the speech resonating chamber to a musical brass instrument illustrates several important points. For example, just as the vibration of the lips in the mouthpiece of a trombone creates the source of sound, so too does the vibration of the vocal cords in the neck. With the trombone, aspects of the sound source are either amplified or damped (sometimes called "dampened") by the length, size, texture, and configuration of the brass instrument. With the speech resonating system, the aspects of the sound source created in the larynx are amplified or damped in the resonating tubes of the head and neck, giving each sound its distinctive acoustic qualities. The speech resonating system is called a double Helmholtz resonator.

The velopharyngeal port is an important valving site for resonance (see Figure 15.2). The velopharyngeal port is where the soft palate contacts the back of the throat (pharynx) to close off the nasal passageways. In English, there are three sounds that have the velum lowered, thus opening the velopharyngeal port: /m/, /n/, and "ng" (as in long). These sounds are called nasals. (Other languages such as French and Navajo have more nasal sounds.) When the velum is lowered, and the velopharyngeal port opened, air and increased acoustic energy is transmitted through the nasal cavities. When the velopharyngeal port is partially or completely opened on non-nasal sounds, or there is a hole or cleft in the palates, speech is hypernasal. Conversely, when there is obstruction of the nasal passageways or the velopharyngeal port is closed on nasal sounds, hyponasality occurs.

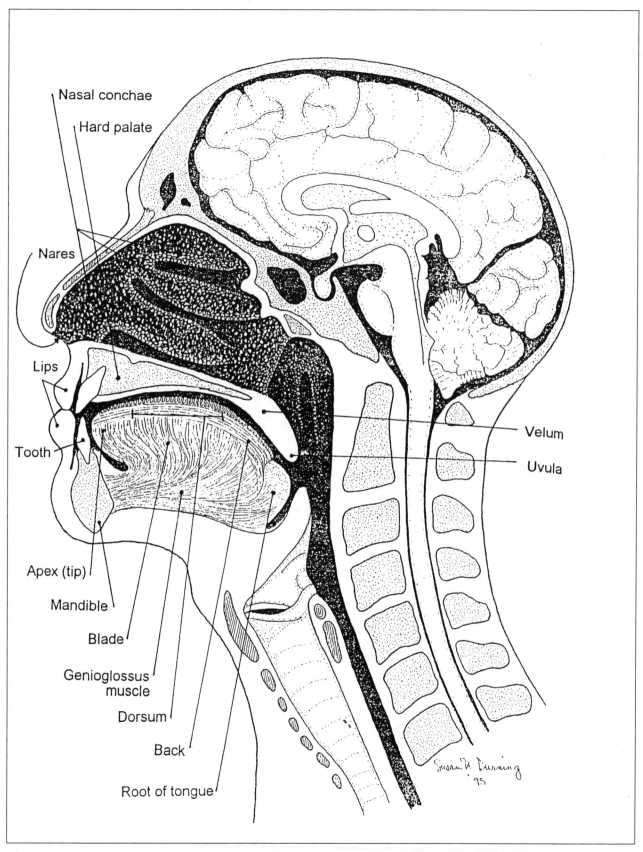

Figure 15.2 *Cross section of the head showing the articulators*

15.8 Prosody

Prosody is the rhythm and flow of speech. It includes acoustic patterns such as stress, intonation, and melody of speech production. Prosody also includes the fluency, cadence, inflection, and emphasis aspects of speech. Speech fluency is the act of producing connected speech without interruptions, interjections, and unnecessary pauses. It also includes the fluent organization of speech into thoughtful utterances. Intonation is the rise and fall of pitch during speech, and can provide information about meaning. For example, the rise of pitch at the end of an utterance can signal that a question has been asked. Stress primarily involves the loudness of a particular sound in a word compared with the adjacent sounds. Speech prosody is highly individualized, and there are a variety of individual prosodic aspects of speech. Integral to normal speech prosody is feedback where the output is evaluated at its source and modifications made if necessary, a servosystem. Table 15.1 shows the processes of communication, physiological functions, and the physical laws and theories associated with speech acoustics.

15.9 International Phonetic Alphabet and Phonetic Transcription

This section addresses general phonetics which includes the transcription of speech sounds. Phonetic transcription is an important aspect of using speech patterns for forensic purposes. In General American English, there are forty-four sounds and only twenty-six letters in the alphabet to represent them. Consequently, listing sounds using conventional letters of the alphabet is fraught with error. The same letters can stand for two different sounds, and some letters do not have corresponding sounds. For example, the "th" letters can represent two similar but different sounds: "th" as in "that," and "th" in "thought." Also for example, when using the alphabet to represent sounds, there is difficulty knowing what speech sounds the letters "c" and "k" represent. Scientists created the International Phonetic Alphabet (IPA) to address these transcription problems and other issues. The International Phonetic Association is the oldest representative organization for phoneticians and was established in 1886 in Paris (IPA, 2006).

A phoneme is the speech sound and a grapheme is the letter used to represent it. With the International Phonetic Alphabet, one phoneme is represented by only one grapheme (phonetic symbol), and vice versa. It eliminates transcription confusion. Small variations in phoneme production may be represented by diacritic markers placed near a phonetic symbol.

Table 15.1
Communication Processes and Acoustics

Communication Process	Physiological Function	Speech Acoustics: Physical Laws and Theories
Respiration	Air Compression for Speech Production	Boyle's Law and the Kinetic Theory of Gases
Phonation	Energizing Speech for Speech Production	Myoelastic-Aerodynamic Principle of Voice Production
Articulation	Shaping Compressed Air for Speech Production	Serially-Ordered Speech Acts
Resonance	Nasal Coupling and Nasality During Speech Production	Double Helmholtz Resonator
Prosody	Speech Rhythm and Flow	Closed-Loop Feedback (Servosystem)

15.10 English Consonants

The consonants of the English language are classified in two ways: manner and place of production. Manner of production is classification of speech sounds by the type of air modification produced by the articulators. In the manner of production classification system, consonants are divided into stops and continuants. A stop (plosive) consonant is one where the air stream is completely occluded by the articulators, and a continuant results from partial occlusion. Nasals are speech sounds where the soft palate is lowered, and there is increased nasal resonance. Also, in the production of nasals, the oral cavity is constricted by the lips or tongue to direct the air flow and energy through the nasal cavities. Glides are sounds produced by a gliding motion of the articulators. In the production of a glide, the articulators move from one position to another. Fricatives are sounds produced by constricting the air stream, and affricates are combinations of stops and released air flow and energy. Plosives are sounds produced by occluding the air stream with the articulators and releasing it. Figure 15.3 shows the continuants consonants of the English language by manner of articulatory contact, the IPA graphemes, and words containing the phonemes.

Place of articulation classifies consonants by the point of articulatory contact in the oral tract where the sounds are produced. Bilabials are sounds produced by both lips, labio-dentals—lips and teeth; lingua-dental—tongue and teeth; lingua-alveolar—tongue and alveolar ridge; lingua-palatal-tongue and palate; lingua-velar—tongue and soft palate; and glottal—vocal cords.

Figure 15.4 shows the stop consonants of the English language by point of articulatory contact, IPA graphemes, and words containing the phonemes. According to Ladefoged and Maddieson (1988), there are approximately sixteen different places of consonant articulation in the world's languages.

15.11 English Vowels

Vowels depend on the height and front-to-back position of the tongue in the oral cavity, and the rounding of lips during their production. Vowels are classified as high, mid, and low depending on how elevated is the tongue, and whether it is toward the front, middle, or back of the oral cavity. For example, some vowels are classified as low-back, high-back, or low-front sounds (see Figure 15.5).

A diphthong is a vowel produced by a gliding action of the articulators, and there is a noticeable change in the acoustic properties from beginning to end of its gliding motion. Rhotic vowels have an "r" sounding or flavor to their production. Figure 15.6 shows several English diphthongs and gives examples.

Type of Phoneme	Phoneme	Examples
nasal	m	"motion" "come"
nasal	n	"now" "done"
nasal	ŋ	"going" "gong"
glide	j	"yellow" "you"
glide	r	"ran" "carrot"
glide	l	"litigation" "mall"
glide	w	"water" "way"
fricative	ʒ	"beige" "garage"
fricative	z	"zipper" "buzz"
fricative	ð	"that" "other"
fricative	v	"verdict" "shove"
fricative	ʃ	"shoot" "bush"
fricative	s	"summons" "bus"
fricative	θ	"think" "bath"
fricative	f	"forensic" "cuff"
fricative	h	"hat" "house"

Figure 15.3 English continuant consonants

Type of Phoneme	Phoneme	Examples
affricate	dʒ	"jury" "jump"
affricate	tʃ	"church" "bench"
plosive	g	"gun" "mug"
plosive	d	"drill" "hood"
plosive	b	"bang" "cab"
plosive	k	"kill" "bilk"
plosive	t	"terror" "hat"
plosive	p	"pill" "up"

Figure 15.4 English stop consonants

Tongue Height	Tongue Front/Back	Phoneme	Examples*
high	front	I	"h<u>i</u>t" "b<u>i</u>t"
low	back	ɑ	"m<u>o</u>b" "b<u>o</u>b"
low	front	æ	"pl<u>a</u>nt" "c<u>a</u>t"
high	front	i	"f<u>ee</u>" "s<u>ee</u>"
mid	front	ɛ	"f<u>e</u>deral" "cr<u>e</u>dible"
mid	back	o	"<u>o</u>ver" "<u>o</u>kay"
mid	back	ʌ	"m<u>o</u>ther" "<u>u</u>p"
mid	back	ɔ	"<u>a</u>ll" "f<u>a</u>ll"
high	back	u	"s<u>ue</u>" "bl<u>ue</u>"
high	back	ʊ	"b<u>oo</u>k" "c<u>oo</u>k"
central	rhotic (unstressed)	ɚ	"moth<u>er</u>" "lawy<u>er</u>"
central	rhotic (stressed)	ɝ	"b<u>ir</u>d" "h<u>ear</u>d"
mid	front	e	"f<u>a</u>ke" "b<u>a</u>ke"

Figure 15.5 *English vowels (Lowe 1994). *Examples added*

Dipthong	Examples
ai	b<u>uy</u>, m<u>y</u>, s<u>igh</u>
aʊ	h<u>ow</u>, n<u>ow</u>, c<u>ow</u>
ɔi	b<u>oy</u>, t<u>oy</u>, j<u>oy</u>
Iɚ	d<u>ee</u>r, st<u>ee</u>r, f<u>ear</u>
ɔɚ	d<u>oor</u>, m<u>ore</u>, st<u>ore</u>
ɑɚ	c<u>ar</u>, st<u>ar</u>, b<u>ar</u>
ɛɚ	c<u>are</u>, st<u>air</u>, d<u>are</u>
ʊɚ	p<u>oor</u>, j<u>ury</u>

Figure 15.6 *English diphthongs (Lowe 1994).*

The syllable is the basic physiologic and acoustic unit of speech. Syllables consist of a vowel that can stand alone or be surrounded by one or more consonants. There are several types of syllables, and they are designated with the letters "C" (consonant) and "V" (vowel). For example, CCV represents the consonant-consonant-vowel occurrence in the word "sleigh." "Man" is a CVC syllable, and "up" is a VC syllable.

15.12 Summary

Speech and language are related but different aspects in the communication chain. Speech is one modality of language, one avenue of communication. The speech program includes the neurological commands for the five basic motor speech processes: respiration, phonation, articulation, resonance, and prosody. The International Phonetic Alphabet provides a way of representing speech sounds in a clear and concise way.

Suggested Readings and Resources

Culbertson, W., Cotton, S., and Tanner, D. (2006). *Anatomy and Physiology Study Guide for Speech and Hearing.* San Diego: Plural Publishing. This study guide provides an in-depth examination of the anatomy and physiology involved in speech and hearing.

Tanner, D. (2006). *An Advanced Course in Communication Sciences and Disorders.* San Diego: Plural Publishing. This book proposes the Unified Model of Communication Sciences and Disorders and explores the communication chain from speaker to listener.

References

The International Phonetic Association (2006). Phonetic symbols. Retrieved September 23, 2006 from the World Wide Web: http://www.arts.gla.ac.uk/IPA/ipa.html (Author).

Ladefoged, P. and Maddieson, I. (1988). *Language, speech and mind: Studies in honour of Victoria Fromkin* (pp. 49-61). London: Routledge.

Chapter 16

The Acoustic Foundations to Voice Prints

16.1 Chapter Preview

This chapter provides the acoustic foundations for speech pattern detection using voice prints. There is a review of Fourier's law for analyzing and synthesizing speech sounds and a discussion of sound waves to give the reader a basic understanding of speech acoustics. Resonance, the foundation to speech pattern recognition, is detailed. Shimmer, jitter, and voice onset time are also described.

16.2 Speaker Recognition

Listeners engage in speaker recognition, the detection of speech patterns, all of the time. Whether it is the matter-of-fact reporting of a nightly news anchor, a relative's message on voice mail, or a friend's voice in a crowd of partygoers, the human ear provides a very reliable way of knowing who is speaking. Pitch, loudness, rate of speech, emphasis, and a host of subtle cues are processed by the listener and judgments made about the speaker's identity. Most of the time, these cues are dealt with subconsciously and the listener is unaware he or she is doing it.

Not only does the human ear recognize familiar voices, it provides subjective information about how the speaker feels about what is being said. A person can tell whether the speaker is emotionally distraught, relaxed, tired, happy, sad, and so forth, based on speech cues. The words spoken provide objective information, and "how" they are spoken gives information about the speaker's frame-of-mind. Humans are marvelous sensing creatures and a speaker's speech and voice provides ongoing valuable information about his or her identity and psychological condition. Titze and Story (2002, p. 1) comment on verbal and nonverbal multiple messages:

> We send multiple messages when we speak. Some are linguistic and some paralinguistic, meaning that they are independent of the words that we utter. Such paralinguistic messages concern our health, our mood, our genetic makeup, and our upbringing. Many of them are encoded in voice quality, which in the most general sense is everything in the acoustic signal other than overall pitch, loudness, and phonetic contrast (vowels and consonants).

Besides being able to recognize people by their voices, the human ear also registers whether the speaker's speech and voice are consistent with his or her physical appearance. If the speaker is male, the listener expects a lower pitch than if she is female. A large-framed person should have speech and voice typical of his or her physical appearance. A tiny person should have the speech and voice typical of his or her diminutive stature. A male or female with excessive masculine or feminine physical characteristics should project them in their speech and voice traits. When a person's speech and voice are substantially different from expectations, the listener senses that something is awry. This difference between speech expectations and reality creates cognitive dissonance (Tanner, 2003). As used here, cognitive dissonance refers to listener anxiety, disquiet, and apprehension when speech and voice characteristics differ from expectations. Cognitive dissonance is common when listeners are confronted with a disabled person's speech symptoms that are inconsistent with his or her expected intelligence. For example, many people expect a person in a wheelchair with drooling and slowly produced, distorted speech to be mentally deficient. However, there are individuals with those physical limitations who are not mentally deficient and some are mentally superior. Listener cognitive dissonance is created when there are these disparities between expectations and reality. Factors contributing to speech and voice expectations in normal people include gender, height, weight, and age.

16.3 Speech Analysis and Synthesis

Expressive communication is encoding or synthesizing a message and listening is decoding or analyzing it. Speech analysis is the process of breaking down an acoustic signal into its component parts and speech synthesis is the reverse process. Both processes can now be done by computers and they have revolutionized the telecommunication industry and services for the disabled. Today, most cell and car phones can use speech and voice commands to recognize the speaker and dial telephone numbers. These telephones breakdown the speech signal into its component parts, compare them to previously stored information, and permit verbal commands. Synthesis allows segments of the speech signal to be combined. Speech synthesis technology has progressed dramatically and type-to-speech, automatic closed-captioning, and other forms of augmentative communication are providing disabled individuals with opportunities to interact with the verbal population that were unavailable previously. Advances in these technologies show no signs of relenting, and the future promises even more inventions to accommodate the communication disabled (Culbertson and Tanner, 2002; Tanner and Culbertson, 2002; Tanner, 2001; Wade, Petheram, and Cain, 2001).

16.4 Fourier's Law

In the 1800s, Joseph Fourier, a French mathematician, discovered that any complex sound can be broken down into its simple sound waves. Any nonsinusoidal wave, a complex wave, can be represented as the sum of a number of sinusoidal waves, simple waves, of different frequencies, amplitudes, and phases. This mathematical principle is Fourier's law and allows for speech synthesis and analysis. Speech synthesis involves adding acoustic segments to create a complex wave. Complex sound waves are analyzed into simple sine waves revealing their frequencies and amplitudes. The Fourier transform allows speech to be seen as a spectrum (Tosi, 1975; 1979). The Fourier law is the basis by which the sound spectrogram or "voiceprint" is produced. The comparison of a sound spectrogram to a fingerprint is common but inaccurate. A fingerprint is static and unchanging. A spectrogram represents speech patterns that change from utterance to utterance and from speaker to speaker. However in this text, speech sound spectrograms will be referred to as voice prints due to the widespread use of the label. The Fourier mathematical expressions are provided below for illustrative purposes:

Source: Tosi 1975; 1979, 23–25.

Fourier expansion

$$v(t) = c_0 + \sum_{n=1}^{\infty} c_n \sin n\omega t + \varphi_n$$

or alternatively

$$v(t) = c_0 + \sum_{n=1}^{\infty} a_n \cos n\omega t + \sum_{n=1}^{\infty} b_n \sin n\omega t$$

where

$v(t) =$ values of the successive vertical ordinates v (amplitudes, intensities, pressures and so on) of a complex periodic wave, expressed as a function of time t;

$c_0 =$ a vertical axis constant term (amplitude, intensity, pressure and so forth); if the complex wave is symmetrical in reference to the horizontal axis of time, then $c_0 = 0$;

$c_n =$ peak ordinate (amplitude, intensity, pressure and so on) of the nth harmonic in the sin Fourier expansion;

$\sum_{i=1}^{n} =$ summation of a series of similar terms that differ from each other only by the value n; for the first term it is $n = 1$, for the second term $n = 2$, and so on until the last term is added to the series;

$n =$ number of the harmonic considered;

$w =$ angular frequency of the periodic complex wave $w = 2F_0$;

$\varphi_n =$ phase of the nth harmonic, or the time or equivalent angle (period $\int$ 360) obtained by shifting the sinusoidal wave along the horizontal axis to obtain a zero ordinate at zero time;

$a_n =$ peak ordinate of the nth harmonic in the cosine term of the cos-sin Fourier expansion; and

$b_n =$ peak ordinate of the nth harmonic in the sine term of the cos-sin Fourier expansion.

Also

$$c_n = \sqrt{a_n^2 + b_n^2}$$

and

$$\varphi_n = \frac{\tan^{-1} b_n}{a_n}$$

where

$$c_0 = \frac{1}{\tau} \int_{-\frac{\tau}{2}}^{\frac{\tau}{2}} v(t)\, dt ,$$

$$a_n = \frac{2}{\tau} \int_{-\frac{\tau}{2}}^{\frac{\tau}{2}} v(t) \cos n\omega t\, dt , \text{ and}$$

$$b_n = \frac{2}{\tau} \int_{-\frac{\tau}{2}}^{\frac{\tau}{2}} v(t) \sin n\omega t\, dt .$$

Fourier transforms

$$V(\omega) = \int_{-\infty}^{\infty} v(t) e^{-j\omega t}\, dt$$

where

$V(w) =$ the values of the successive ordinate V of the spectrum of a complex wave as a function of angular frequency w, and

$v(t) =$ the values of the successive ordinates v of the wave expressed as a function of time t.

The Fourier transform provides the value $V(\omega)$ of each ordinate of the spectrum for each angular frequency $\omega (\omega = 2\, f)$ along the horizontal axis.

Similarly, knowing the spectrum $V(\omega)$ of a complex wave, it is possible to convert to the time domain by the use of the inverse Fourier transform:

$$v(t) = \frac{1}{2\pi} \int_{-\infty}^{\infty} V(\omega) e^{j\omega t}\, d\omega$$

Notice that $e^{-j\omega\tau} = \cos \omega t - j \sin \omega t$ and $e^{j\omega\tau} = \cos \omega t + j \sin \omega t$.

16.5 Acoustic Energy

Acoustics is the science of sound. Acoustic energy is the vibration of a mass of particles of air. The earth is surrounded by trillions and trillions of air molecules. Dry air consists of about 20 percent oxygen and 80 percent nitrogen (there are trace amounts of other gases such as hydrogen, carbon dioxide, carbon monoxide, etc.). Because of gravity, the molecules have weight and are more densely compacted the closer they are to the center of the earth. Thus, the atmo-

spheric pressure, on average, is greater at sea level, and decreases with increasing elevation. At sea level, the molecules of air have an average barometric pressure of 29.92 Hg. This reference barometric pressure is the amount of force the air molecules place on mercury in a vacuum tube and is measured by the number of inches the mercury is displaced upward. Air pressure fluctuations are caused by temperature, moisture content, and air mass motion. Air is extremely elastic and thus serves as an excellent medium for the transmission of sound energy. Elasticity is the ability of an object or mass to resume its original shape after being distended. Other media can serve to transmit sound energy such as water and metal, but air is very efficient because of its elastic properties.

16.6 Sound Waves

Sound waves can be likened to water waves. When a ship passes through calm water, it displaces the water next to it causing waves, high crests and low troughs (water peaks and valleys) compared with the surrounding calm water. The wave closest to the ship goes up and down, impacting the water next to it, which goes up and down, affecting the water next to it, and so forth. This continues until waves splash onto the shore. Energy is transferred from the ship to shore through the water. The mass of water next to the ship does not actually reach the shore; it is energy that is transferred through the water. For the most part, the visible water energy transfer is horizontal. Human ears are designed to detect longitudinal waves in which the air particles move back and forth parallel to the wave's direction (Young and Geller, 2007).

Sound waves radiate outwardly 360 degrees and where the waves start is called the starting phase. Starting phase is the mass of molecules when they start to vibrate and is measured in degrees, the starting point of the wave. Sound waves are a series of air vibrations caused by an external force. This force can be a hand clap, a tuning fork flicked with a finger, the vocal cords vibrating, pressure released from a plosive phoneme, and so forth. In simple sound waves, when the force displaces a mass of air particles, they move past their stable neutral position. When they have traveled the maximum distance, they recoil again past the neutral, resting position. Air molecules have mass and because of momentum they are driven back and forth from their resting position. Momentum of an object is the product of mass times velocity. This back and forth movement continues until the elastic force exceeds the opposing force of momentum. When this happens, the vibration stops. Sound waves follow Newton's first Law of Motion: Every object continues in its state of rest or motion in a straight line at constant speed unless forces cause it to change its state.

Compression is when the air molecules are compacted from their neutral or resting position and rarefaction is when the molecules are dispersed from their neutral or resting position. During the compression stage, there is an increase of pressure because the molecules of air are more densely compacted. The air pressure is lower during the rarefaction stage because the molecules are farther apart from their resting or neutral position. Sound moves as progressive points of compression and rarefaction of air molecules. Sound waves are high and low pressure changes traveling through the medium of air. Sound travels at about 1,130 feet per second or about 770 miles-per-hour at sea level (344 meters per second in 20ΥC air). According to Young and Geller (2007), the speed of sound varies greatly relative to the media (in meters per second): helium=999 m/s, hydrogen=1,330 m/s, and steel=5,000 m/s. The graphic sound wave is the representation of this molecular displacement over time and produces a waveform. Acoustic energy is transformed to mechanical energy in the middle ear. The law of conservation of energy deals with the transformation of energy: energy cannot be created or destroyed; it can only be transformed. The idea of entropy also plays a role in energy transformation in a system. Whenever energy freely transforms from one form to another, the direction of the transformation is toward a state of greater disorder or greater entropy.

16.7 Frequency of Vibration and Pitch

One cycle of vibration is the complete movement of the air particles from crest to crest. The number of molecular displacements per second is the frequency (f) of the sound wave. The frequency of these recurrent movements of air particles is measured in Hertz and abbreviated Hz. To know the frequency of vibration, the period (P) must be discerned. The period of a sound wave is the time taken, the duration, to complete one vibratory cycle. There is an inverse relationship between period and frequency. The longer the period, the smaller the frequency; as P increases, f decreases. Conversely, as P decreases, f increases; the shorter the duration, the greater the frequency. The frequency of vibration can be obtained from the following formula: $f = 1/P$ [Hz]. For example, a period of 0.0025 seconds yields 400 Hz, 0.00125 yields 800 Hz, and 0.000625 yields 1,600 Hz. Period can be obtained from this formula: $P = 1/f$ [sec].

The physical property of frequency of air particle vibration is related to the psychological perception of pitch. As air particles vibrate more rapidly during the period, a higher frequency sound is produced, which in turn, creates the psychological perception of a higher pitch. Conversely, as air particles vibrate more slowly during the period, a lower frequency sound is produced, resulting in a psychological perception of a lowered pitch. Frequency of vibration and the psychological perception of pitch are positively correlated, e.g., a unit movement in either direction of frequency of vibration is associated with a unit movement in the same direction in the psychological perception of pitch. Lower frequency vibrations are perceived as lower pitch sounds; higher frequency vibrations are perceived as higher pitch sounds. However, this relationship is not linear. There is not a 1:1 correlation between changes in frequency of vibration and the psychological perception of pitch. For example, doubling the frequency of a particular sound wave does not necessarily result in the doubling of the psychological perception of pitch. Frequency of vibration and psychological perception of pitch are positively correlated, but they are not linearly proportional. Loudness also affects pitch. For example, when a low frequency tone is produced very loudly it seems lower in pitch to the listener. Conversely, higher pitched tones, when played very loudly seem higher in pitch to the listener. A subjective pitch scale for pure tones uses m-e-ls to make pitch and frequency proportional. M-e-l is derived from the word "melody."

The human range of hearing is approximately 20 to 20,000 Hz. Frequencies below 20 Hz are perceived as vibration and those above 20,000 Hz are ultrasonic or above the range of human hearing. Most of the energy of speech lies below 4,000 Hz with 2,000 Hz as the pivotal frequency for speaker identification features. Human ears are very sensitive to vibrations between 1,000 Hz and 4,000 Hz.

The Doppler effect relates to frequency of vibration and the perception of pitch. It occurs when a sound source and a listener are in motion toward or away from each other. (It also occurs with other waves.) It is common occurrence when a sound source passes a listener who is in a stationary position. For example, if a listener is in a stationary position and a car passes him or her at a fixed velocity, the frequency of particle vibration increases, thus causing the sensation of a higher pitch as the car approaches. When the car passes the listener, the frequency of vibration and the perception of pitch decrease. The cycle of vibration, the crest to crest movement of air particles, occurs more frequently because of the car's velocity as it approaches the listener. The result is a compression of the sound waves and the perception of a higher pitch as the car speeds toward the listener. When the car passes the stationary listener, the frequency of vibration of air particles is stretched out, the crest to crest movement of air particles occurs less frequently, resulting in the perception of lower pitch. The magnitude of the change in frequency of air particle vibration depends on the velocity of the car as it approaches and passes the listener. We have all had the experience of sensing a pitch change as objects approach and pass us at various speeds. The magnitude or amount of change in frequency is called the Doppler shift. Motion is movement relative to something and speed is the rate distance is covered divided by time. Velocity is speed together with the direction of travel. Acceleration is the rate at which the velocity is changing with respect to time.

16.8 Amplitude of Vibration and Loudness

The physical property of amplitude of air particle vibration is related to the psychological perception of loudness. If an outside force displaces air particles from their resting position causing vibration, they move back and forth across their neutral positions. Amplitude of vibration is the distance the air particles are dispersed positively and negatively from their neutral or resting position. The maximum displacement in any direction is the peak amplitude and is the intensity or force of the sound wave (measured as the peak sound pressure). The power transmitted along the wave is called the intensity of the sound. It is determined at right angles to the direction of the propagation. Power is the rate or amount of work done in a given time. It is measured in ergs per second or watts such as occurs in light bulbs. Horsepower is a common measure of work used in automobile engines. It is based on the amount of work a horse can do in a given period of time.

Amplitude and the psychological perception of loudness are positively correlated, e.g., the greater the amplitude of air particle vibration the greater the psychological perception of loudness. However, as is the case with frequency of vibration and pitch, there is not a 1:1 correlation between changes in amplitude and the psychological perception of loudness. They are not linearly proportional. The p-h-o-n scale is used to compare loudness levels at different frequencies. The human ear can detect extremely small changes in loudness levels. The strongest sound we can hear is much greater than a just audible one. Loudness of a sound is measured in decibels: one tenth of a Bel or dB (the "B" is capitalized in deference to Alexander Graham Bell). The decibel is a unit expressing the relative intensity of sound on a logarithmic scale (base 10), an intensity ratio. The average intensity of speech as measured about a foot from the lips of a speaker is about 50 dB. The threshold or the minimum power of human hearing is very small, about 10–16 watts. Table 16.1 shows the frequency and amplitude of particle vibration and consequent effects on pitch and loudness.

Vibration can occur whenever mass and elasticity are present. The movement of the mass of air particles from maximum positive to negative position and back to positive position again is called one cycle of oscillation. The oscillations would continue infinitely if not for energy loss in the system such as friction. The movements of the air particles from their extreme positive and negative positions gradually decrease. Vibration amplitudes that decay slowly are lightly damped and those with greater decay are said to be heavily damped. Sinusoidal vibrations are simple movements of mass such as is seen in the movement of a pendulum.

16.9 Wavelength

A wavelength is the distance the wave travels in one cycle of vibration, the distance between two crests, troughs, or some other point. The sound wave will travel a distance of f wavelengths in one second and the velocity is equal to the product of the frequency and the wavelength. The wavelength of a 20 Hz sound wave is about 56 feet: 1,130 feet-per-second/20 cycles-per-second=56 feet. The wavelength of a 1,000 Hz sound wave is about 14 inches: 1,130 feet-per-second/1,000 cycle-per-second=1.13 or 14 inches. The highest frequency of human hearing, 20,000 Hz, yields a wavelength of 0.06 or about 3/4 of an inch: 1130 feet-per-second/20,000 Hz = 0.06 feet. Loudness decreases the farther away a listener is from a sound source. The number of air particles increases with the distance from the speaker and that is why sound dissipates the farther away the listener is. As sound energy moves away from the sound source, it spreads over an increasingly larger area. The inverse-square law says that energy decreases in proportion to the square of the distance from the source. The energy at a person's ear will vary inversely as the square of the ear's distance from the sound source ($I=1/d^2$).

Table 16.1
Particle Vibration and Effects on Pitch and Loudness

Particle Vibration	Pitch
Increase in Frequency of Particle Vibration	Nonlinear Increase in Psychological Perception of Pitch
Decrease in Frequency of Particle Vibration	Nonlinear Decrease in Psychological Perception of Pitch
Increase in Amplitude of Particle Vibration	Nonlinear Increase in Psychological Perception of Loudness
Decrease in Amplitude of Particle Vibration	Nonlinear Decrease in Psychological Perception of Loudness

16.10 Sound Pressure

Each air particle exerts a force on the adjacent one, which exerts a force on the one next to it and so forth. The dyne is the unit of force used in acoustics. One dyne is extremely small. For example, an ounce of sand has about 30,000 dynes of gravitational force. Using dynes, sound pressure can be computed. Sound pressure is the amount of force, dynes, on a surface area, centimeters. One erg is the amount of work done when one dyne force displaces an object by one centimeter. These pressure changes act on the eardrum causing small movements. The smallest pressure changes necessary to produce an audible sound is 0.0002 dynes/centimeter^2.

Sometimes pressure waves cancel each other. This can occur in auditoriums and concert halls. When the sound coming from speakers on the stage meets the sound being reflected from the walls at the back of the auditorium or concert hall, they tend to cancel each other. The pressure waves stand still. This phenomenon is called a standing wave and is used for noise abatement.

16.11 Simple Harmonic Motion, Sinusoidal and Complex Waves

A simple sound wave is produced by recurrent movement when an outside force displaces air particles from their neutral position, and allowing them to be free to oscillate without additional outside influence. As noted above, the mass of air particles will vibrate sinusoidally and the frequency of the oscillations will always be the same. When time is plotted on the horizontal axis, simple harmonic motion is represented by a sinusoidal graph, a sine curve. This vibration of the mass of air particles is called the natural or resonant frequency and is determined by properties such as dimension, texture, and shape. A simple sound vibrates at only one frequency. A pure tone such as is produced by a tuning fork is an example of a simple sound wave. A tuning fork can be tapped and left to vibrate. It will produce only its natural frequency and gradually die out as the energy dissipates. Acoustic energy is lost because of friction when air molecules contact each other. Simple sound waves are very rare and most sounds are complex. Speech is a complex sound wave. Complex sounds have two or more frequencies and result from forced or sympathetic vibration. When graphing complex sound waves, the amplitude spectrum shows the frequencies and amplitudes. Each sinusoidal component is represented by a vertical line whose height is proportional to the amplitude of the component. The height at any frequency shows the energy in the wave at a particular frequency. Frequency is shown on the horizontal line;

the further to the right the higher the frequency. Voice quality and other aspects of speech are a product of resonance. Resonance is the peaking of amplitude at a certain frequency (Young and Geller, 2007).

16.12 Resonance

In the free vibration discussed above, the amplitude of the oscillation is determined by the size of the initial displacement. In free vibration such as occurs with a tuning fork, the amplitude can be no larger than the initial displacement and it will decay slowly as the energy dissipates. In forced vibration, for any source-resonating chamber combination, the amplitude of the total vibration in the system depends on both the amplitude and frequency of the source. For a given amplitude of forcing motion, the vibration of the resonating chamber is largest when the driving frequency equals the natural frequency of the system. When a forcing vibration has the same frequency as the natural or resonant frequency of the resonating chamber, resonance occurs. Resonance is when a body undergoing forced vibration vibrates with the greatest amplitude for frequencies near its own natural frequency. The resonant frequency is the frequency at which the maximum oscillation occurs and it is the same as the system's natural frequency. Optimal resonance occurs when the system vibrates with the most efficiency. With resonance, the amplitude of the vibration can be very large causing the psychological perception of increased loudness at certain frequencies.

Given the above technical discussion of resonance, speech resonance can be explained in a simple way. Suppose that a speaker's neck and head resonating chambers are removed above the level of the glottis. The glottis is the opening of the airway at the level of the vocal cords. If the speaker produces voice, the sound will be a buzz. In a male, the source buzzing sound will be a lower frequency than that of a female. As discussed in Chapter 15, the sound will resemble that of a mouthpiece detached from a trombone or a reed detached from a clarinet. These buzzing sounds are not pure tones and consist of many frequencies.

If the speaker's head is replaced while the source buzzing sound is being produced, certain frequencies in the source buzzing sound will be amplified and others damped. A sound wave at the glottis is changed by the resonance characteristics of the vocal tract. The air columns in the neck and the empty space (about 450 cubic centimeters) in the speaker's head vibrate in response to the source. This gives the speaker his or her distinct voice quality. Changes in the amplitude and frequency of the source interact with the articulatory changes in neck and head resonating chambers to create distinct speech sounds. If another person's head is placed on the source of the sound, because of its different shape and resonance potentials, the voice quality will be different because the source-resonating chambers are different. Titze and Story (2002) examined male and female laryngeal vocal tracts using magnetic resonance imaging (MRI). Through MRI, tubular representations of the vocal tracts were made during the production of four vowel but using different voice qualities and registers. Their results showed that different voice qualities and registers have clearly definable vocal mechanism adjustments.

16.13 Periodic and Aperiodic Sound Waves

All speech sounds are complex waves and each of the simple sinusoidal waves is called a component. The frequency of each component is a whole number multiple of the fundamental frequency. The fundamental frequency (fo) is the basic component of a speech sound wave, the frequency of vibration of the vocal cords. The component whose frequency is twice the fundamental frequency is called the second harmonic. The component whose frequency is three times the fundamental frequency is called the third harmonic, and so forth. Voiceless sounds are aperiodic waves and the duration of each recurrence is random. They have components at all frequencies rather than only at multiples of a fundamental frequency. In theory, periodic waves have an infinite number of identical repetitions during the same period. A quasiperiodic complex wave is one that is partially repetitive. Voiced sounds are generally assumed to be quasiperiodic.

Shimmer (amplitude perturbation) and jitter (frequency perturbation) are related to fundamental frequency. "Shimmer is a measure of the way that the amplitude varies from one period of the fundamental frequency to the next" (Ryalls and Behrens, 2000, p. 75). Ryalls and Behrens (2000, p. 75) note that jitter is a measure of the way vocal cords vary from one cycle of vibration to the next: "Since jitter assesses period-to-period duration variation, it is actually a temporal measure." Shimmer and jitter are not present on voiceless sounds. Shimmer and jitter are variations in amplitude and frequency of a speech waveform, respectively. Frequency instability is used as a measure of speaker stress levels. (See Chapter 22)

16.14 Voice Onset Time

Voice onset time (VOT), measured in milliseconds (ms), is the time it takes for the energy to be released from a stop consonant and for voicing to begin. Voice onset time is relevant to stop consonants. For example, the stop consonant

/p/ has in the initial aspect of its production a buildup of pressure behind the lips. Then, after the release of the pressure, there is initiating of vocal cord vibration: p... --uh. The duration of time between the release of the pressure behind the lips and the start of phonation is the VOT. The /p/ is categorized as a voiceless phoneme, and thus has a relatively long VOT. In contrast, the voiced /b/, the cognate to /p/, differs only by voicing; the tongue and the lips are in similar positions for each phoneme. Voicing is the primary acoustic feature differentiating them. When /b/ is produced, there is a much briefer VOT because the vocal folds begin to vibrate much sooner after the release of the pressure behind the lips. Other phonemes where VOT can be contrasted include /t/ and /k/ and their voiced counterparts /d/ and /g/. In languages other than English, there is occasionally prevoicing where there is voice before the release of the obstructed airflow. Although rare, some English speakers engage in prevoicing.

16.15 Chapter Summary

Speech sound spectrograms, sometimes called voice prints, provide investigators with objective, accurate, and reliable information about speaker identity. A Fourier analysis where a complex sound wave is represented as the sum of a number of sinusoidal waves of differing frequencies, amplitudes, and phases produces the speech spectrogram.

Suggested Readings and Resources

Bell Telephone Laboratories (1958). *The Science of Sound.* New York: Folkways Records and Service Corp. This taped lecture on the acoustics of speech provides examples how sound is produced and analyzed.

Ryalls, J. and Behrens, S. (2000). *Introduction to Speech Science: From Basic Theories to Clinical Application.* Boston: Allyn & Bacon. This brief text addresses the essentials of the speech sciences.

Tanner, D. (2006). *An Advanced Course in Communication Sciences and Disorders.* San Diego: Plural Publishing. Chapter 8 details acoustic and resonance aspects of speech production.

Titze, I.R. and Story, B.H. (2002, Fall). Voice quality: What is most characteristic about "you" in speech. *Echoes,* Vol. 12, No. 2., pp. 1.4. Acoustical Society of America: Melville: New York. This article in the newsletter of the Acoustical Society of America addresses voice quality and several acoustic parameters.

References

Culbertson, W. and Tanner, D. (2002, July-August). The brave new world of the cyber speech and hearing clinic: Treatment possibilities. *Proceedings of the International Conference on Advances in Infrastructure for Electronic Business, Science, Education and Medicine.* L'Aquilla, Italy.

Ryalls, J. and Behrens, S. (2000). *Introduction to speech science: From basic theories to clinical applications.* Boston: Allyn & Bacon.

Tanner, D. (2001, December). The brave new world of the cyber speech and hearing clinic. *ASHA Leader*, 6(22).

Tanner, D. (2003). *Exploring communication disorders: A 21st century approach through literature and media.* Boston: Allyn & Bacon

Tanner, D. and Culbertson, W. (2002, July). The brave new world of the cyber speech and hearing clinic: Diagnostic possibilities. *Proceedings of the 6th World Multi Conference of Systemics, Cybernetics and Infomatics,* Orlando, Florida, USA.

Titze, I.R. and Story, B.H. (2002, Fall). Voice quality: What is most characteristic about "you" in speech. *Echoes,* Vol. 12, No. 2., pp. 1,4. Acoustical Society of America: Melville: New York.

Tosi, O. (1979). *Voice identification: Theory and legal applications.* Baltimore: University Park Press.

Tosi, O. (1975). *Personal Correspondences.* Institute of Voice Identification, Department of Audiology and Speech Sciences, Michigan State University, East Lansing, Michigan.

Wade, J., Petheram, B., and Cain, R. Voice recognition and aphasia: Can computers understand aphasic speech. *Disability and Rehabilitation*, Vol. 23, No. 14, 604-613.

Young, H. and Geller, R. (2007). *Sears & Zemansky's college physics* (8th ed.). San Francisco: Pearson, Addison Wesley.

Chapter 17

The Voice Print and Speaker Identification

17.1 Chapter Preview

This chapter examines the salient features of a voice print for speaker identification purposes. The concept of transitioned speech segments and automatic speech are addressed as is the Tosi Method of Voice Identification. Spectrograms of stops, affricates, fricatives, nasals, glides, vowels, diphthongs, blends, and pauses are provided including composite characteristics. Semiautomatic and automatic voice identification methods and technologies are also discussed.

17.2 Salient Features of the Sound Spectrogram

The sound spectrograph was developed by Kay Elemetrics of Pine Brook, New Jersey, during the 1940s (Potter, Kopp and Green, 1947). The device generated voltage from repeated tracings of an audio tape segment. The early models burned a time-domain image of a speech sample onto a specially coated paper strip. The sound spectrogram (voice print) is a visual representation of speech based on repeating Fourier analyses. There are several salient features of a speech sound spectrogram. The three major aspects of speech represented by the spectrogram are time, frequency, and energy (see Figure 17.1). Time is plotted along the horizontal base of the graph. Older spectrograms were burned onto special sheets of paper attached to a rotating drum and the length of the speech sample was limited to 2.4 seconds. Approximately 250 msec is about 3 centimeters in length on a 2.4 second spectrogram. Frequency of the speech signal is represented on the vertical axis. The lowest horizontal line is the base and the frequencies, extending to at least 4,000 Hz, are plotted in proportional degrees vertically. The relative intensity of sound is portrayed by varying degrees of darkness of the patterns representing the energy of speech signal. Computer-generated spectrographic images allow for the cursor to show relative decibels. According to Borden, Harris, and Raphael (2003, p. 209):

> The sound spectrograph, a free-standing device largely dedicated to producing hard-copy versions of spectrographic displays, has been largely replaced by commercial computer software that is available in several versions. Many laboratories, however, are still equipped with traditional sound spectrographs of various vintages that perform satisfactory analyses. In any event, the types of displays they produce are the same as those generated by the newer technology.

There are several other primary features of the speech spectrogram or spectrographic images. Vertical striations show periodic and aperiodic sound energy. The periodic vertical striations have clearly identified repetitive energy pulses, resonance bars, and correspond to one opening and closing of the vocal cords. Thus, they are visual representations of voiced speech sounds. Unvoiced sounds do not have repetitive resonance bars and appear as random energy bursts. There are three primary formants (F1, F2, F3) important to speaker identification. Formants are bands of acoustic energy and give vowels their perceptual qualities. The lowest formant is F1 and the second formant, F2, is considered the "hub" formant for speaker identification and speech pattern detection. The frequency change in a formant over time is called a formant transition. As can be seen in Figure 17.2, these are rises or drops in the leading or trailing segments of a formant band. They represent the change in the positions of the articulators in connected speech. "In a general sense, the steady-state portion of a formant relates more to the vowel portion of a syllable, while the formant transition relates more to the consonant portion" (Ryalls and Behrens, 2000, p. 72). Plosive sounds, where there is an abrupt release of air pressure, can also be seen on a spectrogram and their typical temporal (time) characteristic determined.

As previously noted, speech patterns are not like fingerprints. A person's fingerprints are static from one sample to the next; they do not vary significantly over time. Acoustic patterns occurring during dynamic (connected) speech change from one speech sample to the next. In dynamic speech, a person may talk faster or slower, with a higher pitch or lower one, and with more or less nasal resonance from one sample to the next. However, there are general acoustic consistencies that serve as identifying factors across speech samples. This is why the human ear can distinguish one speech sound from another and recognize different speakers. The sound spectrogram shows those consistencies. However, because of the variability of dynamic speech, it is necessary to get as many samples of the same utterances as possible. The more samples, the more valid and reliable is the voice identification process. Just as the human ear requires several listening events to be able to recognize the speech and voice of a speaker, so too does the visual voice identification process. The variation of a suspect's speech from one speech sample to the next is called intra-speaker variance and the variance of one suspect's voice sample from several unidentified ones is referred to as inter-speaker variance.

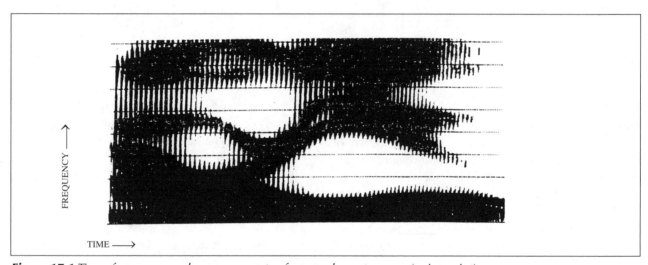

Figure 17.1 Time, frequency and energy aspects of a sound spectrogram (voice print)

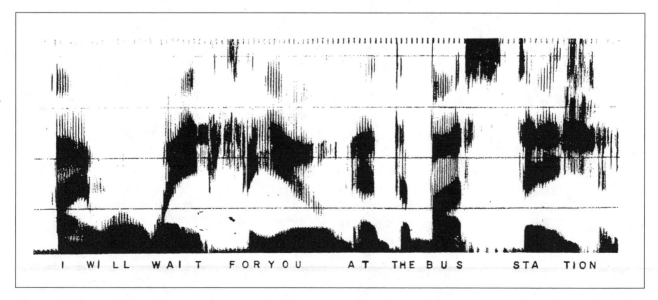

Figure 17.2 Sound spectrogram and primary features (Courtesy Dr. Oscar I. Tosi and the Michigan State University Institute of Voice Identification)

17.3 Transitioned Speech Segments and Automatic Speech

In connected speech, the words run into each other. In Chapter 15, the ideas of coarticulation and assimilation were discussed. Coarticulation is the overlapping of movements during dynamic speech which leads to one sound affecting another or assimilation. In dynamic speech, sounds become more like each other. Because of coarticulation, some acoustic properties of a phoneme may be absent and others distorted as ideal features of a sound. In addition, words and even short phrases blend into one another.

All speech is learned. Children are not born talking; they must learn it. Learning any behavior involves habit strength. The more we engage in a behavior, the more subconscious and uniform it becomes. When possible, subjects' speech samples should be routine, off-the-cuff types of utterances such as "Good morning," "How is it going," "Bye-bye," "You know," and so forth. This is because these utterances are said many times by a particular speaker and the likelihood is great that there is less variance in their acoustic qualities than if the speaker was using a word spoken infrequently by him or her. A neurological explanation for consistency with automatic speech is that new programming is primarily cortical with modifications based on body and auditory feedback. Automatic speech is primarily subcortical and thus the program is relatively established and consistent. Titze and Story (2002, p. 4) comment on vocal tract shape and resonance: "Genetics plays a major role, as does age, culture, dialect, and vocal training. In part, we can control our own voice quality; for example, by maintaining a forward tongue position throughout our speech, by maintaining a lower larynx position (as if yawning), by maintaining our lips somewhat rounded or pursed, or by clenching our teeth." They go on to note that culture, dialect, and vocal training are "firm-wired" whereas the effects of genetics and age are basically "hard-wired."

17.4 Subjective and Objective Methods of Voice Identification (The Tosi Model)

Tosi (1975; 1979, p. 4) was the first physicist and speech scientist to establish a subjective-objective continuum method of voice identification:

> The meaning of the words subjective and objective might vary for different persons. However, for the author, in the context of voice identification they can operationally be defined as follows: subjective methods of voice identification are those in which decisions are produced by the human mind; objective methods are those in which decisions are produced by mechanical or electronic means. However, it is necessary to point out that in these objective methods there still exists a great deal of human interaction, because, for example, the computer has to be programmed and its results have to be interpreted by an examiner.

According to the Tosi Model, the most subjective method of voice identification is using expert listeners, i.e., those who have successfully completed phonetics and voice identification courses, to compare unknown samples with known samples using either short-term or long-term memory. Long-term memory is more subjective than short-term feature comparisons. The second subjective method is voice spectrogram feature comparisons called the visual detection of speech patterns. Objective methods of voice identification include semiautomatic and automatic, with semiautomatic being the most subjective of the two. In the objective semiautomatic method, there is interaction between the examiner and computer during examination. In the computerized method, a computer is programmed to detect salient features and compares them with recently acquired samples or those obtained from a data bank of known speakers. Objective computerized methods are discussed later.

It should be noted that in the Tosi Method, spectrographic voice identification is always done in conjunction with aural analysis. Trained listeners engage in aural identification using the four confidence ratings listed below. When a conflict between spectrographic voice identification conclusions and aural decisions occurred, Tosi frequently relied on the aural results. Tosi often commented: "The human ear is the most sensitive and capable method for voice identification." However, spectrographic voice identification provides an important objective foundation to Tosi Method.

According to the Tosi Method, there are four confidence ratings with each subjective decision:

> Very uncertain that my decision is correct
> Fairly uncertain that my decision is correct
> Fairly certain that my decision is correct
> Almost certain that my decision is correct

These self-confidence ratings can be plotted on a modified Likert scale marking the degree of certainty from left to right and using a 1–4 numerical scale. This is a forced confidence rating and the evaluator must respond to every sample.

17.5 Visual Detection of Speech Patterns

The human eye is extremely accurate in detecting speech patterns on a spectrogram or spectrographic image. Studies have shown that examiners who are untrained and unable to explain the technical aspects of a speech spectrogram can produce highly reliable and accurate voice identification matches. Simply asking untrained observers which spectrogram appears to be similar to another in a sample of several unknowns can provide excellent results in speaker identification. For example, Figure 17.3 shows the same speaker uttering the same statement. The untrained observer can clearly see similarities in the speech patterns. However, training of the examiners significantly improves accuracy.

At the Michigan State University Institute of Voice Identification, the following were salient aspects of a spectrogram to observe in speaker identification cases. Each is discussed in detail below (see Table 17.1).

1. Stops
2. Affricates
3. Fricatives
4. Nasals
5. Glides
6. Vowels
7. Diphthongs
8. Blends
9. Pauses
10. Composite characteristics

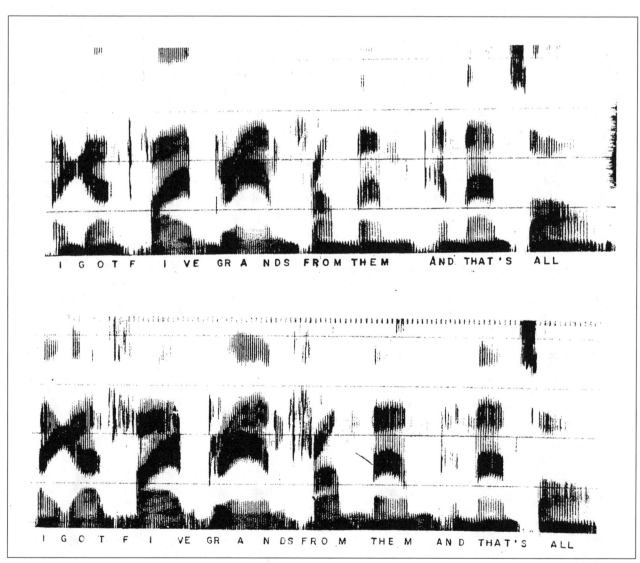

Figure 17.3 One speaker uttering the same statement (Courtesy Dr. Oscar I. Tosi and the Michigan State University Institute of Voice Identification)

Table 17.1
Voice Print Analysis

Salient Feature	Description	Analysis
Stops	Speech sounds made by momentarily ceasing completely the air stream	Voice onset time, length of gaps, frequency, and duration of voiced energy
Affricates	Speech sounds consisting of a plosive and a brief fricative	Duration, frequency, and voice onset time
Fricatives	Speech sounds made by forcing air through a constricted area	Duration and frequency of fricatives, proximity of vertical striations (voiced), voiced energy dispersions
Nasals	Speech sounds produced by lowering the velum to allow airflow through the nasal passageway	Proximity of vertical striations and the frequency of the energy dispersion
Glides	Speech sounds requiring movement of the articulators	Rise and fall of formants
Vowels	A voiced speech sound resulting from relatively unrestricted passage of the air stream through the vocal tract	Midpoint and slope of formant transitions
Diphthongs	Phoneme produced by moving the structures of articulation from one vowel articulatory gesture to another	Transitional features resulting from coarticulatory movements
Blends	Two or more consonants without a vowel separating them (consonant cluster)	Slope of energy release relative to temporal factors
Pauses	Gaps between and within words	Duration between and within words
Composite Characteristics	Overall appearance	Relative intensity of energy dispersion, band width of formants, and their separation

1. Stops (Figure 17.4)

Consonant stops are analyzed by the manner of air stream modulation and the way energy is dispersed on the spectrogram. Consonant stops are created by using the articulators to valve the compressed air coming from the lungs. Stops are made by briefly ceasing completely the air stream and subsequent acoustic energy in the speech tract. Both voiced and voiceless stops involve a buildup of interoral air pressure, release, and voice onset. The voiced stop phonemes are /b/, /d/, and /g/. Voiceless stops are /p/, /t/, and /k/. On the spectrogram, the pressure release, a gap or blank space, is followed by a spike of voiced energy. Factors to observe in speaker identification of stops include voice onset time (see above), length of gaps, frequency, and duration of voiced energy. "The velar /k/ and /g/ have a larger cavity in front of the constriction. This has the effect of concentrating their energy in the midrange of frequencies, around 1500 to 4000 Hz, depending on the tongue position for the following vowel" (Ferrand, 2001, p. 208).

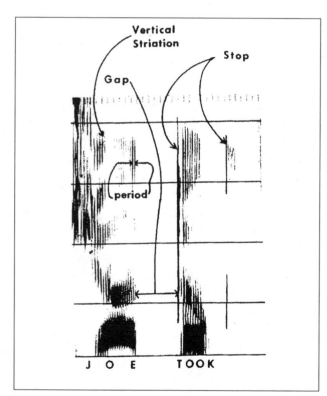

Figure 17.4 Sound spectrogram of the stop consonants /t/ and /k/ (Courtesy Dr. Oscar I. Tosi and the Michigan State University Institute of Voice Identification)

2. Affricates (Figure 17.5)

Technically, affricates are stop consonants, but because they can provide important salient information for speaker identification, they are discussed separately. Affricates are explosions of air shaped into continuents. In English, /tʃ/ ("chur<u>ch</u>") and /dʒ/ ("jump") are the voiceless and voiced affricates, respectively. Factors to consider in speech pattern detection of affricates include their duration, frequency, and voice onset time.

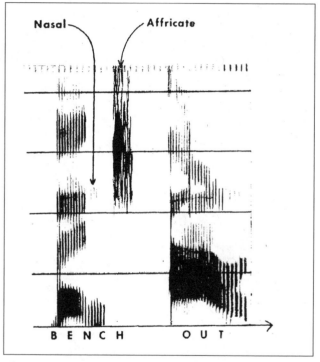

Figure 17.5 Sound spectrogram of the affricate /tʃ/ ("ben<u>ch</u>") (Courtesy Dr. Oscar I. Tosi and the Michigan State University Institute of Voice Identification)

3. Fricatives (Figure 17.6)

Voiced and unvoiced fricatives involve constriction of the air stream and they are typically associated with higher frequencies of acoustic energy. Higher frequency energy can be observed by periodic and aperiodic dispersion of energy toward the top of the spectrogram. Recall that the frequency of the energy of the speech signal is represented vertically with the lower part of the spectrogram indicating low frequencies and higher frequency energy toward the top. In a fricative production, the air stream is constricted but not completely stopped by the articulators. The constricted opening produced by the articulators can occur at several places in the speech tract. As a rule, the more anterior the constriction in the oral cavity, i.e., sounds produced toward the front of the mouth, the higher the frequency of the sound. The fricatives are /ʒ/, /z/, /ð/, /v/, /ʃ/, /s/, /θ/, /f/, and /h/. The duration and frequency of fricatives are salient features to note on the spectrogram. On voiced fricatives, the frequency of vocal cord vibration, as indicated by how close or far apart are the vertical striations, can provide important information for speaker identification. The voiced energy dispersions are also speaker dependent variables.

/ng phonetic symbol/ is the result of occluding the air stream at the level of the tongue and palate and directing the air stream through the nose. Salient features of nasals on a spectrogram include frequency of vocal fold vibration as noted by the closeness of the vertical striations and the frequency of the energy dispersion. Antiresonances are created by the opening of velopharyngeal port and are discussed in the vowel section below.

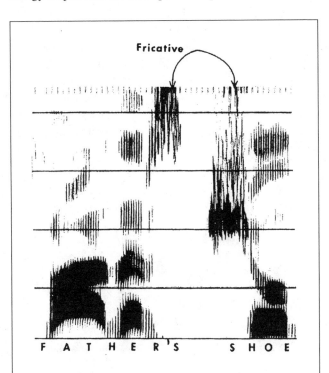

Figure 17.6 *Sound spectrogram of the fricatives /s/ and /ʃ/ ("shoe") (Courtesy Dr. Oscar I. Tosi and the Michigan State University Institute of Voice Identification)*

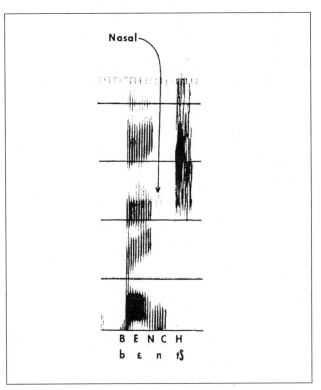

Figure 17.7 *Sound spectrogram of the nasal / n / ("bench") (Courtesy Dr. Oscar I. Tosi and the Michigan State University Institute of Voice Identification)*

4. Nasals (Figure 17.7)

The English language has three nasals, /m/, /n/ and /ŋ/; see page 36 of book/, and they are all voiced. Nasals are produced in a binary manner where the oral and nasal cavities are either connected or separated by the velum (soft palate) and the posterior pharyngeal wall. Although there are coarticulation and assimilation in the production of all sound in dynamic speech, there are no phonetic degrees of nasality: the velopharyngeal port is either opened or closed in the production of nasal sounds. The /m/ nasal is produced by occluding the oral air stream at the level of the lips and directing the energy through the nose. The /n/ nasal is a result of occlusion of the oral air stream by the tongue and alveolar ridge and directing the energy through the nose. The

5. Glides (Figure 17.8)

The four glides in English are /r/, /l/, /w/, and /j/. They are sometimes called semivowels and produced by a gliding action of the articulators. In the production of a glide, the articulators begin in a stable articulatory position and the vocal cords begin vibration. With continuation of voicing, they move in a smooth articulatory gesture to an ending position. The articulatory transitions are noted on a spectrogram by the rise and fall of formants, particularly the second one. "Glides do not show the steady-state portion of the formant that is seen in diphthongs. They are extremely short in duration and often look like little more than a formant transition between two other sounds" (Ferrand, 2001, p. 202) Speakers have characteristic similarities in producing glides including the rate of the rise and fall of formants, and the total duration of the glide production.

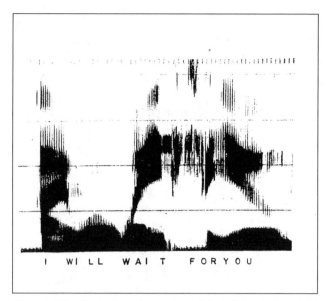

Figure 17.8 Sound spectrogram of the glides /w/ and /j/ ("you") (Courtesy Dr. Oscar I. Tosi and the Michigan State University Institute of Voice Identification)

6. Vowels (Figure 17.9; Figure 17.10)

All vowels are voiced. They are classified by the front-to-back position of the tongue and its relative height in the oral cavity. Lip rounding also plays a role in producing the acoustic properties of vowels. (See Figure 15.5 for English vowels categorized by tongue height and front-to-back position.)

Although vowels provide many clues to speaker identification, three features are of primary importance. First, the relative positions of the first, second, third, and occasionally the forth formant, are speaker dependent variables. The relative positions of these formants are primary indicators of resonance patterns, and are typically similar from one utterance to the next. The frequencies of the formants are usually discerned by using their midpoints. A horizontal line can be drawn in the middle of the energy dispersion of the vowel from the beginning to end of its production. This line represents the frequency midpoint, the mean frequency, of the vowel's particular formant. Second, the relative slope and spacing of the individual formants provide speaker identification information. With some vowels, the slope of the formants is from a low to higher frequency, and with others, the slope is from high to low. Third, as noted above, the frequency of vocal cord vibrations, as indicated by how close or far apart are the vertical striations, can signal fundamental voice frequency. In visual inspection of the formants, their intensity can be observed by how dark or

light they are. Although the relative intensity of the formants are speaker dependent variables, it is less reliable of speaker identity than relative formant frequency and slope.

In connected speech, sometimes the nasal port is partially opened during vowel production. This is a result of coarticulation and assimilation. This phenomenon is more common in non-English languages especially French. Partial opening of the velopharyngeal port during the production of vowels produces negative resonances or antiresonances. The resonance of the particular vowel in a format is diminished by damping factors. In effect, because of the shape of the oral-nasal cavity, certain sound waves cancel or attenuate each other. These are also called zeroes and they are in contrast to positive resonances or poles. The nasalization of vowel sounds is highly individualized and apparent on spectrograms by the width and frequencies of formants.

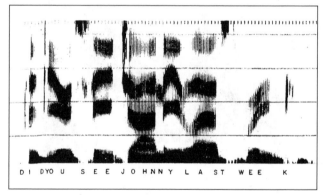

Figure 17.9 Sound spectrogram of several vowels (Courtesy Dr. Oscar I. Tosi and the Michigan State University Institute of Voice Identification)

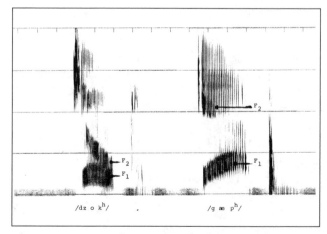

Figure 17.10 Sound spectrogram of the vowels /o/ and /æ/

7. Diphthongs (Figure 17.11)

Diphthongs, also called vowel combinations, are sounds produced by moving the structures of articulation from one vowel articulatory gesture to another. All diphthongs are voiced and thus have the periodic vertical striations. Eight English diphthongs are listed in Figure 15.6. Like consonant blends (see below), the movement of the articulators shows up on a spectrogram as rising and falling slopes of acoustic energy. Diphthongs have the distinct features of each vowel and the transitional features on the spectrogram resulting from coarticulatory movements.

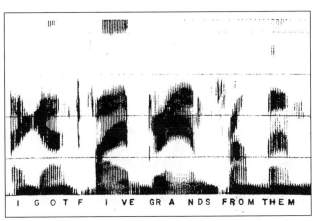

Figure 17.12 Sound spectrogram of the blend /gr/ (Courtesy Dr. Oscar I. Tosi and the Michigan State University Institute of Voice Identification

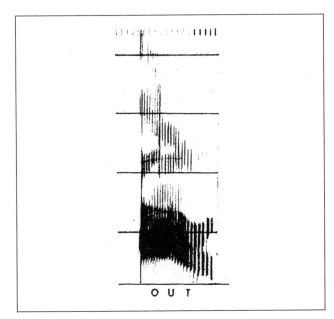

Figure 17.11 Sound spectrogram of the diphthong "ow" (Courtesy Dr. Oscar I. Tosi and the Michigan State University Institute of Voice Identification)

8. Blends (Figure 17.12)

Blends, also called consonant clusters, are two or more consonant sounds without a vowel separating them. Examples of blends include /br/ as in "brush," /sk/ as in "skill," /dr/ as in "drum," and /gr/ as in "grand." The slope of energy release and temporal (time) factors related to each consonant blend's production are speaker dependent variables. Typical voice onset patterns can also provide information about the speaker's identity as can the relative intensity of each consonant in the blend.

9. Pauses (Figure 17.13)

The spectral characteristics of a speaker's voice are not limited to energy dispersions on a spectrogram. The gaps or pauses also provide important speaker identification and rate of speech information. The habitual rate of speech is learned and is highly individualized. Three factors are important when analyzing speech spectrograms for speaker dependent variables related to pauses and consequent rate of speech. First, the length of the pauses is examined both between and within words. Second, the duration of the syllable gives information about typical phoneme production and overall speech rate. Third, the number of pauses, important for overall speech rate, can give basic information about respiratory support, the speed of programming, and the sequencing and production of dynamic utterances. Tosi developed a device known as a pausimeter which measures speech sound interwave gaps (Tanner, 1976).

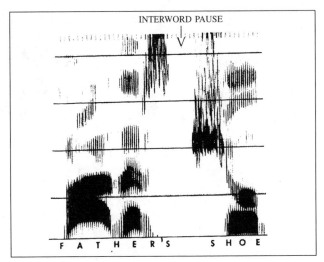

Figure 17.13 Sound spectrogram showing pauses between and within words (Courtesy Dr. Oscar I. Tosi and the Michigan State University Institute of Voice Identification)

10. Composite characteristics (Figure 17.14)

Just as some speakers' voices sound strong and full to listeners, general resonance characteristics can be gleaned from spectrograms. Several composite factors go into observing general resonance characteristics on spectrograms: relative intensity of energy dispersion, band width of formants, and their separation. Assessing relative intensity requires that loudness of the input signal be controlled. Relative intensity of segments of the speech sample is displayed by the darkness of the pattern energy bursts. Band widths and interformant separation give vowels and voiced consonants their distinctive acoustic properties. These factors are related to the size, shape, and texture of speech mechanism cavities and are an interplay between the source of the sound in the larynx and the resonant chambers. Other important composite characteristics include plosive spikes, slopes, and patterns of fricative energy dispersions. Factors related to extreme variation in fundamental frequency as measured by formants and proximity of vertical voiced energy dispersions, and speech disorders such as sound substitutions, additions, and distortions can also be noted from spectrograms. Typical accent and dialectical variations also show up in spectrograms and are speaker dependent patterns.

17.6 Semiautomatic and Automatic Voice Identification

Dr. Oscar I. Tosi at the Michigan State University Institute of Voice Identification addressed the "objective" computerized or automatic speech recognition in the early 1970s. In the 1980s and 1990s, he also developed algorithms for computerized assessments of speech articulation disorders (Tanner, 2001). The algorithms provide acoustic parameters for normalcy of individually produced phonemes. Tosi's work into computerized speech assessment set the foundation for computer evaluation of clinical speech samples, and automatic flagging of phonemes that do not meet the speech parameters for normalcy. "Type to speech" devices now permit speech pattern recognition even in some brain-injured subjects (Wade, Petheram, and Cain, 2001).

Although automatic speaker recognition requires little interaction with the examiner, it is often not optimal for most forensic cases (Culbertson and Tanner, 2005, p. 18):

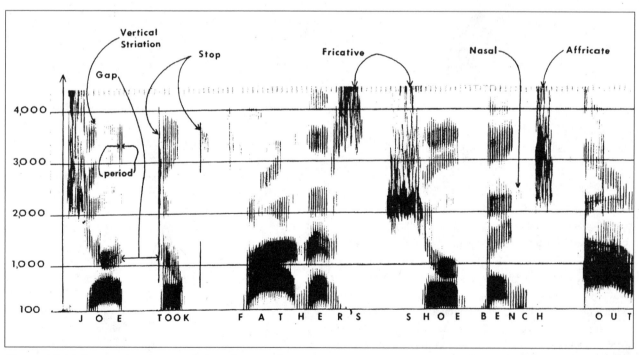

Figure 17.14 *Composite characteristics of a sound spectrogram (Courtesy Dr. Oscar I. Tosi and the Michigan State University Institute of Voice Identification)*

Automatic objective speaker recognition requires little interaction with the examiner. The most common model is a comparison of stored speech samples with the speech sample to be examined to determine the extent to which the sample in question matches one or more stored samples. A computer compares speech parameters of the utterances in this closed-set paradigm. The automatic method would seem to occupy the objective extreme of the subjective-objective continuum, but its use sacrifices utility for objectivity. Automatic matches can only be made reliably when stored known samples are compared with a single specified speaker. Further, comparisons must be made between specified standard utterances, that is, both speech samples to be matched must be of speakers uttering the same passages or words. Thus, the automatic method has its greatest utility in situations where it was important to verify the identity of a specified individual, such as in security clearance applications, but would not be commonly encountered in most forensic situations.

For a computer to deal with speech, the signal must be converted into numbers. This process is completed by a specialized board or device, and involves measuring, filtering, sampling, and converting voltages into digits (Kewley-Port, 1999). Musical computerized disks use the same analog-to-digital conversion principle but with much higher sampling rates than is required for speech. According to Ryalls and Beherns (2000), high quality analog-to-digital conversion for music requires about 44kHz sampling rate which means the sample is read from the continuous original signal at 44,000 times per second. Speech sampling requires a lower rate than music because in speech there is less required information. The music signal has information at frequencies well above 4,000 Hz. Most energy for speech is located below 6,000 Hz.

According to Kewley-Port (1999), an acoustic processor codes the digital waveform into a small set of coded samples for each second of speech, permitting information about time, energy, and frequency to be greatly reduced from the original digital signal. The foundation to this process is the Fourier analysis: "A Fourier analysis reveals the fundamental frequency and indicates the location of formant frequencies. However, typically an additional mathematical procedure, known as linear predictive coding (LPC) is used to indicate the exact frequency location of formants" (Ryalls and Beherns, 2000, pp. 139-140). For forensic speaker identification, specialized algorithms may be written to address the ten salient spectrographic features discussed above. Voice onset time variables may also be addressed on certain phonemes.

17.7 Admissibility of Voice Prints

With few exceptions, voice prints and expert testimony about them have been admissible in the courts. According to the United States Department of Justice (2006): "The majority of the courts which have considered the question have ruled that voiceprint evidence is admissible. See *United States v. Smith*, 869 F.2d 348, 351 (7th Cir. 1989); *United States v. Williams*, 583 F.2d 1194 (2d Cir. 1978), cert. denied 439 U.S. 1117 (1979). Although the District of Columbia Circuit has held that voice print evidence is inadmissible, see *United States v. Addison*, 498 F.2d 741 (D.C. Cir. 1974), the continuing validity of that determination is questionable in view of the Supreme Court's subsequent decision addressing the admissibility of scientific evidence in *Daubert v. Merrell Dow Pharmaceuticals, Inc.*, 509 U.S. 579 (1993)."

17.8 Summary

Speech sound spectrography, sometimes called voice printing, provides investigators with accurate and reliable information about speaker identity. The speech spectrogram is produced by a Fourier analysis where a complex sound wave is represented as the sum of a number of sinusoidal waves of differing frequencies, amplitudes, and phases. There are subjective and objective methods of voice identification. Detection of speech patterns involves stops, affricates, fricatives, nasals, glides, vowels, diphthongs, blends, pauses, and composite characteristics.

Suggested Readings and Resources

Hollien, H. (2002). *Forensic Voice Identification*. San Diego: Academic Press. This book addresses the history of voice prints and introduces the concept of "earwitness lineups."

Tosi, O. (1979). *Voice Identification: Theory and Legal Applications*. Baltimore: University Park Press. This is the classic textbook on speaker identification using voice prints.

Young, H. and Geller, R. (2007). *Sears & Zemansky's College Physics* (8th ed.). San Francisco: Pearson, Addison Wesley. This textbook addresses all major physics issues related to voice prints.

References

Borden, G., Harris, K, and Raphael, L. (2003). *Speech science primer: Physiology, acoustics, and perception of speech.* Philadelphia: Lippincott Williams & Wilkins.

Culbertson, W. and Tanner, D. (2005). Forensic phonetics: Perspectives on subjective and objective approaches to speaker identification. *4ᵗʰ Annual Hawaii International Conference on Social Sciences, Honolulu, Hawaii.*

Ferrand, C. T. (2001). *Speech science. An integrated approach to theory and clinical practice.* Boston: Allyn & Bacon.

Kewley-Port, D. (1999). Speech recognition by machine. In J.M. Picket (Ed) *The acoustics of speech communication: Fundamentals, speech perception theory, and technology.* Boston: Allyn & Bacon.

Potter, R., Kopp, G., and Green, H. (1947) *Visible Speech.* New York: Van Nostrand. Reprinted (1966). New York: Dover.

Ryalls, J. and Behrens, S. (2000). *Introduction to speech science: From basic theories to clinical applications.* Boston: Allyn & Bacon.

Tanner, D. (1976). Spectrographic, pausimetric, and intelligibility factors related to Parkinsonian dysarthria. *Doctoral Dissertation.* East Lansing: Michigan State University.

Tanner, D. (2001, April 3). Hooray for Hollywood: Communication disorders and the motion picture industry. *ASHA Leader*, 6(6).

Titze, I.R. and Story, B.H. (2002, Fall). Voice quality: What is most characteristic about "you" in speech. *Echoes*, Vol. 12, No. 2., pp. 1,4. Acoustical Society of America: Melville: New York.

Tosi, O. (1979). *Voice identification: Theory and legal applications.* Baltimore: University Park Press.

Tosi, O. (1975). *Personal Correspondences.* Institute of Voice Identification, Department of Audiology and Speech Sciences, Michigan State University, East Lansing, Michigan.

United States Department of Justice (2006). Admissibility of spectrograms (voice prints). Retrieved from the World Wide Web June 4, 2006: http://www.usdoj.gov/usao/eousa/foia_reading_room/usam/title9/crm00258.htm (Author)

Wade, J., Petheram, B., and Cain, R. (2001). Voice recognition and aphasia: Can computers understand aphasic speech. *Disability and Rehabilitation*, Vol. 23, No. 14, 604-613.

Part IV
Speaker Profiling

Chapter 18

The Art and Science of Speaker Profiling

18.1 Chapter Preview

This chapter examines the forensic art and science of obtaining information from speakers based on what they say and how they say it. In this chapter, there is a definition of speaker profiling and a brief history of behavioral-criminal profiling. Intuitive, deductive logic, and scientifically based speaker profiling are defined and reviewed.

18.2 The Concept of Speaker Profiling

Humans are marvelous sensing creatures. Every day, people make hundreds, if not thousands, of subjective and objective judgements about what a speaker says and how he or she says it. People make speaker inferences about issues ranging from the inane to the profound, often not giving a moments thought to their accuracy or the mental processes involved in reaching them. Whether it is a mother analyzing the truthfulness of her child's denial of responsibility for spilled milk or the President of the United States assessing the sincerity of a terrorist's recorded statement, the speech act per se carries an infinite number of objective and subjective information bits. And most people believe they have an intuitive ability to sense underlying information based on what is said and how it is said. In effect, everyone engages in speaker profiling and some persons are more adept at it than others.

Lord Alfred Tennyson addressed the power of words to conceal and reveal the personality of the speaker: "For words, like nature, half reveal and half conceal the soul within." Speaker profiling is the art and science of deter-

mining the identity and characteristics of a speaker, and inferring and deducing the veracity, embedded meaning, and implications of his or her verbal statements. Speaker profiling is broader in its intent and analysis than criminal-behavioral profiling which is the study of the abnormal personality of an offender. Speaker profiling addresses normal and abnormal speakers in a variety of contexts and is a systematic method of analysis yielding logical and scientifically based conclusions as well as conjecture and informed speculation based on the semantics, grammatical constructions, accompanying nonverbal acts, and the motor speech variabilities of the speaker.

Criminal-behavioral profiling also addresses what a speaker says and how he or she says it when speech samples are available during an investigation. In recent years, there has been an increase in public awareness and interest in criminal-behavioral profiling. Several movies and television programs use crime scene investigation and criminal-behavioral profiling for plot and storyline development. They focus on the dynamics of the investigative process and the methods and procedures profilers use to reach logical conclusions and informed speculation about the crimes. Hicks and Sales (2006) note that literature's first criminal profiler was C. Auguste Dubin in Edgar Allan Poe's *The Murders in the Rue Morgue*. Poe gives the character an intuitive ability to profile: "In addition to providing the first profiling prototype, Poe may have been the first to expose the American public to the lore of 'profiling intuition'—the sixth sense that modern profilers are popularly thought to possess" (Hicks and Sales, 2006, p. 4). Sir Arthur Conan Doyle's sleuth, Sherlock Holmes, is another fictional profiler who used his highly developed perceptual abilities to solve crimes.

> The fictional sleuth Sherlock Holmes was famous for his highly developed perceptual skills. While both Sherlock Holmes and Dr. Watson would both be present when questioning a suspect in a crime,

Holmes would come away from the meeting knowing much more than Dr. Watson. Both Watson and Holmes would see the same person, but Sherlock Holmes would perceive much more. The suspect's slight accent, aftershave, red clay on his shoes, and uneven suntan would all spark meaning in the sleuth's mind. Sherlock would know where the person was born, where he vacationed, his annual salary, and his preferred mode of travel. It was "elementary" that Sherlock Holmes perceived more and better than the average detective (Tanner, 1999, pp. 86-87).

"The Whitechapel Murders" in London in 1888 provided the first departure of profiling from the realm of fiction (Hicks and Sales, 2006). The investigation involved a forensic medical specialist, Thomas Bond, and speculations about the offender's behavioral and psychological characteristics. However, because "Jack the Ripper" was never apprehended, the accuracies of Bond's speculations could not be confirmed. Pierce (2002) reports that during World War II, the United States Office of Strategic Services provided a psychological profile of Adolph Hitler to estimate his vulnerabilities. According to Hicks and Sales (2006), profiling expertise was first used by law enforcement in 1956 and the Mad Bomber case in New York City. The Mad Bomber set off more than fifty homemade bombs over the course of seventeen years and the criminal profile was helpful in capturing him. In the 1970s, the Federal Bureau of Investigation (FBI) began training investigators in identifying similar patterns of offender behaviors. In 1985, the FBI trained five investigators in analytical approaches to criminal investigation. "These investigators, after completing a yearlong fellowship with the FBI's Behavioral Science Unit, were certified as Criminal Investigative Analysts. They returned to their jurisdictions and began to provide criminal personality profiles and investigative assistance to the city, state and federal agencies within their geographic areas" (Pierce, 2002, pp. 113-114). Today, police, military, and intelligence organizations use formal or informal profiling, including speaker profiling, and the procedure has widespread application.

18.3 Deductive Logic and Intuitive Speaker Profiling

In the chapters that follow, there is a clear distinction between profiles of speakers based on science and those reached from conjecture. Information about a speaker generalized from scientific studies involves "probable" conclusions that can be "induced" from the scientific literature on speech and language production. Conjecture, although far less empirical, also has value when the profiler understands its applications, strengths, and weaknesses. Scientifically based speaker profiles are a result of inductive logic while the so-called "sixth sense of profiling" is largely intuitive and based on deductive logic.

Intuition is knowing something instinctively, without apparent conscious thought, and usually accompanied by emotion. The mental representations of intuition usually take the forms of hunches, suspicions, and feelings of insight. The emotions associated with intuition can range from a sense of euphoria to impending doom. Conjecture profiles based on intuition are largely arrived at automatically and occur at the perceptual level of mental processing. According to Lum (2002), the basis of intuitive logic is often unknown, implicit, and frequently not communicable to others. The "sixth sense" of speaker and other types of profiling are a result of informal and often unconscious (or partially conscious) intuition and deductive logic.

Whereas scientific-based speaker profiling is founded on inductive logic, the scientific method, and probabilities, conjecture profiles are based primarily on deductive logic. Deductive logic results in conclusions that are just as certain as the premises, and the conclusions are either valid or invalid. The following shows deductive reasoning concerning pitch rise as an indicator of increased tension of a speaker during interrogation.

A. Deductive Reasoning
- Increased tension causes pitch rise in all speakers.
- This speaker shows increased pitch during questions about the crime.
- Therefore, the speaker is experiencing increased tension during questions about the crime.

As can be seen by the above logical argument about pitch and tension, in deductive reasoning, it would not be possible for the conclusion to be false if the premises were true. A valid argument is one where the conclusion logically follows the premise. At the core of conjecture speaker profiling using deductive logic are the truthfulness and robustness of the premise or premises and whether or not it is valid argument. In speaker profiling using deductive logic, the profiler assesses the truthfulness of the premise or premises and determines whether the argument is valid. In the above profile information bit about the pitch of a suspect's voice and an increase in tension, if it is true that pitch and body tension are always positively correlated, then it is logical for the profiler to believe that the speaker is experiencing increased tension during interrogation. The increased tension could be a result of anxiety associated with making deceptive statements.

In any logical argument, consistency is important; if the argument is true, it must always be true. Conversely, if an argument is false, it must always be false. More specifically, if an argument proposes that two or more relationships exist in a speaker, it must always be true that this relationship exists. This consistency statement is based on a historical truism about logic; nothing can be said to exist and not to exist at the same time. "Fuzzy" logic usually involves a lack of consistency.

B. Scientifically Based Speaker Profiling

As noted above, scientifically based speaker profiling is based on inductive reasoning and the scientific method. With regard to the above reasoning concerning pitch rise as an indicator of increased tension of a speaker during interrogation, inductive reasoning results in probabilities that the conclusion is correct.

C. Inductive Reasoning

- Increased tension causes pitch rises in most speakers.
- This speaker shows increased pitch during questions about the crime.
- Therefore, the speaker is experiencing increased tension during questions about the crime.

It is probable that the speaker is experiencing tension during questions about the crime, and inferences about his or her physiological state and uttering deceptive statements can be made.

Canter (2000) provides a scientifically based model of profiling derived from questions addressing behavioral salience, distinguishing between offenders, inferring characteristics, and linking offenses. Behavioral salience concerns the behavioral features of a crime important to identifying the perpetrator. Distinguishing between offenders involves analyzing differences between crimes, linking offenders and looking at the commonalities. Inferring characteristics address methods of identifying multiple offenses by the same offender. Canter proposes that psychological research assess the above categories to provide useful profiling methodologies for law enforcement.

The most powerful and robust profiles about speakers are also scientifically based. The forensic information that can be gleaned from speakers' accent and dialect is substantial (see Chapter 19). Levels and types of intoxication can also be surmised from the speech of suspects (see Chapter

20). During a forensic interview and interrogation, what is said and how it is spoken can provide information about truth, deception, anxiety, and involvement in criminal activities (see Chapter 21). Voice stress analysis, using instruments to assess the veracity of a speaker, while far less accurate than a polygraph, can be used to prompt confessions and for forensic interviewing and interrogation (see Chapter 22). Valuable forensic information about persons with communication disorders can be gleaned by the nature and severity of their speech, voice, language, and hearing impairments (see Chapter 23).

Vast amounts of information about a speaker's neurology, emotions, and personality can be obtained based on decades of research conducted on people with normal and disordered communication. The discipline of communication sciences and disorders has accumulated a large body of scientifically based information about the neurology, emotions, and personality of speakers based on their speech fluency, rate-of-speech, word selection, linguistic structures, respiratory-laryngeal functioning, articulatory precision, and so forth. Chapter 6 details three types of empirical research methods in communication sciences and disorders: catalog-epidemiologic, descriptive, and experimental. All three methods provide a strong scientific basis for speaker profiling.

Speaker profiling scientific information based on catalog-epidemiologic research concerns identifying and cataloging the number of entities or factors associated with normal and abnormal speech. These types of studies involve the frequency, incidence, and prevalence of normal speech and language patterns or communication disorders in a population or subpopulation. Data derived from catalog-epidemiologic research are usually obtained from large-scale incidence and prevalence studies.

Speaker profiling scientific information derived from descriptive research involves observations and recordings of speech and language production behaviors and providing a systematic method of analyzing them. Data obtained from descriptive research are not from large scale incidence and prevalence studies and do not address formal cause and effect manipulation of variables. These types of studies involve single subjects or small groups of subjects with limited inferences to larger populations. However, relationships are discovered as well as systematic methods of presenting them.

The most powerful scientifically based speaker profiling information is obtained from experimental research. As reported in Chapter 6, the experimental scientific method is systematic. In this research design, there is a review of the literature giving the scientist and reader relevant background information about the topic under investigation, clear definitions of relevant terms, and detailed hypotheses or research questions. In this type of research, variables are manipulated to reach conclusions that can be generalized to a larger population. The power of the study to generalize is based on the research design and the size of the sample drawn from the larger population. The results and discussion sections explain the limits of the conclusions that can be drawn and any weakness of the study. In addition, the scientist suggests areas of future research to give guidance to succeeding researchers to build on the theme of the study. All experimental research has a margin of sampling error.

In communication sciences and disorders, there are two general types of experimental research: pure and applied. In pure research, the scientist conducts a study with no practical goal other than to quench the human need for knowledge and understanding; there is no search for a pragmatic solution to a problem. For example, in theoretical physics, scientists developed and launched the Hubble Telescope to question the origin of the universe. Knowledge of the origin of the universe does not have an immediate benefit for humans nor does it solve practical problems such as renewable energy sources or cures for diseases. However, pure research often provides the background and theoretical bases for applied research. In applied research, the scientist has a clear question or problem that will be partially or completely answered by the research. An example of applied

research in theoretical physics was the splitting of the atom that provided the science necessary for the development of the atomic bomb. In communication sciences and disorders, pure research may be conducted to find areas of the brain responsible for producing grammatically correct sentences while applied research may discover treatments or therapies helpful in overcoming communication disorders associated with strokes.

Both pure and applied research in communication sciences and disorders, and related disciplines, support the art and science of speaker profiling. Pure and applied research provide the basis for understanding normal and disordered communication such as the muscles involved in pitch elevation, tongue movements, or the effects of paralysis on speech sound production. These facts may provide the perceptual information for intuition or truthfulness of the premises used in deductive logic. Further, scientific research directly may show the effects of intoxicants on speech production or define geographic boundaries for speaker profiling using accent and dialect. During forensic interviews and interrogations, pure and applied communication sciences and disorders research may provide the interrogator with underlying information about a suspect's speech patterns such as the psychological implications of increased disfluencies, decreased rate-of-speech, lisping, or so forth. Table 18.1 shows speaker profiling methods and their features.

Table 18.1
Speaker Profiling Methods

Intuitive Profiling	Deductive Logic Profiling	Scientifically Based Profiling
Perceptual information processing	Conclusion are *true* if the premise or premises are true and vice versa	Most powerful and robust method of speaker profiling.
Attributable to a "sixth sense" in some persons	Logical arguments about the relationship must be consistent	Based on scientific studies with probable conclusions
Mental representation in the form of hunches, suspicions, and feelings of insight	A *valid* deductive logical statement is one where the conclusion logically follows the premise	Always a margin of error associated with the research results
Accompanied by an emotional response ranging from euphoria to a feeling of impending doom	Value of deductive logic in speaker profiling is dependent on the relative truthfulness of the premise or premises	Power and the ability to generalize is related to the size of the sample and research design

18.4 Summary

Intuition, deductive logic, and scientifically based speaker profiling can provide a wealth of information about speakers. Speaker profiling is not limited to the analysis of the speech of offenders, it is also applicable to normal and disorders speakers. Speaker profiling provides a valuable forensic tool for investigators and others needing additional information about the speech of suspects or subjects.

Suggested Readings and Resources

Canter, D. (2000). Offender profiling and criminal differentiation. *Legal and Criminological Psychology*, 5, 23-46. This article discusses the "Canter Model" of scientific profiling.

Hicks, S. and Sales, B. (2006). *Criminal Profiling: Developing an Effective Science and Practice*. Washington, D.C.: American Psychological Association. This text addresses nonscientific and scientific profiling methods today and in the future.

Pierce, R. (2002). "Profiling for corporate investigators." In R. Montgomery and W. Majeski (Eds), *Corporate Investigations*. Tucson: Lawyers & Judges Publishing Company. This chapter addresses criminal personality profiling in the corporate world and includes profiling for threats and workplace violence prevention.

References

Canter, D. (2000). Offender profiling and criminal differentiation. *Legal and Criminological Psychology*, 5, 23-46.

Hicks, S. and Sales, B. (2006). *Criminal profiling: Developing an effective science and practice*. Washington, D.C.: American Psychological Association.

Lum, C. (2002). *Scientific thinking in speech and language therapy*. Mahwah, New Jersey: Lawrence Erlbaum Associates.

Pierce, R. (2002). "Profiling for corporate investigators." In R. Montgomery and W. Majeski (Eds), *Corporate Investigations*. Tucson: Lawyers & Judges Publishing Company.

Tanner, D. (1999). *The family guide to surviving stroke and communication disorders*: Austin: Pro-Ed.

Walters, S. (2003). *Principles of kinesic interview and interrogation* (2nd ed.). Boca Raton: CRC Press.

Yeschke, C. (1993). *Interviewing: A forensic guide to interrogation* (2nd ed.). Springfield, Ill.: Charles C. Thomas Publisher.

Chapter 19

Speaker Profiling Using Accent and Dialect

19.1 Chapter Preview

This chapter explores the forensic information that can be gleaned from accent and dialect. Accent and dialect, while often used interchangeably, refer to different linguistic behaviors and are explored in this section. Provided in this chapter are phonological and grammatical structures, and examples of word derivations of English dialects. There is also a discussion of accent and dialect as reflective of social class, education, occupation, and ethnicity.

19.2 Speaker Profiling Using Accent and Dialect is Not Racial Profiling

Investigating a speaker's accent and dialect, and attending to ethnic cues are not disguised racial profiling. A person's race is a biological determinant where skin color, body type, facial features, and other physical attributes are passed genetically from one generation to another. Race and culture are not synonymous. Culture refers to the values, beliefs, and actions of a community, and transcends the race composition of its members. Some beliefs and actions of the cultural community are reflected in its clothing, food preparation and preferences, customs, religious rituals, family roles, and so forth. The list of cultures is so great as to be forensically meaningless. For example, in the Native American general population, there are hundreds of tribes,

and within each tribe, there are groups of people who are traditionalists, nontraditionalists, educated, uneducated, native speakers of the language, and rural, urban, or reservation dwellers. According to Westby and Vining (2002), there are approximately 700 native groups and about 550 were formally recognized as sovereign nations. Conceivably, each constitutes a culture with behaviors and customs that are substantially different from each other, the larger tribe, and other groups of Native Americans. It has been said that there is a "police culture" where law enforcement personnel share similar attitudes, values, and customs. Profiling using accent and dialect addresses the ethnicity of the suspect or suspects. Ethnicity is more clearly delineated and is the shared belief in a recognized culture and adhered to by substantial number of individuals. What is most important, ethnic groups often share political agendas.

> Ethnicity refers to a shared culture that forms the basis for a sense of peoplehood based on the consciousness of a common past. Race, language, and ancestral customs constitute the major expressions of ethnicity in the United States. Ethnicity is not passed genetically from generation to generation. Rather, ethnicity is constructed and reconstructed in response to particular historical circumstances and changes. In its most intimate form, an ethnic group can be based on face-to-face relationships and political realities that mobilize its members into political self-determination (Battle, 1998, p. 4).

Communication, in all of its forms, defines and propagates ethnicity. "Some linguistic forms and communicative behaviors are so characteristic of certain ethnic groups that, when used, they immediately mark the speaker as either being from that group or as having a great deal of interaction with the group" (Payne and Tayor, 1998, p. 124).

Speaker profiling using accent and dialect can provide information about a person's region, state, or country of origin. Since September 11, 2001 and the worldwide war on terrorism, identifying a person's ethnicity has taken on urgency, and can be one of many factors used to prevent future terrorist acts. Besides providing valuable information about a suspect's homeland, these speech patterns also suggest his or her socioeconomic status and can be used in creating a composite profile of a person or persons.

19.3 Accent and Dialect

Accent and dialect overlap, and the terms are often used interchangeably, but technically, they are different. Dialect refers to the use of an identifiable pronunciation and vocabulary spoken in a particular geographical area. Dialect also suggests a person's ethnicity, culture, religion, and socioeconomic status. Accent, on the other hand, is having the speech sound traits of the speaker's native language carried over into a second language. There are no "substandard" dialects and accents in the sense that they are below acceptable standards for human communication; all rule-governed cultural variations in the production of speech and language are normal. Dialects and accents are not communication disorders; they are "nonstandard" patterns of speech and language. According to Haynes and Pindzola (2004), speech-language pathologists must consider dialectical variations when evaluating articulation disorders, but there are few clinical tests taking dialect into consideration. Everyone speaks with a dialect that is detectible by people from a different region, culture, religion, and socioeconomic status. In the United States, most people speak the Standard American Dialect, which is the type of pronunciation and vocabulary used by news anchors on the major television networks. However, local television programs often have speakers that use the speech patterns and vocabulary typical of the geographical region.

Obviously, accents and dialects are more common in regions where many immigrants have settled and English is a second language. Some regions have large populations of nonnative English speakers such as is seen in the Southwest. Other accents and dialects can be found in smaller geographic areas such as Asian-American speakers in San Francisco, California and Cuban-American speakers in Miami, Florida.

Battle (1998) notes that there have been three "waves" of immigration to the United States. The first wave of immigration occurred between 1841 and 1890 and took place when many Europeans came to the United States in search of a better life. During the first wave, nearly 15 million immigrants came to the United States especially from Ger-

many, Ireland, Britain, French Canada, Scandinavia, Mexico, and Asia. The second wave occurred between 1891 and 1920 during the industrial revolution. During this time, 18 million people immigrated to the United States including those from Italy, Asia, Austria-Hungary, and Russia. The third wave of immigration occurred between 1965 and 1990, and consisted mainly of immigrants from Asia and Latin America. Many of those from Latin America are undocumented immigrants. Currently, the Hispanic/Latino population accounts for the greatest increase to the U.S. population. A fourth wave of immigration has occurred more recently. Between the 1990s and 2005, more than 10 million people primarily from Mexico illegally immigrated to the United States. This influx of illegal immigrants through the porous southern United States border was significantly reduced when national guard troops were deployed to assist border patrol agents in 2006. According to Alvarez and Kolker (1987), accents and dialects are more varied and apparent in the eastern part of the United States because that is where many immigrants first settled.

19.4 Regional Accent and Dialectical Variations in the United States

Broeder and Extra (1999) reviewed 1990 census data about immigration and current language usage published by the Census Bureau in several separate reports. Almost 25 percent of the nearly 20 million Americans who were born abroad immigrated between 1985 and 1990. The main countries of origin (contributed at least 500,000 inhabitants) were, in descending order, Mexico, Philippines, Canada, Cuba, Germany, Great Britain, Italy, South Korea, Vietnam, and China. Approximately one-third of California's population was of foreign extraction, followed by New York, Florida, Texas, New Jersey, and Illinois. Broeder and Extra also found that nearly 32 million people said they speak a language other than English at home. The non-English language most frequently spoken at home is Spanish, followed by French, German, Italian, and Chinese. Sixty percent of the non-English speakers reported that they spoke English very well with more Asians declaring that they did not speak English or spoke it badly. It is likely that most of the speakers, even the ones reporting that they spoke English well, did so with an accent and dialect that clearly signaled their ethnicity. According to the 2000 census, of the approximately 20 million Mexican-Americans, about 14 million speak a language other than English (United States Census, 2000).

Currently, there is no consensus on the number of regional dialectical variations in the United States nor their geographic boundaries. According to Nist (1966), at least ten regional dialects exist: Southern, Eastern New England, Western Pennsylvania, Appalachian, Central Midland, Middle Atlantic, and New York City. Carver (1987) identifies several more general regional dialect areas in the United States, and further divides larger regions into smaller dialectical groups such as Lower South, Upper South, Hudson Valley, Western New England, and so forth. When accent and dialect are broadly defined, more than twenty-five discernable types can be observed in the United States (see Table 19.1). Broeder and Extra (1990, p. 19) note, "From the census experiences in the reviewed non-European English-dominant immigration countries, it becomes clear that nation-wide population data on ethnicity and (home) language use are valuable instruments for indicating the multicultural composition of societies." The Linguistic Atlas (**A**rchitecture and **T**ools for **L**inguistic **A**nalysis **S**ystems) Projects (2006) provide a current database about dialectology, the study of dialects. The Linguistic Atlas Projects are a collection of studies on dialects conducted during the past eighty years around the country by various individuals and is being updated regularly. Delaney (2006) provides a map of twenty-six regional American dialects including Hawaii.

A person's accent sometimes results from differences between "meaningful" sounds. For example, in Spanish, the difference between "sh" and "ch" is not enough to signal difference in meaning between any two words. However, in English, "sh" and "ch" have significant semantic differences. For the speaker whose first language is Spanish and the second English, he or she will have trouble perceiving differences between the two sounds. The speaker is likely to say "I found my 'chew' in the closet" for "I found my 'shoe' in the closet." The "ch" and "sh" substitution signals Spanish as a first learned language when a person speaks English.

19.5 Accent, Dialect, and Vowels

According to Eisenson (1979), regional pronunciation differences are more likely to involve vowel variations than consonants.

For American-English speakers, the pronunciation of Harry and hairy may or may not be different, depending on region and social class. Similarly, there may or may not be differences in vowel choice for Mary, merry, and marry. The words class, not, hot, orange, creek, coffee, candy, nurse, first have vowel variation according to region (Eisenson, 1979, p. 143).

Additional vowel dialectical variations include the "aw" sound in words, such as "caught" and "coffee," to be produced as "cawht" and "cowffee." Rural dialects often result in "wire" being produced as "war" as in the utterance: "The cowboy fixed the barbed-war fence." "Krik" for "creek" is a common rural dialectical variation. According to Wolfram (1986), other examples of vowel variations include "tam" for "time," "fellers" for "fellows," and "sody" for "soda."

19.6 Accent, Dialect, Consonants, and Phonological Rules

Major regional dialectical consonant variations involve the "ng" phoneme such as occurs in be<u>ing</u> and go<u>ing</u> (Eisenson, 1979). For example, in Arizona many speakers use the "ng" phoneme instead of "ing" in words such as "going" and "running"; they are said: "goin<u>gh</u>" and "runnin<u>gh</u>." Eisenson notes that greatest regional variation in consonant pronunciation is for words with the letter "r" in the middle or final positions of words.

Table 19.1
Partial List of Accents and Dialects in the United States

African-American	Dutch-American	Queens
Appalachian	Eastern	Southern
Boston	Hillbilly	Texas
Boston Brahmins	Kentucky	Upstate New York
Bronx	Korean-American	Vietnamese-American
Cajun	Manhattan	Virginia
Canadian	Mexican-American	Wisconsin
Chicago	Mississippi	Yonkers
Cowboy	New England	
Dakota	Ohio	

Wolfram (1986, pp. 99-102) provides additional phonological structures and word derivations of vernacular English dialects based on a review of several sociolinguistic studies. The phonological structures and word derivations are socially significant in terms of the standard-vernacular continuum, but not exclusive to a particular region (Wolfram, 1986).

Final Cluster Reduction: This dialectal variation is common when certain languages such as Vietnamese and Spanish are carried over into English and is common in the African-American English dialect. It is the omission of the word-final consonant such as in "find," "cold" and "act" to produce the dialectical variation of "fin. . " "co. ." and "ac . ." The speaker with final cluster reduction may produce the utterance, "It is co. . outside" for "It is cold outside."

Plurals Following Clusters: Speakers who produce plurals following clusters alter words such as "desk" and "test" to produce "desses" and "tesses." According to Wolfram, this dialectical variation is probably a function of overlearning standard English plurals.

Intrusive "t": This dialectical variation is common in rural regions and is the addition of the "t" consonant to words such as "cliff" and "across." The speaker using the intrusive "t" says "clift," and "acrosst."

"th" Sound Variations: Several dialectical variations involve the voiced (as in t̲h̲at) and voiceless "th" (as in t̲h̲ink") sounds. These variations appear to be sensitive to the position of the "th" sounds in words, i.e., the initial, medial, or final parts of words. Examples of "th" variations include: "aritmetic" for "arithmetic," "efer" for "ether," "toof" for "tooth," and "broder" for "brother." It is common in many dialects to produce "heith" for "height," which is probably related to generalizing the "th" in "width" to "height."

"r" and "l" Sound Variations: In several dialectical variations, the "r" sound may be reduced or lost. This results in words transformations such as "Ca'ol" for "Carol," "sto'y" for "story," "p,ofessor" for "professor," and "sec'etary" for

"secretary." Sound variations for the "l" include "woof" for "wolf" and "hep" for "help."

Initial "w" Reduction: Southern-based and rural dialects often reduce the "w" sound such as in "young'uns" for "young ones."

Unstressed Initial Syllable Loss: Loss of the initial syllable results in dialectical variations such as "cause" for "because," "round" for "around," "taters" for "potatoes."

Initial "h" Retention: This dialectical variation occurs in rural dialects such as occurs in "hit" for "it," and "hain't" for "ain't." Another "h" variation is "Uston" for "Huston."

Other Consonants: According to Wolfram (1986), other consonant variations include the speaker saying "aks" for "ask," "chimley" or "chimbley" for "chimney," "skreet" for "street," and "skring" for "string."

19.7 Accent, Dialect, Word Usage, and Grammatical Structures

Dialectical word usage also varies greatly with interesting regional examples. According to Alvarez and Kolker (1987) calling a "milk shake" a "cabinet," "rubber band," a "gum band," "schlep," for "to carry," and "snickelfritz" for a "rowdy child" are examples of regional word usage dialectical variations. Calling farming work shoes "clodhoppers," a skunk a "polecat," and a glove compartment a "jockybox" are also examples of regional word usage dialects.

Wolfram (1986) notes that many socially significant grammatical structures involve the verb phrase and provides dialectical grammatical variations (Table 19.2). Wolfram (1986, p. 114) comments on the complexity of dialects:

One of the ironies of our understanding of linguistic variation is the fact that this complex behavior has so often been reduced to simplistic and uninformed explanation, being attributed to ignorance and simplicity. Nothing could be farther from the truth; instead, linguistic variation deserves our utmost respect as a representation of the complex workings of the human mind and human social adaptive mechanism.

Table 19.2
Selected English Grammatical Dialectical Variations

Grammatical Category	Grammatical Structure	Examples
Verb phrase	Irregular verbs	"I had went to the police." "He seen the policeman." "She come to the cop." "They knowed it was wrong."
Verb tense	Omission of past tense	"The cops mess up."
Subject-verb	Subject-verb agreement Irregular verbs	"The cars was followed." "Me and him gets in an argument." "They throwed rocks at the cops."
Verb addition	Completive "done" Habitual "be"	"They done took him to the police station." "I be itching for a fight."
Pronouns	Changes to case	"Me and him took the money." "Y' all took my statement." "I don't like them there cops."

Table 19.2 shows several English dialectal variations by grammatical category, verb phrase, verb tense, subject-verb, verb addition, and pronouns.

Attention to regional accent and dialect variations provides important investigative tools for law enforcement agencies. Most informants can identify people speaking with a regional accent and dialect. Speaker profiles of accent and dialect can be valid and reliable investigative tools for determining a person's region of origin.

19.8 Accent, Dialect, and Socioeconomic Status

"In addition to correlating with ethnicity, linguistic behavior tends to reflect social class, education, and occupation" (Payne and Taylor, 1998, p. 125). In the United States, social class, education, and occupation can be combined into one category: socioeconomic status. Unlike what is observed in many other countries, rarely do people in the United States achieve uneven social class, education, and occupation levels. Although there are exceptions, in the United States, people with less education have occupations of lower prestige and earning power, and are considered members of the lower class strata. Conversely, people with higher educations have occupations of higher prestige and earning power, and are members of the upper class strata. Because the United States has a large middle class, these distinctions are not as clearly defined as they are in many other countries. However, even in America, high, middle, and low socioeconomic distinctions can often be made based on a person's speech and language behavior. Concerning speech and language behaviors, the greatest linguistic socioeconomic distinction is apparent between the extreme upper and lower strata of society. According to Wyatt (2002), the effects of accent and dialect on a person can be assessed by eliciting information about the perceived impact of English communication difficulties in social interaction, and assessing current and future occupational or educational goals.

Many reasons have been given for speech and language behavior differences between socioeconomic levels. Payne and Taylor (1998) list home environment, child-rearing practices, family interaction patterns, and travel and experience as chief factors for language variation relative to social class. Research has shown that mother and child interaction in lower socioeconomic families is less desirable than what is observed in higher socioeconomic families. Hart and Risley (1995), and other researchers, have found substantial variation in language stimulation and learning in young children from low socioeconomic levels when compared to those reared in families with more education and higher income levels. Generally, children reared in families in lower socioeconomic levels tend to receive fewer stimulating language learning opportunities. In addition, other factors that are associated with low income such as malnutrition, dental problems, and other health factors may also contribute to suboptimal conditions for speech and language development. Families from middle and upper socioeconomic levels also have more opportunities for travel, and thus are exposed to a greater variety of languages, accents, and dialects.

19.9 Accent, Dialect, and Terrorism

Although Middle Eastern Arab speakers do not sponsor all terrorism, today, the majority of terrorist acts are conducted by radical Muslims who speak the Arabic language. Often, there are verbal threats of impending terrorist acts and audios accepting responsibility for them once they occur. The forensic value of profiling the accent and dialectical patterns of these speakers are threefold. First, by analyzing the accent and dialect of the speakers, determination can be made as to the region of the Middle East the speakers reside. Second, the veracity of pre and post terrorist reports can be ascertained by comparing the accent and dialect patterns of the speakers for consistency. If two terrorist speakers provide pre and post verbal threats and reports, accent and dialect can provide information about their ethnicity. Third, accent and dialect analysis of speakers can provide screening information to help detect terrorists who may be entering the United States through ports-of-entry. Accent and dialect analysis can provide information about homeland and region of origin. As Mansfield (1992) notes, one useful method for classifying Middle Easterners is by the languages they speak.

"The land of the Arab world lies in northern Africa and southwestern Asia. It ranges from Mauritania in the west to Oman in the east. The Arab countries from Egypt and Sudan eastward comprise the region of the world known as the Middle East" (Battle, 2002, p. 114). Wilson (1998) reports that 160 million people speak Arabic or dialects of Arabic, and they can be grouped into North African, Egyptian/ Sudanese, Syrian/Levantine, Arabian Peninsular, and Iraqi. According to Wilson, the North African dialects, those spoken by Moroccans, Algerians, Tunisians, Libyans, and Mauritanians were influenced by the Berbers and the languages of the colonists from other North African countries. The Egyptian/Sudanese dialect is understood by most Arabs because it is the dialect used in movies, television, and radio. Syrian/Levantine and Arabian Peninsular dialects are

mutually comprehensible by Lebanese, Syrians, Jordanians, Palestinians, Saudis, Yemenis, Adendis, Kuwaitis, Gulfs, and Omanis. The most prestigious of all the Arab dialects are the Arabian Peninsular dialects spoken in Saudi Arabia, Yemen, Aden, Kuwait, Gulf, and Oman because they are considered by Arabs to be the closest to the language of the Koran. "Arabs from Pakistan, India, and Iran speak Urdu, Hindi, and Farsi, respectively" (Wilson, 1998, p. 201). According to Wilson (1998), between 90 percent and 94 percent of the Arab world are Muslims, and most speak Arabic.

According to Mansfield (1992) and Lamb (1987), roughly two million Arabs live in the United States. Like English speakers, Arabic speakers' social class, education, and nationality can be gleaned by accent, dialect, and other social-communicative behaviors. For example, Parker and Riley (1994) observe that native speakers of Arabic dialects typically break up speech sound clusters with the /i/ ("ee" as in "see") differently. "Egyptian Arabic speakers insert /i/ between members of a consonant-liquid cluster, while Iraqi Arabic speakers insert /i/ before a consonant-liquid cluster" (Parker and Riley, 1994, p. 229). The differences between Egyptian Arabic and Iraqi Arabic dialects are shown on the words "floor" and "Fred." In Egyptian Arabic, the words would be pronounced /filor/ and /fir d/. In Iraqi Arabic, "floor" would be pronounced /iflor/ and "Fred" pronounced /ifr d/.

In addition to accent and dialect, there are several non-verbal and communication-cultural variables related to Arab speakers. Wilson (1996), Nydell (1997), and Wilson (1998) note several cultural practices with Arab speakers including not showing the soles of ones shoes when sitting with legs crossed, prolonged hand shakes when greeting and parting, and some Arab males will not shake hands with a female. They go on to note that Arabs are frequently late for appointments or do not keep them at all, maintain steady eye contact with the listener, and that the use of the left hand is considered rude. Personal space during a conversation with Arabs is usually less than what is customary with Americans. Finally, they note that the Arabic language is rich with metaphors, similes, and proverbs.

19.10 Automatic Language Accent and Dialect Profiling

It is currently possible for computerized, automatic accent and dialect analyses of subjects at ports-of-entry into the United States. Current speech pattern recognition technology gives homeland security a means of screening foreigners as potential terrorists. A speech sample could be taken without the subject's knowledge at ports-of-entry and automatically analyzed to provide information about his or her ethnicity. Algorithms can be written to analyze general speech patterns, word usage, other salient features of high-risk ethnic groups previously associated with terrorist acts. These speech analyses would flag accent and dialect patterns suggesting high-risk ethnic groups entering the United States for further investigation.

As Figure 19.1 shows, the objectives of accent and dialect profiling are to obtain geographic, socioeconomic, and ethnic information for investigative and screening purposes. By using knowledgeable informants and real-time or recorded speech samples, law enforcement personnel and screeners at ports-of-entry to the United States can glean important information about identified or unidentified sub-jects based on their accents and dialects. While profiling using accent and dialect is not a definitive nor a foolproof method of obtaining information about criminal acts or the potential for them, it can provide valuable forensic information.

19.11 Summary

Accent, dialect, and other communication patterns can be important investigative tools. The way a person communicates suggests his or her ethnicity, culture, country and region of origin. It also provides information about socioeconomic status. There are predictable features involving vowels, consonants, and word usage that can provide valuable information.

Accent and Dialect Profile Objectives

From subject's accent and dialect, obtain geographic, socioeconomic, and ethnic information.

Profiling Procedures

By using knowledgeable informants and real-time or recorded speech samples, assess speaker's accent and dialect patterns suggesting the following:

> homeland and region of country
> education
> employment
> socioeconomic status
> urban or rural dweller

Determine whether speech patterns are accent-carryover of first learned to a second language, or effects of a regional dialect, or both. Analysis addresses phonological rules, habitual use of vowels and consonants, and word usage.

Profile Results

Based on accent and dialect profile information, identified or unidentified subject's likely country and region of origin are presumed including ethnicity. Also presumed are the subject's likely general education level, employment status (trade, business, or professional), and whether he or she is a rural or urban dweller.

Figure 19.1 Accent and dialect profiling objectives, procedures, and results.

Suggested Readings and Resources

Alvarez, L. and Kolker, A. (1987). *American Tongues*: A Film. New York: Center for NewAmerican Media. This video reviews the history of accents and dialects in the United States and provides examples.

Architecture and Tools for Linguistic Analysis Systems (AT-LAS) (2006). NIST ATLAS Project Home. Retrieved September 24, 2006 from the World Wide Web: http://www.nist.gov/speech/atlas/. This website provides a vast amount of accent and dialect information.

Battle, D.E. (2002). Middle Eastern and Arab American Cultures. In D.E. Battle (Ed) *Communication Disorders in Multicultural Populations* (3rd ed.) Boston: Butterworth Heinemann. This chapter addresses multiple issues in addressing communication in Middle Eastern and Arab American cultures.

Delaney, R. (2006). Dialect Map of the United States. Retrieved September 25, 2006 from the World Wide Web: http://www.geocities.com/yvain.geo/dialects.html This website provides a colorful dialectal map of the United States with descriptions for each region.

References

Alvarez, L. and Kolker, A. (1987). *American Tongues*: A Film. New York: Center for NewAmerican Media.

Battle, D.E. (2002). Middle Eastern and Arab American Cultures. In D.E. Battle (Ed) *Communication disorders in multicultural populations* (3rd ed.) Boston: Butterworth Heinemann.

Battle, D.E. (1998). Communication disorders in a multicultural society. In D.E. Battle (Ed) *Communication disorders in multicultural populations* (2nd ed.). Boston: Butterworth-Heinemann.

Broeder, P. and Extra, G. (1999). *Language, ethnicity and education.* Philadelphia: Multilingual Matters Ltd.

Carver, C.M. (1987). *American regional dialects: A word geography.* Ann Arbor: University of Michigan.

Delaney, R. (2006). Dialect Map of the United States. Retrieved September 25, 2006 from the World Wide Web: http://www.geocities.com/yvain.geo/dialects.html.

Eisenson, J. (1979). *Voice and diction* (4th ed.). New York: Macmillan.

Hart, B., and Risley, T. (1995). *Meaningful differences in the everyday experience of young American children.* Baltimore: Paul H. Brookes.

Haynes, W.O., and Pindzola, R. (2004). *Diagnosis and evaluation in speech pathology.* Boston: Allyn & Bacon.

Lamb, D. (1987). *The Arabs: Journeys beyond the mirage.* New York: Random.

Linguistic Atlas Projects (2006). About the Site. Retrieved September 24, 2006 from the World Wide Web: http://us.english.uga.edu/information/about.

Mansfield, P. (1992). *The Arabs.* New York: Penguin.

Nist, J. (1966). *A structural history of English.* New York: St. Martin's Press.

Nydell, M. K. (1997). *Understanding Arabs: A guide for westerners.* Yarmouth, ME: Intercultural Press.

Parker, F. and Riley, K. (1994). *Linguistics for non-linguists: A primer with exercises* (3rd ed.) Boston: Allyn & Bacon.

Payne, K. T. and Taylor, O. L. (1998). Communication differences and disorders. In G. Shames, E. Wiig, and W. Secord (Eds.), *Human communication disorders: An Introduction* (5th ed). Boston: Allyn & Bacon.

United States Census (2000). Census 2000 Demographic Profile Highlights: Selected Population Group: Mexican. Retrieved from the World Wide Web June 10, 2006: http://factfinder.census.gov

Westby, C. And Vining, C. (2002). Living in Harmony: Providing Services to Native American Children and Families. . In D.E. Battle (Ed) *Communication disorders in multicultural populations* (3rd ed.) Boston: Butterworth Heinemann.

Wilson, M.E. (1996). Arabic speakers: Language and culture, here and abroad. *Topics in Language Disorders.* 16(4), 65-80.

Wilson, F. W. (1998). Delivering speech-language and hearing services in the Arab World: Some cultural consideration. In D.E. Battle (Ed.) *Communication disorders in multicultural populations* (2nd ed.) Boston: Butterworth-Heinemann

Wolfram, W. (1986). Language variation in the United States. In O. L. Taylor (Ed) *Nature of communication disorders in culturally and linguistically diverse populations.* San Diego: College Hill Press.

Wyatt, T. (2002). Assessing communicative abilities of clients from diverse cultural and language backgrounds. In D.E. Battle (Ed), *Communication disorders in multicultural populations* (3rd ed.) Boston: Butterworth Heinemann.

Chapter 20

Speaker Profiling and Intoxication

20.1 Chapter Preview

This chapter addresses speaker profiling and individuals who are intoxicated. There is a review of motor speech production associated with levels of neurological functioning. Language and motor speech production are discussed with an emphasis on how intoxicants can impair speech production. The effects of intoxicants are discussed concerning speech programming, cerebellar functioning, extrapyramidal irregularities, and the language of confusion. There is also a section on neurological diseases and disorders that produce symptoms similar to the speech patterns of intoxicated persons.

20.2 The Forensic Aspects of Intoxication and Speech Patterns

Law enforcement personnel are frequently called upon to investigate, detain, and arrest intoxicated individuals. Lawyers, when litigating cases, must sometimes address statements made by individuals who were under the influence of intoxicating substances during the commission of crimes. Judges and juries may be required to make judgments about levels of intoxication and their influence on verbal reports and criminal behavior. In this chapter, intoxication is broadly defined as "temporary acute poisoning" caused by intoxicating agents and includes the effects of alcohol, illegal substances, and prescription medications. Speech patterns are valuable indicators of intoxication and can suggest the intoxicant and level of impairment. In addition, people with certain neurological diseases and disorders can have speech symptoms similar to those of people in intoxicated states.

Aristotle was the first philosopher to study the speech patterns of intoxicated individuals (O'Neill, 1980). People in intoxicated states may have the level of intoxication and the type of intoxicant revealed by "what" they say and the "way" they say it. There are two distinct functional categories of communication concerning the speech patterns of intoxicated individuals: language and motor speech production. Language involves the use and understanding of symbols whereas motor speech production concerns the neuromuscular activities of speaking. Although discussed separately, they are interconnected and overlapping systems.

Language is a system of symbols, a process for communicating thoughts and feelings from one person to another. Language is defined as the "multimodality ability to encode, decode, and manipulate symbols for the purposes of verbal thought and/or communication." Modalities are avenues of communication. They are ways people share thoughts and feelings. The primary language modalities are speaking, auditory comprehension, reading, writing, and gesturing. People also send and receive information through the language of mathematics. According to Davis (2007), language and mental processes are interconnected; those factors that affect language also affect mental processes and vice versa. The information presented herein primarily concerns verbal language and the use of speech to express thoughts and feelings. Speech is the most common means of expression and understanding, and is the channel through which most communication takes place. People under the influence of various intoxicants will have certain speech and language aspects affected or disrupted.

Neuromuscular speech production involves the physical act of producing speech sounds. It also includes feedback the person receives about the muscles and structures of speech production. When discussing motor aspects of speech production, the level of neurological functioning disrupted by the intoxicant causes specific types of output. Attention to the neuromotor speech production of intoxicated individuals can provide important forensic information.

20.3 Intoxication, Neurological Organization, and Motor Speech Production

The nervous system is composed of the brain and spinal cord, and all other associated nerves and sense organs (Zemlin, 1998). According to Zemlin, there are eleven recognized systems in the human body (a system is two or more organs combined to exhibit a functional unity): skeletal, articular (joints and ligaments), muscular, digestive, vascular, nervous, respiratory, urinary, reproductive, endocrine (glands of the body), and integumentary (skin, hair, nails). The nervous system operates holistically; no single part functions completely independent of other systems. This is particularly true during communication. "With just a moment of thought it becomes apparent that no one of these systems is independent of the others. The speech mechanism draws heavily on some systems and less heavily on others, but either directly or indirectly, it is dependent upon all of the systems of the body" (Zemlin, 1998, p. 30). However, there are certain levels of neurological organization that are important to speech functioning and intoxication can result in specific types of impaired output.

As reviewed in Chapter 15, there are five distinct but overlapping aspects to motor speech production: respiration, phonation, articulation, resonance, and prosody. Respiration is the breath support necessary for speech production. Phonation is the vibration of the vocal cords and consequent energy produced in the larynx, and articulation is the use of the tongue, lips, teeth, and other structures of the mouth to shape speech sounds. Resonance is the amount of nasality present in speech, and prosody is the rhythm and cadence of utterances. Neurological disruptions caused by intoxicating agents can affect these motor speech aspects in different ways creating clusters of unique symptoms. The cluster of symptoms depend, in part, on the level of neurological organization affected by the intoxicant.

Frederic Darley, Arnold Aronson, and Joe Brown of the Mayo Clinic are credited with applying a detailed hierarchy of motor organization levels and their corresponding speech movements. Although scientists before them linked certain speech patterns to neurological levels of organization, Darley, Aronson, and Brown (1975) provided a detailed review of motor speech organization and resulting communication deficiencies. The levels of motor speech organization are 1) conceptual programming, 2) cerebellar, 3) upper motor neuron, 4) extrapyramidal, 5) vestibular-reticular, and 6) lower motor neuron (Darley, Aronson, and Brown, 1975). Review of the available literature on intoxication and motor speech production suggests they can be analyzed by primarily addressing conceptual programming, cerebellar, and extrapyramidal levels of organization. Although extreme intoxication can damage and impair the six levels of motor organization provided by Darley, Aronson, and Brown, the speech patterns of intoxicated individuals typically affect language, motor speech programming, coordination, and automatic aspects of speech muscle movement. The intoxicants discussed herein are separated into stimulants and depressants resulting in differing speech and language patterns. Stimulants tend to increase speech irregularities while depressants tend to suppress speech fluency and precision.

20.4 Disruptive Effects of Anxiety on the Speech Production of Intoxicated Persons

Intoxicants can have various effects on a person's anxiety levels. Decades of fluency research have shown that moderate to severe anxiety disrupts the fine motor coordination necessary to produce speech. When speakers experience higher levels of anxiety, they tend to produce speech with more dysfluencies. They repeat, prolong, and hesitate more during speech, and the more anxiety they experience, the more dysfluent are they. Detainment, arrest, and interrogation result in increased speaker anxiety and likely increases in the number and severity of speech dysfluencies. However, speakers under the influence of depressants rarely show anxiety-based struggled speech.

There are three levels of anxiety to consider when examining its disruptive effects on speech fluency. Relatively low levels of anxiety may actually result in the speaker being more fluent and articulate because he or she consciously compensates for the increased stress. The speaker's anxiety level causes him or her to monitor output and purposefully produce speech more fluently. Increased but relatively low levels of anxiety cause improved speech fluency and precision in some speakers during questioning because the speaker can deal efficiently with the anxiety. Higher levels of anxiety have disruptive effects on speech fluency and precision because the speaker cannot consciously compensate. He or she does not think clearly and the speech dysfluencies reflect attempts to organize and sequence utterances. Extreme levels of anxiety can cause speakers to be functionally unable to produce comprehensible speech due to their disruptive effects. Of course, not all people react to anxiety in the same way, but as a rule, higher levels of anxiety tend to increase speech dysfluencies and reduce precision.

20.5 Intoxicants and Motor Speech Programming

All five aspects of speech production (respiration, phonation, articulation, resonance, prosody) can be disrupted by the effects of intoxicants on motor speech programming, but articulation is the most conspicuous and prominent. Motor speech programming is where the idea behind the purposeful utterance is formulated and the articulatory plan is created. During motor speech programming, the entire articulatory act, from beginning to end, is planned including each articulator's timing, speed, and strength of movements. "The timing, speed, strength, and precision of the motor speech act in general, and the articulatory plan in particular, are generated at the planning phase. At this phase, all the motor speech requirements necessary to produce the utterance is created including the specific muscular movements related to each voluntarily produced speech sound production" (Tanner, 2006, p. 125). Neurologically, the areas important to motor speech articulatory programming are Broca's area, and the tracts leading to and from it, located in the left frontal lobe of most people. In addition, the articulatory plan may occur in other areas of the left hemisphere of the brain, specifically the anterior insula and lateral premotor cortex (Wise, Greene, Büchel, and Scott, 1999).

An intoxicated individual showing irregularities of motor speech programming has the linguistic representation of the utterance. The speaker has the word or words for the utterance in his or her mind; the speech irregularities do not result from amnesia for words. Also, speech patterns indicative of intoxication-induced programming impairments are not a result of paralysis or paresis (weakness) of the speech musculature. In addition, the person has the intent to produce speech. He or she wants to utter a statement, but is unable or impaired in doing so because motor speech programming has been affected by the intoxicant.

When motor speech programming is disrupted or impaired, speakers produce utterances with complications (Darley, Aronson, and Brown, 1975). Complications of the speech act involve additions, substitutions, fillers, revisions, and visible signs of speaker struggle. The speech of people with disrupted speech programming can be characterized by groping (Owens, Metz, and Haas, 2000). An ad-

dition is the insertion of an unnecessary sound or syllable to a word. For example, a person may say, "I do not have a (s)gun," for "I do not have a gun." He or she adds an unnecessary sound to the word "gun." Another example of an insertion is the schwa vowel "uh." The speaker may say, "I left the (uh) scene of the accident. The substitution of one sound for another occurs when the suspect says, "I do not have a (t)un, for "I do not have a gun." He or she has substituted the /t/ for the /g/ sound in the initial position of the word.

Complications of the speech act include the use of fillers, revisions, and visible signs of speaker struggle. A filler is the insertion of a sound, syllable, or word during a pause. It is usually an attempt by the speaker to prevent interruptions. Typical fillers include "and," "uh," and "you know." For example, a suspect may say, "I take medications for (uh, uh, uh) diabetes." Revisions are the speaker's attempts to correct a motor speech programming error or to appear more articulate: "No officer, I was not steeding, uh, sdeeding, uh speeding." Visible signs of struggle to program an utterance are usually apparent on the speaker's face. They are facial grimaces, eye-squints, jaw and lip tremor, and other indications that the suspect is forcing speech. They are similar to the facial expressions of people who are engaging in strenuous activities.

Speakers under the influence of stimulants are likely to have motor speech programming irregularities and deficits, and complicate the speech act. The accuracy of motor speech programming is diminished by increased rate of speech. Speakers talking rapidly, more than 500 words per minute, tend to sacrifice speech precision. Rate of speech can be affected by the number and length of the pauses. Pausing several times during an utterance has the effect of slowing the rate of speech as does having fewer but longer pauses. Rate of speech is also dependent on the duration of the syllable. Speakers who prolong the syllable or "stretch out" the word also speak fewer words per minute.

20.6 Intoxicants and Motor Speech Coordination

Like motor speech programming, all five motor speech processes can be impaired due to the effects of intoxicants on speech coordination. However, in motor speech coordination deficits, articulation and prosody are the most conspicuous and prominent involved processes. Motor speech coordination is a result of several areas of the nervous system working in an integrated manner. However, the cerebellum is a fundamental brain structure for coordinating speech acts. It does not initiate speech movements, but imposes control over them (Duffy, 1995). It is so important to coordination that it is called "the great modulator" of muscular movements.

Movements come from the motor cortex with excessive range and force. If not for the cerebellum, these muscle movements would overshoot and undershoot their targets. For example, overshooting and undershooting are seen when an intoxicated person tries to pick up a pencil. Because the commands coming from the motor cortex are not modulated and coordinated appropriately, the person's hand misses the pencil, hits the desk on which it is lying, and generally is imprecise in the simple act of grasping and retrieving it.

In speech, the lack of modulation and coordination is seen in articulatory overshooting and undershooting. For example, in speech sounds where the tip of the tongue touches the alveolar ridge (where the tip of the tongue touches the tissue just behind the upper incisors in the production of /t/, /d/, and /l/ sounds), without the coordinating effects of the cerebellum, there would be ill-coordinated speech. The tongue would hit the alveolar ridge with too much force and overshoot and undershoot its target. The result would be explosive, distorted, imprecise speech.

Prosody is a major area of deficit in the speech of intoxicated individuals when the cerebellum has been affected. Prosody includes stress and emphasis, intonation, rhythm, melody, pitch and voice quality of speech. Intoxicated individuals may produce sounds and syllable with too much or too little syllable stress. Their speech also may lack the loudness and pitch variability seen in individuals not under the influence of intoxicants. "Scanning" and "measured" have been used to describe ill-coordinated speech. Because of the lack of modulation and coordination, intoxicated persons produce imprecise consonants and vowels often with a slow rate of speech.

20.7 Intoxicants and Automatic Motor Speech

The extrapyramidal system is involved in inhibiting unwanted movements, maintaining posture, and changing body position. Intoxicant-induced deficits or irregularities of the extrapyramidal system cause unwanted movements such as tremor, body jerks, and tics. These unwanted movements occur on a continuum ranging from slow to quick. All body muscles can be affected by deficits or irregularities of the extrapyramidal system including those of respiration, voicing, and articulation.

"By purist definition, the extrapyramidal system comprises all higher motor mechanisms other than those arising from the pyramidal cortex and traveling in the pyramidal tracts" (Darley, Aronson, and Brown, 1975, pp. 48-49). The extrapyramidal system consists primarily of the basal ganglia which is at the base of the brain hemispheres but includes all of the brain structures associated with automatic movements.

Normal tremors are rhythmic modulations of muscles and can occur during rest and movement. Excessive tension and a sudden ballistic movement are necessary to set off tremors. These tremors are observable modulations of speech muscles and are different from the micro-tremors described in Chapter 22. Normal tremors of the speech mechanism are usually indicative of excessive muscular tension due to anxiety and forced speech.

Abnormal tremors occur because of a breakdown of the normal steadiness of neural muscular control and are a result of a disease state or are characteristic of a particular disease (Darley, Aronson, and Brown, 1975). Intoxicant-induced tremors may cause speech to be produced with a 'quivering' quality including excessive audible voice modulations. Voice modulations are caused muscle tremors of the larynx affecting pitch and loudness.

Tics, sudden uncontrolled contraction of the muscles of the speech mechanism, cause changes in speech patterns because they move the articulators abruptly. These unwanted movements during speech result in unwanted sounds. Prolonged and excessive use of drugs can cause tardive dyskinesia where the speaker has muscular jerks, tremors, and writhing-twisting movements of the speech muscles. These movements result in the production of unwanted and abnormal sounds interjected during utterances. Table 20.1 summarizes prominent speech patterns and the likely site of neurological involvement of intoxicated speakers. As a rule, intoxicants involve multiple motor systems affecting programming, coordination, and automatic speech. Depressants tend to result in diminished motor speech acts whereas stimulants cause complications errors (see Table 20.2).

20.8 The Language of Intoxication

Confusional states are commonly seen in patients with traumatic brain injuries and dementia, and the same diagnostic parameters used in medicine can be applied to intoxicated individuals. The language of individuals under the influence of intoxicants reflects their confusional states. The content of their utterances suggests the nature and severity of the confusional states. Generally, a confused person has two primary factors contributing to his or her confusion: memory deficits and disorientation.

Table 20.1
Speech Patterns of Intoxicated Individuals

Neurological Organization	Speech patterns
Motor speech programming	Speech sound additions Speech sound substitutions Interjections Facial contortions Eye squints Rapid rate of speech
Motor speech coordination	Speech sound distortions Speech sound omissions Slow rate of speech
Automatic motor speech	Tremor of jaw Tremor of the lips Tremor of the tongue Eyelid tremor Muscular jerks of the jaw, lips, tongue, larynx

Table 20.2
Stimulants and Depressants Effect on Speech Patterns

Speech Parameter	Speech Pattern	Stimulants	Depressants
Rate-of-speech	Words-per-minute	Increases number of words spoken per minute	Decreases number of words spoken per minute
Injections	Insertion of sounds, syllables, words, and short phrases	Increases number of injections	Decreases number of injections
Production errors	Complication errors; simplification errors	Increases number of substitutions and additions	Increases number of omissions and distortions
Accompanying nonverbal communication	Associated facial expressions and gestures	Facial and general body tension; increased use of descriptive and reinforcing gestures	Facial sag; decreased use of descriptive and reinforcing gestures
Automatic speech	Hypokinetic and hyperkinetic movement disorders	Tics, jerks; jaw, lips, tongue, and eyelid tremors; tardive dyskinesia	Drooling

The memory defects seen in intoxication-induced confusional states include retrograde and anterograde amnesia. In retrograde amnesia, speakers cannot recall people and events occurring before the intoxication. They may not be able to provide information about what they were doing and with whom they were doing it before becoming intoxicated. Anterograde amnesia is a memory deficit and the consequent inability to retain information while under the influence of the intoxicants. Severely intoxicated individuals cannot remember requests and commands nor can they attend to and store new information due to amnesia. Some individuals who suffer brain injury because of chronic intoxication may be permanently impaired in acquiring new information.

In confusional states, there are typically four types of disorientation: time, place, person, and situation. Some intoxicated individuals are primarily disoriented to one facet of reality while others are globally disoriented. The memory deficits suffered by intoxicated individuals are related to the disorientation they experience because of the relationship between being unable to remember facets of one's life and being disoriented.

Disorientation to time is when the speaker is confused about the hour, day, week, month, or longer aspect of time. Intoxicated individuals may believe it is morning when it is evening or may erroneously report the day of the week. Disoriented people may also not accurately perceive the passage of time. They may believe that several hours have transpired when, in fact, only a few minutes have passed. Disorientation to place is manifest when the speaker incorrectly reports a street, city, or state.

Disorientation to person is when the speaker cannot correctly identify family, friends, coworkers, and acquaintances. He or she does not appreciate previous relationships. Disorientation to person can also extend to loss of identity where the speaker is confused about his or her occupation, marital status, level of education, and so forth. In cases of extreme intoxication, the person may be confused about his or her gender. When a person is disoriented to situation, he or she does not appreciate what is happening to him or her. The speaker may not concede that he or she is being arrested or has been incarcerated. During extreme intoxication, the person may be oblivious to the events surrounding criminal conduct.

Table 20.3
Language Patterns of Intoxicated Speakers

Function	**Deficit**	**Type**
Memory	Retrograde amnesia Anterograde amnesia	Memory loss of events before intoxication Memory loss of events since intoxication
Orientation	Disorientation to time Disorientation to place Disorientation to person Disorientation to situation	Confusion about time events Confusion about location Confusion about people, identity or both Confusion about predicament
Receptive language	Auditory comprehension deficits Reading comprehension deficits	Difficulty following verbal commands (slow rise time and auditory fade) Difficulty following written commands (slow rise time and auditory fade)
Expressive language	Confabulation Tangential speech	Remarking about events without regard to truthfulness or accuracy Digressing and divagating speech

The receptive and expressive language of intoxicated speakers can include spoken and written impairments. Intoxicated individuals may be unable to follow verbal commands due to the effects of the intoxicants. They may only follow the first in a series of requests owing to auditory fade. In auditory fade, because of impaired concentration, only the former in a series of requests are attended to. The opposite of auditory fade is slow rise time. In slow rise time, the final aspects of a series of commands are followed and the person neglects the initial requests. This behavior is due to the intoxicated individual's gradual uptake of attention due to distractibility and loss of concentration. These patterns of behavior are also seen in reading and following written instructions.

Expressively, intoxicated individuals may confabulate. Confabulation is the remarking about events without regard to their accuracy—chronic lying. The confabulation is usually verbal, but can also be written. Expressively, intoxicated individuals also are tangential in their speech and writing. One thought leads to another less relevant thought, which leads to another, and so forth. The tangential behavior of intoxicated individuals described above may also be manifest in the graphic mode; the deficits are seen in writing. Table 20.3 shows the typical language patterns of intoxicated individuals.

20.9 Neurological Diseases and Disorders Resembling Intoxication

There are three categories of neurological disease and disorders that can produce speech symptoms similar to those seen in intoxication. First, speakers with strokes and traumatic brain injuries may display memory, orientation, receptive and expressive language symptoms that may be confused with intoxication. Strokes and traumatic brain injuries can be mild and only minimally affect memory, orientation, and language, and the speech symptoms only negligibly apparent. Traumatic brain injuries can also be severe and result in profound deficits with the speaker producing obvious, conspicuous, and discernible language and cognitive symptoms.

Second, neurological disorders such as Parkinson's disease, multiple sclerosis, and amyotrophic lateral sclerosis (Lou Gehrig's disease) can cause speech disorders resembling intoxicated states, particularly in their late stages. Depending on the level of neurological organization involved in the disease process, patients with the above progressive diseases will speak with imprecise articulation, tremors, impaired rate, and so forth.

The third category of neurological diseases and disorders affecting speech and language is dementia. Primarily occurring in the elderly, Alzheimer's disease and other forms of dementia can impair the fabric of language, speech production, and memory-orientation. In early stage dementia, the symptoms may not be readily apparent, but in middle and late stages, the patient will usually have conspicuous behaviors suggesting impaired mental and neurological functioning.

20.10 Speech and Language Factors to Consider When Distinguishing Intoxication from Neurological Diseases and Disorders

In some cases, it may be difficult to distinguish intoxication from certain neurological diseases and disorders. In both conditions, speech and language may be incomprehensible and unintelligible. However, the following can suggest when the speaker's behaviors are a result of neurological disease or disorder rather than intoxication:

1. Speakers with impaired speech and language resulting from neurological diseases or disorders often present with hemiparalysis or hemiparesis (weakness) on one side of the body. Because, in most people, the major speech and language centers are located on the left side of the brain, the right side of the body will be affected in strokes and focalized traumatic brain injuries. (The left side of the brain controls the right side of the body and vice versa.) Some patients suffering from strokes and focalized traumatic brain injuries may require canes, walkers, or wheelchairs.

2. Speakers with impaired speech and language resulting from neurological disease or disorder may also have facial sag, a drooping of the eyes and mouth, due to paralysis. They may also drool. These impairments are usually not present in intoxicated individuals.

3. Speakers with Parkinson's disease, multiple sclerosis, amyotrophic lateral sclerosis, and other progressive neuromuscular disorders will usually not present with mental and cognitive impairments. Especially in early onset stages, they will only have the motor speech patterns that resemble intoxication.

4. Patients with neurological disease and disorders may have explanatory cards describing their impairments. These cards are supplied to the patients by doctors and therapists for those who are functionally unable to communicate. They will usually be kept in wallets, purses, or glove compartments of automobiles.

5. Particularly with alcohol consumption, there will be an odor associated with the intoxication. Patients with neurological diseases and disorders will not have the breath odor of alcohol.

6. The kinds of word-finding problems experienced by stroke patients usually have "rhyme or reason." A patient with difficulty remembering names due to stroke often supplies a word that is phonetically or semantically associated with the desired word. However, some stroke patients produce jargon with sounds that do not constitute words or use words improperly with regard to meaning.

7. Nystagmus, the rapid involuntary rocking and rapid-slow moving of the eyes, may be an indicator of intoxication, or a symptom of neurological impairments.

20.11 Summary

The speech patterns of intoxicated individuals can provide information about levels of neurological organization affected by the intoxicants. Although all levels of neurological organization can be affected during intoxicated states, breakdown of speech programming, and cerebellar and extrapyramidal functions typically can be seen in speech patterns. In addition, the receptive and expressive language functions can be impaired, and intoxicated individuals typically have discernible speech and language behaviors due to the intoxicants.

Suggested Readings and Resources

Darley, F., Aronson, A., and Brown, J. (1975). *Motor Speech Disorders*. Philadelphia: Saunders. This textbook addresses neurological systems applicable to understanding the effects of intoxication on speech production.

Tanner, D. (2006). *An Advanced Course in Communication Sciences and Disorders*. San Diego: Plural Publishing. Chapters 6 and 7 of this text examine motor speech planning and production.

Zemlin, W. (1998). *Speech and Hearing Science* (4th ed.). Boston: Allyn & Bacon. This textbook addresses all of the major neurological aspects of speech production.

References

Darley, F., Aronson, A., and Brown, J. (1975). *Motor speech disorders*. Philadelphia: Saunders.

Davis, G. A. (2007). *Aphasiology: Disorders and clinical practice* (2nd ed.). Boston: Allyn & Bacon.

Duffy, J. (1995). *Motor speech disorders*. St. Louis: Mosby.

O'Neill, Y.V. (1980). *Speech and speech disorders in western thought before 1600*. Westport, Connecticut: Greenwood Press.

Owens, R., Metz, D., and Haas, A. (2000). *Introduction to Communication Disorders*. Boston: Allyn & Bacon.

Tanner, D. (2006). *An advanced course in communication sciences and disorders*. San Diego: Plural Publishing.

Wise, R.J.S., Greene, J., Büchel, C., and Scott, S.K. (1999). Brain regions involved in articulation. *Lancet*, 353: 1057-61.

Zemlin, W. (1998). *Speech and hearing science* (4th ed). Boston: Allyn & Bacon.

Chapter 21

Speaker Profiling, Forensic Interviewing, and Interrogation

21.1 Chapter Preview

In this chapter, there is a discussion of the principles of speaker profiling as they pertain to forensic interviewing and interrogation. An overview of the psychology of speech is presented including the physiological dynamics associated with stress. Several theories about fluency disruption are examined to show the possible underlying psychological and emotional conflicts experienced by disfluent speakers. The forensic value of attending to rate-of-speech is examined as are loudness, pitch, voice quality, and nasality, word choice and grammatical construction, and nonverbal cues.

21.2 Speech: The Ego on Display

The speech and language patterns of a subject can provide valuable forensic information during an interview and interrogation. Although some criminologists consider forensic interviewing and interrogation the same information-gath-

ering process, technically they differ. According to Yeschke (1993), interviewing is the general task of gathering testimonial evidence. Interrogation is more specific with regard to goals and objectives: "An interrogation is a face-to-face meeting with the distinct task of gaining an admission or confession in a real or apparent violation of law, policy, regulation or other restriction" (Yeschke, 1993, p. 3). Regardless of the goals and objectives of interviewing and interrogation, the subject's speech patterns and language constructs can provide a remarkable window into the human psyche.

Speech is "the ego on display," sending cues about a person's intelligence, emotions, and personality to the listener. A person's intelligence is revealed by the use and understanding of language. People with larger vocabularies and precise grammar tend to be perceived as more intelligent than those with smaller vocabularies and imprecise grammar. Slow talkers are perceived as mentally slower in cognition whereas those who talk faster appear to process information more rapidly. Soft-spoken people seem more timid and reticent whereas loud talkers appear more self-assured and dominant. People with speech disorders are also stereotyped. Stuttering persons are sometimes perceived as dim-witted and anxious, lisping males are stereotyped as effeminate, and women with breathy voices are thought to be sexy (see Chapter 23).

The motion picture industry appreciates the power of speech to define characters. Actors use speech patterns to accentuate and amplify characters. They often use speech stereotypes which may or may not be accurate depictions of personality traits (Tanner, 2001; Tanner, Culbertson, and Secord, 2001). Accurate or not, people make a plethora of judgments about the speaker's emotions and personality based on speech patterns.

What a person says and how he or she says it is a window into the speaker's personality, opening many subtle and not so subtle cues about truthfulness, involvement and detachment, and emotions associated with a crime. A knowledgeable, perceptive interviewer and interrogator can use the speaker's speech patterns to cut through irrelevant and deceptive information and get to the truth about a crime or incident. Certainly, listening to what the speaker says is important, but how he or she says it often more revealing.

"How you speak shouts louder than what you say" is a common statement made by professors of speech communication when discussing nonverbal communication. Nonverbal communication is the use of facial expressions, gestures, proxemics, clothing and accessories, tone of voice, loudness, emphasis, fluency, and rate-of-speech to express information beyond the meaning of the spoken words. It has long been known that nonverbal communication can carry more than 70 percent of the meaning during communication. Words carry objective and subjective meaning, and nonverbal communication shows the feelings, emotions, and attitudes associated with them. And what is most important, when there is a conflict between what is spoken and the associated nonverbal communication, the listener usually believes the latter. For example, during an interrogation, a suspect may state: "I am happy to tell you all that I know about the crime." Certainly the words and sentence structure tell the interrogator that the suspect will willingly reveal all of the information he or she knows about the events related to the crime. However, if the suspect utters the words with legs and arms crossed, not making eye-contact, and in a low, harsh monopitched voice, the nonverbal communication may suggest the opposite.

Mixed messages may play a role in the investigation of alleged rape. Certainly, "No means no" should clearly express a woman's intent not to engage in sexual intercourse with a man. Unfortunately, the word "no" can be uttered in such a way as to cloud its intent and sometimes negate its meaning. If the word is uttered softly, with a breathy voice quality, and a pitch rise at the end of the statement, rightly or wrongly, the listener may perceive that "no" may not be an absolute indicator of the woman's desire. The verbal message is further confused if the woman wears provocative clothing and moves closer to the man while uttering the word "No." In fact, the so-called notion of "seduction" is that the male may manipulate a tentative woman into sexual intercourse due to his powers of persuasion: "Her voice said no, but her eyes said 'yes'." Again, the above is not to justify forced sexual intercourse on any woman, only to suggest that there can be ambiguity when the word "No" is stated.

As can be seen by the above discussion, the examination of speech patterns and language has multiple forensic applications during forensic interviews and interrogations. Interviewers and interrogators can assess a subject's anxiety levels yielding information about his or her culpability and knowledge of a crime. Consistency of responses to questions, including habitual word usage and sentence structures can be cues regarding whether or not the subject has been coached and rehearsed about the events related to a crime. A subject's speech can provide information about his or her level of involvement with a crime; speech can suggest high levels of involvement or detachment. Dominance, submission, anger, fear, grief, contempt, and pleasure can also be revealed by what the speaker says and how he or she says it. However, by far, the most important and forensically valuable use of speech patterns analysis is for lie detection. Knowing or having cues about statements that are true or false, sincere or insincere, accurate or inaccurate, leading or misleading, based on the speaker's speech patterns during an interview and interrogation can be valuable forensically.

21.3 Principles of Speaker Profiling

Walters (2003, pp. 10-18) provides nine Basic Practical Kinesic Principles useful for avoiding interviewing and interrogation pitfalls and getting to a suspect's truthfulness or deceptiveness. These principles are applicable to speaker profiling and are discussed in detail below.

1. No single kinesic behavior, verbal or nonverbal, proves a person is truthful or deceptive.

The most important principle of effective interviewing and interrogation is that conclusions drawn from the interview and interrogation must not be based on one factor. No single speech pattern or language construct can provide a definitive speaker profile about the suspect. The speaker's truthfulness, candor, contempt, sincerity, and so forth, are the result of astute observation and perception, intuition, logical deduction, scientific induction, and conjecture (see Chapter 18). Profiling in general, and speaker profiling in particular, are far from exact sciences. Conclusions drawn from what a speaker says and how he or she says it must be tempered by the fact that all profiling inherently involves error; the question is the degree of significance that can be attached to any speech pattern.

2. Behaviors must be relatively consistent when the stimuli are repeated.

Behavioral consistency is important in speaker profiling. Speaker profiling involves assessing the significance of many verbal and nonverbal behaviors. The speaker's consistency of responses and behaviors suggest whether they are random stress reactions or indicative of significant cognitive and emotional responses. In speaker profiling, the information obtained during the interview and interrogation by a speaker's speech pattern is drawn from consistent responses and behaviors, and the degree of their consistency suggests the power of the conclusions that can be drawn by them.

Basic Practical Kinesic Principles 3, 4, and 5 address feelings, moods, emotional states, and physiological status of subjects and are discussed together as they pertain to speaker profiling.

3. The interviewer must establish what is the normal, or "constant," of behavior for each subject. Accurate assessment of a person's behavior can be made only after establishing this reference point.

4. Once the constant has been established, the observer then looks for changes in the subject's constant of behavior.

5. Changes in a subject's behavior are reliable for diagnosing deception only if they appear in clusters.

Walters (2003) notes that approximately 65 percent of communication involves body language; 7 percent can be attributed to verbal content; quality of voice carries 12 percent of meaning; and the remaining 16 percent is a mixture of miscellaneous symptoms such as odors and signals that are difficult to identify. During interviews and interrogations, the speech profiler must establish the normal pattern of speech behavior and identify cluster changes before conclusions can be drawn about their significance.

6. Behaviors that are significant must be timely.

When connecting clusters of behaviors to stress stimuli, the same interval used in polygraph examinations is used: the 3–5 second rule. Timely analyses of behaviors require that the cluster of behaviors must occur roughly 3–5 seconds from the time of the stress prompt. However, some subjects are slower or faster to respond to stress, and this individual variable is determined during the basal analysis. With regard to speaker profiling, the speaker's rate-of-speech must also be considered; slow talkers will take more time to show stress reactions that those who habitually speak faster.

7. The interviewer should monitor his own behaviors in order to avoid contamination of the subject's behavior.

There are many other sources of stress which can contaminate the interview and interrogation and lead to false or misleading speaker profiles. According to Walters (2003, p. 17):

The strongest sources of stimuli in the interview room should be the content of the interviewer's questions or the presentation of physical evidence. They should not be the outward verbal and nonverbal behaviors of the interviewer. Such negative influences can be caused by inappropriate professional behavior from the interviewer, but there can be other, more subtle behavioral phenomena. Leading questions, a loud voice, finger pointing, exaggerated facial expressions, insults, and similar behaviors often create reactions from a subject.

Walters notes that the above behaviors usually occur when the interviewer or interrogator has already developed preconceptions, is unprepared and ill-trained for the interview, or has some personal agenda.

8. Observing and interpreting behavior is hard work.

Walters (2003) notes that delaying an important interview or interrogation does an injustice to the victim, witnesses, and the suspect. Although interviewing takes a great deal of concentration, and observing and interpreting are hard work, it should be done in a timely manner and given the necessary energy. "That means watching, listening, and diagnosing the significance of the subject's kinesic behaviors" (Walters, 2003, p. 18). Majeski (2002, p. 258) also comments on observing and interpreting behavior as hard work: "In the author's expert opinion, there is a direct correlation between the ability to listen and comprehend and the expenditure of individual effort."

9. Kinesic interviewing is not as reliable with some groups as with the general population.

As noted in Chapter 20, persons under the influence of intoxicants present atypical speech patterns and the type of intoxicant suggests its effect on speech production. Besides persons under the influence of intoxicants, Walters (2003) notes that the mentally deficient, children, adolescents, and psychotics respond differently to the interview. Mentally deficient individuals are easily led by those with higher intelligence. Interviews of children have come under much scrutiny recently given that they are easily led by interviewers with agendas. Adolescents may have a great deal of random body language and are more susceptible to peer pressure. Interviewing and interrogating psychotics is wrought with error of interpretation because psychotic persons are, by definition, separated from reality.

21.4 The Art of Listening in Speaker Profiling

Effective listening is important to all criminal profiling, but it is essential to speaker profiling. The forensic interviewer and interrogator must possess the basic abilities to hear what is said, perceive and understand the salient aspects of the verbal and nonverbal messages, and interpret meaningfully their implications. Yeschke (1993, pp. 162-163) observes that forensic interviewing involves the total person in the process: "Always be alert for signals of their mental processes, look for clues of motivation and hidden needs. As you listen attentively to what interviewees have to say, continually observe the ways they act. Through mannerisms, gestures, recurrent phrases and modes of expression, interviewees signal their thinking, hidden needs, and possible deception."

Majeski (2002) classifies investigators into three categories of listeners: poor, indifferent, and good. Poor investigative listeners would not prefer to expend the energy necessary to absorb important information during the interview. Indifferent investigative listeners tune out too much information and tend to ask the same questions or listen to old information as though it were new information. Good investigative listeners are very successful in obtaining all of the essential information most of the time. Majeski (2002, p. 258) summarizes the importance of good investigative listening: "If you don't concentrate, you will not hear. If you do not hear, you will not know. Without knowledge, you cannot understand and understanding is essential in helping distinguish between the truth and a lie."

Although active listening is essential to speaker profiling, knowledge of phonetics and a working ability to use phonetic symbols are equally important. The competent speech profiler must know the differences between speech and language so as to distinguish between speech patterns and phonology, semantics, and grammar aspects of language. Knowledge of how the five basic motor speech process of respiration, phonation, articulation, resonance, and prosody combines to produce speech enables the speech profiler to analyze and dissect the speaker's fluency, voice parameters, articulation, language constructs, and so forth.

To accurately and actively listen to a subject's speech, and to effectively perceive, classify, describe, and interpret his or her speech patterns for profiling purposes, a working understanding of The International Phonetic Alphabet (IPA) is also required. This information is provided in Chapter 15: Speech Production and Phonetics.

Speaker profiling involves attending to the speaker's (1) disfluencies, (2) rate-of-speech, (3) voice loudness, pitch, and quality, (4) nasality, (5) word choice and grammatical construction, and (6) nonverbal cues. Attending to the speaker's disfluencies provides information about general stress and specific psychological and emotional reactions to questions and statements, and gives insight into underlying psychological and emotional conflicts.

21.5 Speaker Profiling Using Speech Disfluencies

All speakers have normal disfluencies: repetitions, prolongations, and hesitations in their ongoing speech. Some individuals have a speech disorder, stuttering, and the number and type of their dysfluencies are abnormal. (When referring to normal repetitions, prolongations, and hesitations, "disfluency" is used; when referring to stuttering, "dysfluency" is used.) During an interview and interrogation, the frequency and type of speaker's disfluencies can provide information about his or her anxiety levels, conflicts, thought organization, and learned negative emotions.

Normal repetitions involve sounds, syllables, words, and phrases. Sound repetitions include both vowels and consonants such as "I was n-n-n-not, uh, uh, at the scene of the crime." A syllable repetition may result in this type of statement: "That is not my pis, pis, pis, pistol." Word and phrase repetitions involve single or multiple words such as "I, do, do, do understand my rights," and "I do not want, I do not want, I do not want to talk to a lawyer." Normal prolongations usually involve speech sounds that have a continuous air stream and energy emission such as the consonants "s," "th," and "v," and vowels. "I did not sssshoot that person" is an example of prolongation of the "s" speech sound. Hesitations occur in normal speech disfluenices and blocks are a result of stuttering. Hesitations usually occur when the speaker is trying to select the most appropriate word or is delayed in remembering the correct one. Blocks are a stuttering symptom of hypertense speech musculature that interrupt the flow of air through the speech tract.

In the profiling literature, there is considerable confusion about stuttering, stammering, and cluttering. For example, Walters (2003, p. 41) erroneously observes: "Stammering occurs because the subject may be trying to verbalize a large or important thought line at a faster rate than the mouth and other associated speech organs can function to form speech. Stuttering occurs because the person hasn't made up his mind before he speaks as to know how he is going to express an idea." This confusion in the profiling literature about stuttering, stammering, and cluttering is understandable given that these fluency disorders are often ill-defined in the discipline of communication sciences and disorders. Stuttering and stammering are essentially the same speech disorder; the term "stuttering" is used in the United States and "stammering" is used in some European countries. As can be seen from Table 21.1, in normal disfluency, there are fewer sound, word, and phrase repetitions than what is seen in the speech disorder of stuttering. Stutterers have frequent and longer prolongations of speech sounds. In normal disfluency, the speaker has infrequent hesitations usually while trying to remember words, and stutterers block between and within word boundaries. As noted above, a block is the momentary cessation of airflow during speech due to one or more constricted speech valves. Struggle and excessive muscular tension is seen in stuttering while in normal disfluency, there are few forced attempts to improve speech fluency. People who stutter, particularly children, frequently insert the "uh" vowel during the moment of stuttering while normally disfluent speakers seldom utter the speech sound while searching for words or while rearranging a thought for expression.

People who clutter are often stereotyped as being scatterbrained and disorganized in their thinking. Table 21.2 delineates stuttering from cluttering. As can be seen from the table, while both stuttering and cluttering are fluency disor-

ders, cluttering also involves disorganized verbal thought processes. Cluttering is a thought-organization communication disorder characterized by a short attention span, excessive rate-of-speech, and omissions and substitutions of speech fragments.

During an interview and interrogation, it is necessary to figure out the typical number and types of disfluencies a suspect displays during nonthreatening discussions. Nonthreatening discussions can include topics related to sports, recreation, and the weather. During this time, the interviewer and interrogator gains an understanding of the speaker's overall fluency levels during emotionally neutral discussions. Basal disfluency determination is necessary for three reasons. First, all speakers have normal disfluencies and there is a high degree of variability from person to person in the number that normally occur during nonthreatening discussions. As a group, males tend to have more disfluencies than females, and young children between the ages of three and seven have the highest number. Additionally, medications and drugs can affect speech fluency as can certain neurological conditions. Second, there is a high degree of speaker fluency variability on a day-to-day basis. Because of such variables as sleep, exercise, caffeine intake, nutrition, and so forth, speakers can significantly vary their fluency from one day to the next. Third, upwards of 5 percent of population may have the fluency communication disorder of stuttering (Bloodstein, 1995). Although several behaviors are involved in stuttering, it primarily consists of more frequent and severe repetitions, prolongations, and blocks.

Table 21.1
Normal Disfluencies and Stuttering

Normal Disfluency	Stuttering
Few sounds, words, and phrase repetitions	Many sounds, words, and phrase repetitions
Infrequent and short prolongations of consonants and vowels	Frequent and longer prolongations of consonants and vowels
Infrequent hesitations usually while trying to remember words	Frequent blocks between and within word boundaries
Lack of awareness and concern about disfluencies. No struggle to produce speech	Awareness and concern about dysfluencies Struggle present to produce speech
Few occurrences of the vowel "uh" during disfluencies	Vowel "uh" often present during dysfluencies
Little muscular tension present during disfluencies	Excessive muscular tension present during dysfluencies

Table 21.2
Stuttering and Cluttering

Stuttering	Cluttering
A fluency disorder	A fluency disorder involving verbal thought-organization
Speaker is aware of the problem	Speaker is unaware of the problem
Usually a slow rate of delivery	Usually a rapid rate of delivery
Dysfluencies related to specific sounds, words, and people, and situations	Dysfluencies not related to specific sounds, words, people, situations
Speaker has normal concentration and attention span	Speaker may have poor concentration and reduced attention span

Factors to consider in determining the basal disfluency level of a suspect include informal assessment of 1) overall fluency levels, 2) suspect's awareness of disfluencies, 3) number and extent of repetitions, 4) number and length of prolongations, 5) number and duration of hesitations, and 6) visible features accompanying disfluencies.

Informal assessment of overall fluency levels can be done by placing the speaker's fluency level on a 1–10 continuum. Disfluent speakers, those with many and severe disfluencies, receive high numbers and those who speak easily and smoothly receive low ratings. The speaker's awareness of his or her disfluencies is important in distinguishing normal disfluencies from stuttering. People producing normal disfluencies are generally unaware of their repetitions, prolongations, and hesitations, and consequently do not struggle to overcome them. People who stutter, on some level, are aware of the speech disorder and usually engage in visible and audible avoidance and escape behaviors to rid themselves of it.

Although it is difficult to provide descriptive data about normal repetitions, prolongations, and hesitations in all speakers, as a rule, fewer than two syllable repetitions per word are within the range of normal especially when airflow is not interrupted and they are done rhythmically. Additionally, people with atypical disfluencies often prolong on the schwa vowel "uh" and when doing so, tend to have a pitch rise toward the end. Hesitations and gaps between words are typical of normal speakers while pauses, gaps, and blocks within word boundaries are atypical. Also, people producing atypical disfluencies may show strain and struggle in their faces during the disfluencies and may be afraid to talk because of them. Signs of speaking strain and frustration should be noted when determining basal speech fluency patterns.

Having determined the typical number and type of disfluencies of the suspect during nonthreatening discussions, the interviewer and interrogator has a sense of the speaker's usual fluency patterns. Significant departures from the speaker's basal fluency patterns tied to his or her statements and answers to questions can provide important forensic information. Speech disfluency during an interview and interrogation is a gauge of the speaker's general anxiety levels, and more importantly, variations of his or her anxiety associated with specific statements and questions.

21.6 Speaker Profiling Conjecture: Disfluencies

The act of speaking fluently is a highly complex neurological and muscular event. Thousands of neurological impulses and more than 100 muscles are involved in producing speech. It is not surprising that anxiety can disrupt the process causing an increase in the number and severity of speech disfluencies. For the purposes of speaker profiling, anxiety is the subjective psychological reaction of worry, angst, fear, and apprehension resulting in decreased feelings of well-being, or in the extreme, a sense of impending doom. Anxiety leads to increased muscular tension which causes an increase in the number and severity of repetitions, prolongations, and hesitations. Therefore, speech disfluencies are a barometer of a speaker's anxiety levels.

That increased speech disfluenices are associated with or caused by conflicts is a well-accepted fact in the literature on stuttering. Sigmund Freud first postulated conflicts to be at the core of stuttering in his early writings about the treatment of a stutterer, Frau Emily. Freud eventually concluded that psychoanalysis was not an appropriate treatment for the communication disorder. During the mid-1900s, some stuttering authorities advanced conflict theories about the core reason speech fluency disintegrates in some persons. The conflict theories ranged from the bizarre to commonsense explanations for stuttering. The most bizarre theories advanced during that time involved psychosexual conflicts and fixations. For example, one theory proposed that stuttering was the result of an oral fixation where the stutterer symbolically nursed an illusionary nipple during the stuttering moment. Perhaps the most bizarre psychosexual conflict and fixation theory ever advanced was the anal projection theory. According to its proponents, the anal sphincter function was displaced orally and the stutterer was symbolically smearing his audience with feces during the moment of stuttering. Today, few authorities in stuttering consider the cause of stuttering to be psychosexual conflicts or that the goal of treatment be a resolution of them. However, most authorities on the nature and treatment of stuttering, either formally or informally, recognize the fact that stutterers are confronted with speaking conflicts. In stuttering, there are the drives to speak and the need to remain silent (Sheehan, 1953). Speaking with significant disfluencies involves a double approach-avoidance conflict from the perspective of the speaker. Although several other factors may be involved in the speaker's disfluent output during an interview and interrogation, he or she may be experiencing a double approach-avoidance conflict. What follows is conjecture regarding significant increases in the basal number and severity of disfluencies during the interview and interrogation.

Conflicts are at the core of indecision and the source of anxiety. They occur when a person is prompted simultaneously to respond to two or more incompatible response alternatives. Obviously, some conflicts are less anxiety-generating than others. However, all conflicts generate anxiety and it is reduced only when the quandary is resolved. The typical conflicts experience by humans are the approach-approach, avoidance-avoidance, simple approach-avoidance, and the double approach-avoidance quandaries.

An approach-approach conflict involves two desirable options, but the decision-maker can only select one. An example of the approach-approach conflict is an informant receiving a cash reward for information about a crime or have a minor offense dismissed. To the informant, both cash and dismissing of the minor offense are equally desirable options; briefly, the informant is placed in an approach-approach conflict. This type of conflict is the least distressing of all conflicts, but it is anxiety generating nonetheless and the anxiety is reduced only when a decision is made. The avoidance-avoidance conflict, on the other hand, involves two equally undesirable decisions. An example of the avoidance-avoidance conflict occurs when a criminal must choose between two methods of execution. Both are undesirable, but the person must decide; he or she is in a trap situation. The simple approach-avoidance conflict involves one goal that has both desirable and undesirable aspects to it. For example, a witness may be motivated to testify against a mobster to get the suspect incarcerated. The undesirable aspect of the decision involves fear of retaliation; the witness may risk harm for testifying. Because human decision-making is usually complex, the double approach-avoidance conflict is the most common type of quandary experienced by a subject during an interview and interrogation. In the double approach-avoidance conflict, the subject is confronted with both approach and avoidance tendencies each with positive and negative aspects to them. These types of conflicts generate anxiety during the interview and interrogation often resulting in increased speech disfluencies. As can be seen in Table 21.3, the subject during an interview and interrogation has the tendency to speak and to remain silent, and each option has both positive and negative components.

In the double approach-avoidance conflict, silence is both approached and avoided. Silence is approached because it is a refuge from danger. As long as the subject remains silent, there is no possibility of making incriminating statements. Silence is also approached to await attorney counsel as per the subject's Miranda rights. Conversely, silence is avoided by the subject because remaining silent when asked direct questions about the crime suggests he or she is concealing something. To add to the concealment perception, the interviewer and interrogator may state that if the subject has nothing to hide, he or she would be more open and provide information about the crime. In summary, for the subject during an interview and interrogation, silence is approached as a refuge from danger and simultaneously avoided so as not to suggest that he or she is hiding something about the crime.

Speech, like silence, is also both approached and avoided in the double approach-avoidance conflict. Speaking is approached because it suggests that the subject is cooperative and willing to participate in the investigation. By speaking during the interview and interrogation, the subject verbally interacts with the investigators providing the essential foundation for building relationships and continuing the investigation. By speaking, the subject projects his or her innocence and desire to cooperate. However, speech is avoided because there is the risk the subject may inadvertently incriminate himself or herself. If the subject is concealing something, during speech, he or she may let incriminating information slip to the investigators. If the subject has nothing to hide, he or she may misspeak, bringing on suspicion and accidently causing him or her to be a suspect or person of interest in the crime. In summary, for the subject in an interview and interrogation, speaking, like silence, is approached to show cooperation while simultaneously avoided as a risk to safety.

Walters (2003), Davis, Connors, and Walters (1999), and others report that deceptive subjects demonstrate more speech disfluencies than truthful ones, and that the presence of disfluencies, when it is not a habitual pattern of speaking, indicates an approximately 90 percent probability of deception. The deception may take the form of omissions of truthful information or misleading statements. In the double approach-avoidance paradigm, increased disfluencies during an interview or interrogation can be a barometer of anxiety associated with the conflict situation and the disfluencies are a manifestation of the magnitude of that anxiety.

21.7 Speaker Profiling Using Rate-of-Speech

Although there are several ways of determining rate-of-speech, the number of words per minute uttered by the speaker is the most convenient. Typically, an average speaker, in a relaxed situation and during a casual conversa-

tion utters about 150 words per minute. All other things being equal, if a speaker is discussing a complex or technical topic, there is a decrease in the number of spoken words per minute. Also, as the complexity of the topic under discussion decreases, there is a subsequent increase in the number of words spoken per minute. Several other factors are involved in the speaker's rate-of-speech including the language spoken, caffeine intake, general alertness, agitation, libido, and perceived tolerance and acceptance of listeners.

Speakers of certain languages and dialects typically convey more information per minute than do others. For example, a Spanish speaker generally speaks faster than do speakers of other languages. Dialectal variances also exist. For example, speakers of the Southern and Western dialects tend to talk slower and more deliberately than do New Englanders. An excessive caffeine intake causes most speakers to talk more rapidly and other stimulants can also cause an increase in the number of spoken word per minute. (See Chapter 20 for a discussion of the effects of stimulants on speech production.) Alert speakers tend to talk faster than those just arising from sleep or resting, and agitation increases the number of words spoken per minute. The rate-of-speech of a speaker is also related to his or her libido.

Libido, as commonly used in the Freudian sense, signifies the reproduction urge and sexual energy. However, Carl

Table 21.3

Speaker Double Approach-Avoidance Conflict During Forensic Interviews and Interrogations

Approach-Avoidance Tendencies	Conflicts	Examples
Silence	Silence (approach) is a refuge from interview and interrogation threats.	By not talking about an alibi, there is no risk of incrimination.
	Silence (avoidance) suggests concealment.	By not verbally providing an alibi, there is a suggestion that none exists.
Speech	Speaking (approach) suggests cooperation.	By verbally providing an alibi, interviewee or suspect shows cooperation.
	Speaking (avoidance) creates risk of incrimination.	By discussing an alibi, there is the risk of misspeaking about a factual alibi or disclosing incriminating information about a false alibi.

Jung broadened the definition to include overall psychic energy. In the broader definition of the libido, a person's psychic energy is reflected in his or her rate-of-speech. An example of a common misunderstanding about stuttering shows the relationship of libido to rate-of-speech. Parents of young children who stutter often comment that their child is speaking too fast and needs to slow his or her rate-of-speech. Speech clinicians are often called upon to provide therapies to slow the rate-of-speech of a young child. Increasing the length of syllables can cause reductions in a person's rate-of-speech, e.g., stretching out each word. Also, increasing the number and duration of pauses during utterances can cause slower speech. In rare instances, this type of therapy is appropriate and successful; however, most of the time, a child's rate-of-speech simply reflects his or her libido. Trying to slow the rate-of-speech of a very active child is counterproductive. The child who rapidly jumps from one topic of conversation to another, is physically active, and enthusiastically exploring his or her environment is simply showing high psychic energy levels. It would be abnormal for such a child to speak very deliberately and with a greatly reduced rate-of-speech. Effecting such a basic change in behavior would be futile because libido and rate-of-speech are usually strongly tied and resistant to modification.

The perceived tolerance and acceptance of listeners plays an important role in a speaker's rate-of-speech. Professors of public speaking frequently note that students in their courses tend to speak very rapidly during the delivery of a speech. The reasons for a more rapid rate-of-speech during public speaking concern the perception of time during stress, and a behavioral phenomenon known as negative reinforcement. Both reasons are applicable to speaker profiling using rate-of-speech during a forensic interview and interrogation.

Several years ago the London Sunday Times surveyed a sample of the United States public about their fears. In the survey, as expected, the respondents placed fear of death, snakes, and separation from loved ones high on the list. Most notably, however, was the number one reported fear: public speaking. Several reasons are given for the universal fear most people have about public speaking including being unprepared, laughter from the audience, making an embarrassing statement, and so forth. However, the underlying reason for fear of public speaking relates to rejection. People know that as the size of the audience increases, there is a greater likelihood of the speaker being rejected. Rejection during public speaking, and during a forensic interview and interrogation is a basic fear because most people strive for tolerance and acceptance about what they are saying and how they say it. Speakers scan their audience for signs of rejection and indications of tolerance and acceptance. If during speaking, the speaker notices signs of rejection from the audience, the perception of the passage of time is greatly reduced. During stressful speaking situations, time seems to pass slower. In addition, speakers often provide fillers such as "You know," "Uh," and other injections of verbiage and speech sounds to reduce the slowed perception of time. Filled pauses in speech appear to pass time more quickly than unfilled pauses during the presentation of information in a stressful situation.

With stressful speech comes the need to escape from the aversive situation. Speakers under stress talk more rapidly to reduce how much time they experience stress. Most people engage in this type of escape behavior, and it can become habitual because of the reinforcement associated with the escape from the stressful situation. By increasing rate-of-speech, the speaker reduces the perception of slowed passage of time, and completes the imparting of information more rapidly, thus more quickly ending the potential for rejection. Further, the speaker is rewarded by the elimination of fear, tension, and anxiety by the feelings of relief when speaking is concluded. This increases the likelihood that this behavior, speaking more rapidly, will recur in the future.

21.8 Speaker Profiling Conjecture: Rate-of-Speech

Rapid rates of speech are associated with happiness and joy, fear, anger, confidence, and indifference (Aronson, 1990; Markel et al., 1973; Scherer, 1973; Costanzo et al., 1969; Huttar, 1968; Davitz, 1964; Eldred and Price, 1958; Fairbanks and Hoaglin, 1941). Slow rates of speech are associated with sadness, grief, contempt, and boredom (Aronson, 1990; Markel et al., 1973; Williams and Stevens, 1969; Huttar, 1968; Davitz, 1964; Eldred and Price, 1958; Fairbanks and Hoaglin, 1941).

If a speaker significantly alters his or her rate-of-speech during the forensic interview and interrogation, there are two forensically relevant underlying reasons. First, the subject could be confidently presenting well-rehearsed statements about a case or related evidentiary information. As noted above, as the complexity of information being presented by a speaker increases, there is a subsequent decrease in the rate-of-speech. When presenting memorized information, particularly if that information is complex, involving dates, times, and locations, and when presented in a stressful situation such as during an interrogation, speakers usually talk more slowly and deliberately. If the interviewer and interrogator ask the same question to the subject at different times and in different ways, the speaker is even more likely to reduce the rate-of-speech to preserve the consistency of his or her story.

The second reason a speaker may significantly alter his or her rate-of-speech during the forensic interview and interrogation relates to perceived threats to safety and associated anxiety and negative emotions. As discussed above, the subject may feel threatened by the interview and interrogation. To reduce the threat, and to minimize the anxiety and associated negative emotions (fear or anger) associated with it, he or she speaks more rapidly. By speaking more rapidly, the subject completes the required presentation of information and responses to questions quickly. At the end of the speaking episode, the speaker feels relief, which is rewarding and increases the likelihood he or she will continue to use rapid rate-of-speech as an escape behavior. Sometimes, the increased rate-of-speech is barely perceptible and at other times, it may be dramatic. An example of increased rate-of-speech during legal anxiety-provoking and threatening situations is witness testimony during a deposition. Sometimes during depositions, attorneys require witnesses to count to ten before beginning to respond to a question, and to slow the rate-of-speech sufficiently so that court reporters can adequately transcribe the information.

Of course, some speakers are aware that during an interview and interrogation they are being observed about their rate of speech delivery, and they consciously slow it. Normal or reduced rate-of-speech may also be part of a subject's attempt to project a calm and relaxed persona, and thus to appear innocent. Aronson (1990, p. 117) observes: "An increased speaking rate prompts testers to increase their ratings of competence. A decreased rate encourages them to evaluate the individual as being less competent, but more benevolent." During a forensic interview and interrogation, a slower rate-of-speech typically projects the innocence of the speaker, while a faster rate-of-speech suggests that the speaker has adequate knowledge of the crime or the events surrounding it. The slower speaker may also be sad or clinically depressed. Newman and Mather (1938) notes that during the manic phase of manic-depression, patients tend to "press speech" and have "vigorous articulation" characterized as "lively." As these patients become less manic, more pauses and hesitations occur thus slowing the overall rate-of-speech.

In medicine, patients usually come to a physician with a "presenting story." These are very well thought-out descriptions of the patient's medical condition uniquely from his or her perspective. Physicians know to let the patient have time for his or her presenting story to get the relevant information from the patient, and to make him or her feel listened to. Forensic interviewers and interrogators should also allow witnesses and suspects the opportunity to present information about the crime or case from their perspectives. The forensic verbal presenting story takes the form of a "statement as to the crime" and accompanies the written statement analysis which may include handwriting analysis. The verbal presenting story about the crime should be taken early in the investigation and without leading the subject. This can be done by simply asking such questions as, "Tell me about the facts about the case as you see them," and "What did you see and hear?" The interviewer and interrogator should also give sufficient time for the subject to present the information about the case or crime without interjection or interruption. According to Brown (2002, p. 214), a crime scene statement is invaluable in solving a crime and being able to prove who did it: "Although the statement may not have the yellow security area ribbon around it to keep others out and prevent contamination, it should be treated and reviewed just as carefully and expertly as any other crime scene. The investigator must understand that the statement can be contaminated just as any other crime scene."

21.9 Speaker Profiling Using the Voice

A speaker's voice, his or her loudness, pitch, quality, and nasality have important value during the forensic interview and interrogation. Dr. Arnold Aronson at the Mayo Medical School, in an exhaustive compilation of research spanning several decades and citing nearly forty studies on the psychology of the voice, notes that the voice may provide clues to the underlying personality in normal persons. "The extrinsic and intrinsic laryngeal muscles are exquisitely sensitive to emotional stress, and their hypercontraction is the common denominator behind the dysphonia and aphonia in virtually all psychogenic voice disorders" (Aronson, 1990, p. 121). Extrinsic laryngeal muscles are those with their origin outside the larynx and intrinsic laryngeal muscles have both their origin and attachment within the larynx. Extrinsic laryngeal muscles, and particularly intrinsic laryngeal muscles, play an important role in a speaker's voice loudness, pitch, quality, and to a lesser extent, nasal resonance.

In Chapter 22, there is a detailed discussion of the fight or flight response and the important role it plays in the human voice. The fight or flight response may be prompted by an external threat such as occurs during a mugging. The flight or fight response may occur because of an internal threat, such as a psychological conflict or a symbolic threat to family, or job. The flight or fight response is an unconscious (subconscious) survival instinct. Both fleeing and fighting involve an increase in musculoskeletal tension as well as several other biological responses. The increased musculoskeletal tension affects the respiratory, laryngeal, and articulatory speech mechanisms potentially causing several voice changes. During a forensic interview and interrogation, the subject is confronted with both external and internal threats. The external threat involves fear of incrimination and possible incarceration for criminal involvement in an offense, lying to investigators, or perjury. The internal threat experienced by non-sociopaths and non-psychopaths concerns conflicts to tell the truth or lie, the human conscience, and the sense of right and wrong. Sociopaths and psychopaths do not have the psychological integrity to be conflicted. Aronson (1990, p. 119) details the fight or fight response with regard to the voice:

Clinical and instrumental studies prove that otherwise normal voice perceptibly and measurably changes under emotional stress. A smooth, well-modulated voice signifies cortical control over the emotionally primitive, phylogenetically older nervous system. During subcortical emotional release, phonatory and respiratory control disintegrates. Massive automatic fight-or-flight reactions prepare the organism for increased physical work—fixing the upper extremities to the thoracic cage for combat, requiring firm adduction of the vocal folds and wide abduction to facilitation an increased volume and flow of oxygen in order to meet the body's increased metabolic demands.

Table 21.4
Voice Parameters, Personality Traits and Discrete Emotions

Voice Parameter	Personality Traits and Discrete Emotions
Breathy voice quality	Neurotic tendencies, anxiety, low dominance, high introversion
Harsh/metallic voice quality	High dominance, emotional instability
Nasal whine	Emotional instability, low dominance
High loudness-low pitch	High dominance
Hoarseness	Reticence, self-consciousness
Decreased variations in fundamental frequency	Decreased ratings of competence/benevolence
High pitch	Happiness, joy, confidence, anger, fear
Low pitch	Indifference, contempt, boredom, grief, sadness
Wide pitch ranges	Anger, fear, contempt
Narrow pitch ranges	Indifference, boredom, grief, sadness
Extensive pitch variability	Happiness, joy, anger, fear
Diminished pitch variability	Indifference, grief, sadness
High loudness levels	Happiness, confidence, anger, contempt, joy
Low loudness levels	Boredom, grief, sadness
Increased mean fundamental frequency	Decreased ratings of competence/benevolence

Such emergency physiologic states are incompatible with fine voice pitch, loudness, and quality control.

Table 21.4 lists several forensically significant indicators of the psychology of the voice. Based on voice parameters, personality traits, and discrete emotions provided by Aronson (1990), a deceptive person may have one or more of the following at any given time during a forensic interview and interrogation: breathy voice quality, nasal whine, hoarseness, higher pitch, variations in fundamental frequency, and extensive overall pitch variability. Each is discussed below and the conclusions that can be drawn from them. The forensic value of these speech patterns is related to their occurrence relative to specific questions and topic changes during the interview and interrogation. Additionally, changes in voice pattern behaviors are reliable for diagnosing deception only if they appear in clusters.

21.10 Speaker Profiling Conjecture: The Voice

A. Loudness

Aronson (1990), Costanzo, et al. (1969), Williams and Stevens (1969), Huttar (1968), and Zuberbier (1957) report that high loudness levels are associated with happiness, joy, contempt, and confidence. When high loudness is associated with low pitch, the speaker is also projecting high levels of dominance (Aronson, 1990; Mallory and Miller, 1958; Moore, 1939).

To effect an increase in loudness, a speaker must generally increase abdominal, thoracic, and laryngeal muscle tension. These changes in musculoskeletal tension occur when a person is threatened from without (external), such as occurs in the presence of a physical threat, and also when the tension is generated from within (internal), such as occurs in a conflict situation. A loud voice accompanied by a low pitch suggests that the speaker is consciously monitoring his or her speech and overriding the natural tendency of the voice to have elevated pitch when there is increased laryngeal musculoskeletal tension. Because anger also generates increased musculoskeletal tension, the loud, low-pitched speaker is likely exercising conscious control over his or her physiological responses. Of course, the high loudness levels and lowered pitch should not be typical and habitual patterns of speech. All other factors being equal in the speech of a subject, a loud speaker may be showing confidence and contempt for the forensic interview and interrogation, and when the loud voice is accompanied by a low pitch, the speaker may be showing dominance over the interviewer and interrogator.

B. High and Low Pitch

Several factors affect the pitch of a subject during the forensic interview and interrogation. When there is an increase in the mass per unit length of the vocal folds, that is, they are thicker, the pitch of the speaker is lower. Conversely, when there is a decrease in the mass per unit length of the vocal folds, that is, they are thinner, the pitch of the speaker is higher. The tension of the vocal cords is also important to pitch; increased vocal cord tension increases pitch while decreased vocal cord tension decreases pitch. Additionally, the speaker's air pressure below the vocal folds affects pitch. Increased respiratory pressure increases pitch while decreased respiratory pressure decreases pitch. Changes in muscular tension is the common denominator in all changes in pitch. Aronson (1990) suggests the term "laryngoresponders" to refer to individuals who react to environmental stress and interpersonal conflict by developing abnormal voices. Rosenman et al. (1964) found voice patterns, among other speech and behavioral reactions, could reliably separate "type A" from "type B" personality types. The "type A" personality displayed an "aggressive" voice quality while the "type B" personality typically produced a voice quality suggestive of "calmness."

High pitch is associated with happiness, joy, confidence, anger, and fear (Aronson, 1990; Levin and Lord, 1975; Scherer et al., 1973; Sedlácek and Sychra, 1973; Williams and Stevens, 1969; Huttar, 1968; Davitz, 1964; Eldred and Price, 1958; Fairbanks and Pronovost, 1939; Skinner, 1935). Low pitch is associated with indifference, contempt, boredom, grief, and sadness (Aronson, 1990; Sedlácek and Sychra, 1973; Williams and Stevens, 1969; Huttar, 1968; Davitz, 1964; Eldred and Price, 1958; Fairbanks and Pronovost, 1939). In addition, low pitch in males has been traced to ancestral male intrasexual competition. Puts, Gaulin, and Verdolini (2006) found that a masculine, low-pitch voice increases ratings of men's physical and social dominance and men who believe they are physically dominant to their competitor lower their voice pitch when addressing him, whereas men who believe they are less dominant raise it.

All other factors being equal in the speech of a subject, a speaker with high pitch is likely to be confident, angry, or fearful. When the pitch change occurs during a specific topic, it may be symptomatic of underlying confidence, anger, or fear associated with it. A speaker with low pitch may be indifferent, contemptuous, bored, or sad. He or she may be indifferent about a particular topic during the forensic interview and interrogation, feeling contempt for the interviewer, interrogator, or situation in general, or simply bored or sad. Moses (1954) found monotonous voice patterns in depressed patients.

C. Pitch Range and Variability

Wide pitch ranges are found during contempt, anger, and fear (Aronson, 1990; Williams and Stevens, 1969; Fairbanks and Pronovost, 1939). Narrow pitch ranges are associated with sadness, grief, boredom, and indifference (Aronson, 1990; Williams and Stevens, 1969; Huttar, 1968; Fairbanks and Pronovost, 1939). There is some evidence that people with wide pitch ranges experience wider ranges of emotional responses than do people with monopitch. Newman and Mather (1938) note that in a group of forty manic-depressive patients, those in the manic stage tend to have wide pitch ranges and frequent gliding pitch changes. As the manic stage subsides, their pitch range narrows. In depressed patients, Newman and Mather (1938) characterize their voice as "dead or listless." Excessive pitch variability is associated with fear, anger, joy, and happiness (Aronson, 1990; Sedlácek and Sychra, 1973; Fairbanks and Pronovost, 1939). Diminished pitch variability is associated with sadness, indifference, and grief (Aronson, 1990; Fairbanks and Pronovost, 1939).

During a forensic interview and interrogation, the subject's pitch range and variability can provide cues about his or her overall affect and the presence of affective disorders. Affect is the subjective aspect of emotions that are observable; the detectable emotions tied to speech. The human voice reflects the subject's overall emotions associated with the interview and interrogation, and can be an accurate gauge of the shear amount of emotional engagement. Subjects with wide pitch ranges may be contemptous, angry, and fearful toward the interview and interrogation, or in the extreme, manic due to mental illness or drug abuse (see Chapter 20 for a review of the effects of drugs on speech patterns). Subjects with wide pitch ranges may also provide more information than those with monopitch. This is because a wide pitch range suggests more openness and willingness to cooperate, and the fact that more information is presented because of overall increased rate-of-speech. Subjects with narrow pitch ranges may be generally more uncooperative because of depression or sadness, and flat affect. As a rule, subjects with narrow pitch ranges provide less information during the forensic interview and interrogation. Subjects with excessive pitch changes may be showing their fear and anger at the forensic interview and interrogation. Those with decreased pitch variability may be projecting unhappiness or nonchalance at the forensic interview and interrogation.

D. Voice Quality and Nasality

The general public uses many adjectives to describe voice quality: masculine, feminine, strong, weak, powerful, tinny, whiny, raspy, breathy, harsh, metallic, throaty, and sexy, to name a few. Most of these adjectives are nondescript and ill-defined. Regardless of the adjectives used to describe voice quality, there are several studies of voice quality applicable to the forensic interview and interrogation. For example, speakers with harsh and metallic voices may be projecting high dominance where as those with breathy voice qualities may be expressing low dominance (Aronson, 1990; Mallory and Miller, 1958; Moore, 1939). Additionally, breathy voice quality has been associated with high introversion, anxiety, and neurosis. A person with a hoarse voice may be reticent and self-conscious (Aronson, 1990).

A speaker's voice quality is a relationship between the function of the larynx and his or her head and neck resonators. As discussed previously, the human voice is analogous to a brass musical instrument. In a brass instrument, the musician produces a buzzing sound in the mouthpiece with the lips. Energy of this sound source is then amplified or damped by the resonating chambers of the brass instrument. The musicial quality of the output is a relationship between the sound-source and the resonance potentials of the instrument. In the human voice, the sound-source is the buzzing created by the larynx and the energy is amplified or damped by the head and neck resonating chambers. Just as a brass instrument's musical quality is dependent on the sound-source and the shape and texture of the resonating system, a person's voice quality varies with the vibration of the vocal folds and the neck and head resonating system's shape and texture. The reasons speakers have unique voices are related to the fact that all speech is learned, and that the shape and texture of people's head and neck resonators differ. The primary sound source for the speech resonating system is the larynx, the buzzing sound produced by the vibrating vocal folds. "Acoustically, this sound is the glottal source for speech resonance before it reaches the resonating chambers of the speech tract. It is from this sound source that certain frequencies within it are amplified and damped by the person's neck and head resonating chambers" (Tanner, 2006, p. 167). The sound source from the larynx can be described on a breathy-to-harsh continuum.

The breathy voice quality occurs when the period of vocal fold closure is shorter compared with the open period. This allows for more air to escape during vibration giving the voice its breathy characteristics. The breathy voice quality is also a result of the force of vocal fold vibration; in breathiness, the force of glottal closure is less than what occurs in harshness. In harsh voice quality, the period of vocal fold closure is longer and more forceful than what occurs in breathiness. Harsh voice quality is also referred to as strident. All voice quality can be placed on a continuum ranging from breathiness to harshness. The degree of nasality superimposes an additional distinct characteristic to a speaker's voice quality.

The typical nasality of a speaker consists of nasal resonance and air movement through the nose because of nasal and oral cavity coupling by the lowering of the soft palate (velum). Three speech sounds in English are produced with the soft palate lowered: /m/, /n/, and "ng." (See Chapter 15 for a review of phonetics.) Hypernasality is too much nasality on non-nasal speech sounds, and hyponasality is too little nasality on nasal phonemes. Some speakers have a distinctly nasal tone or "twang" to their voices due to the natural structure and function of their speech resonating systems. Persons with unrepaired cleft palates also have hypernasality and increased nasal emission due to this cranio-facial birth defect.

Hypernasality has been linked to childhood and adolescent schizophrenia (Aronson, 1990; Ostwald and Skolnikoff, 1966; Goldfarb et al., 1956). When a speaker loses motor speech control during the forensic interview and interrogation to the extent that hypernasality occurs, it suggests a major psychological upheaval. Coupling of the oral and nasal cavities, when compared with other motor speech production actions, is a relatively simple neuromuscular event. Velopharyngeal closure, the elevation and posterior (toward the back of the throat) movement of the soft palate to close the nasal port, operates on a binary function, i.e., off-on. These neuromuscular actions simply open or close the nasal valve during speech. While there are discrete, precise, and minute movements associated with other aspects of motor speech production, the velopharyngeal movements simply open or close the nasal port during nasal valving. During a forensic interview and interrogation, when a speaker has motor speech disruptions so severe as to create unnatural and atypical nasality, he or she is likely experiencing a major psychological stress reaction and conceivably of the magnitude that it affects the perception of reality.

21.11 Speaker Profiling: Word Choice and Grammatical Construction

When analyzed correctly and interpreted properly, the language used by a subject during an interview and interrogation can provide a wealth of forensic information about his or her mind set. The noted author William Gibson observed: "Language is to the mind more than light is to the eye." Language is the "Multimodaly ability to encode, decode,

and manipulate symbols for the purposes of verbal thought and/or communication." The modalities or avenues of language include speech (expressive), auditory comprehension (receptive), writing (expressive), reading (receptive), and gestures (expressive and receptive). Mathematics (expressive and receptive) is considered the universal language. When a subject is speaking during the forensic interview and interrogation, he or she is engaged in expressive language construction and the avenue of expression is speech. The words chosen and the grammatical construction of sentences can reveal the subject's knowledge of a crime, and what is most important, his or her unique interpretation of the events associated with it. As Ben Johnson observed: "Language most shows a man; speak, that I may see thee."

The subject's use of language in the forensic interview and interrogation provides a window into how he or she symbolizes the crime. Language is symbolic; the words used during speech communication are selected by the subject to represent his or her unique perceptions of the crime and the events surrounding it. The subjective truth about a subject's knowledge of a crime lies between the words he or she uses and the actual events that occurred. Words are arbitrary representations of reality, verbal symbols, and that to which they refer are referents, and in the context of the forensic interview and interrogation, the crime. Parts of speech and the language constructs used by a speaker can reveal his or her participation or knowledge of the crime under investigation. From the use of plurals, showing more than one suspect was involved, to past tense sentence structures, suggesting knowledge of the final outcome of the crime, the language used by a subject to express himself or herself can be very revealing.

Gender differences in language acquisition show up early during the developmental period. Decades of research show that girls develop faster and more comprehensively in language than do boys. Women maintain this advantage throughout their lives; they tend to have a greater mastery of language and are more successful communicators. "Females learn to speak earlier, are less likely to have disorders of spoken language, have better chance of recovery from at least some speech disorders, and maintain their linguistic competence more effectively into old age" (Kent, 1997, p. 11). Certainly, there are exceptions to this rule, but during a forensic interview and interrogation, females are likely to be more proficient in expressing themselves than their male counterparts. However, in a study of incarcerated female juvenile delinquents, more than 19 percent had language disorders (Sanger, Moore-Brown, Magnuson, and Svoboda, 2001).

21.12 Speaker Profiling Conjecture: Word Choice and Grammatical Construction

Several aspects of content analysis used in examining the handwriting of subjects also can be powerful tools in speaker profiling. Brown (2002) notes that handwriting mistakes, crossing out and insertions, often provide information about the level of a subject's stress. Analogous behavior in speaker profiling is addressed above in the sections on cluttering and disfluencies. Brown (2002) notes that nouns, pronouns, and verbs are important aspects to handwriting content analysis. They also have application to speaker profiling.

Lack of consistent usage of nouns and pronouns, and using words to obscure the facts, can reveal guilt and motive. For example, in response to the question, "Give us some reasons as to how this could have happened" during the investigation of a check cashing fraud case, a subject answered "He couldn't be trusted" and "They were in dire need of ready money." According to Brown (2002, p. 232):

Every reader should have noted the change in pronouns from 'He' to "They" which raises red flags for sure. But what else is wrong with the second answer? Had the writer said "They needed the money" or something similar, that would have been "normal" response by most honest people. But this person added the terms "dire" need and "ready" money. In those two sentences we have most of the story. "He" was his feeling about himself. "They" referred to the fact that he and his best friend cashed the checks, and the "dire need of ready money" tells us motive."

Brown (2002, p. 231) suggests particular attention be given to the suspect's narration: "… especially how it is divided between minor or insignificant events and the main event, avoidance or concealment of the main event and items that are chronologically out of order."

Walters (2003, p. 44) also notes that repetitive narratives may suggest a need to control speech and to be reassured: "The subject begins to make a comment or express an idea, then repeats the same phrases or words within the same sentence. It is as if the speaker needs to orally reassure himself, as well as the listener, that the correct phrase or word has been chosen to express a particular idea." Yeschke (1993) identifies the "scatterbrain" as a specific interviewee type. These disorganized interviewees, because of their mental and emotional makeup, appear incapable of rationally connected thoughts. These types of interviewees engage in cluttering which is discussed above and in Chapter

12. The scatterbrained interviewee is tense and anxious. Studies of brain-injured patients with language disorders have found that ease of word recall is facilitated by relaxation. Scatterbrained interviewees lack relaxation, concentration, and confidence, and think in uncomplicated terms thus making them less likely to conjure up elaborate lies. Brown (2002) observes that very few subjects will overtly lie; they will avoid and obscure the issue. Both innocent and guilty subjects will deny responsibility or involvement with a crime by answering "No" to direct questions; however, a guilty person will often ask a question in response to the investigator's question. Of course, compulsive liars are exceptions to this rule.

In addition to analyzing nouns and pronouns, Walters (2003) suggests that the subject's use of modifiers can be used to change his or her position on an issue. Words like "ordinarily," "almost," "most of the time," "usually," and "hardly ever" are used by subjects to leave the interviewer and interrogator with a degree of uncertainty, and to give the subject an opening for modification of his or her characterization of the facts. "But" and "however" are the two most common modifiers used during the forensic interview and interrogation.

During the forensic interview and interrogation, Walters (2003) observes that deceptive subjects experience more frequent occurrences of memory lapses than do truthful ones. He identifies three types of memory loss in the forensic interview and interrogation: procedural, episodic, and semantic. Procedural memory primarily involves motor acts, including writing, and recall is done with little or no forethought. Episodic memory involves facts related to the crime: "An interview with a victim, witness, or suspect requires the specific application of episodic recall function" (Walters, 2003, p. 55). Semantic memory involves symbolism and the assigning of words to represent ideas and mental images. The subject's assignment of meaning, word choice, and grammatical construction relates to "vocabulary shifting," and "substitute words," and can provide important information about disengagement from the crime or event .

Vocabulary shifting occurs when the subject changes his or her expressive vocabulary, particularly during stressful aspects of the forensic interview and interrogation and to separate himself or herself from the critical situation mentally or intellectually (Walters, 2003). The most common vocabulary shift is from singular to plural pronouns, suggesting that more than one person was involved in the crime. Verb shift and change of tense can show a subject's knowledge of when a crime occurred: "If an individual is describing what happened in a historical sense, the verb usage should be past tense. Should the subject, however, make a comment about past behavior or conditions, and use a present-tense verb, the implication is that the individual is making up the information as he or she goes along and thus is most likely being deceptive" (Walters, 2003, p. 64). Substitute words involves the subject using "soft" words to give his or her actions a more palatable impression and to minimize them. Examples of using substitute words include a subject attributing lying to "misspeaking" and sexual contact as a "relationship" or "involvement" with another person. Other examples of using soft words include calling embezzlement "borrowing," rape as "hurting" a person, and arrests as "contact with the law."

21.13 Speaker Profiling Using Nonverbal Communication Cues

It has been said that "We cannot not communicate." Nonverbal communication is used and understood by all people all of the time; even silence communicates volumes in certain situations. What is most important, nonverbal communication can negate and contradict the intended meaning of verbal communication. Nonverbal communication accompanies verbal communication and is integral to the meaning exchanged between speaker and listener. Ruthrof (2000, p. vii) observes: "For language to be meaningful, members of a speech community must be able to share, to a high degree, the way in which language and nonverbal readings are to be associated with one another."

There is a high degree of cultural variability in the use and understanding of nonverbal communication. For example, in some gang cultures, members avoid staring people straight in the eyes. Direct eye contact can be considered a threat. "Lack of eye contact may be a telling sign of a language disorder, but it is also one of the key communicative devices in gang culture" (Mosheim, 2005, p. 7). Essential nonverbal communication cues addressed in the forensic interview and interrogation include facial expressions, gestures, proxemics, and clothing, touch, and smell.

Facial expressions, particularly the eyes and lips, are powerful in expressing human emotion. According to Adler and Towne (1978), there are at least eight distinguishable positions of the eyebrows and forehead, ten for the lower face, and eight for the eyes and lids. While bodily gestures can reveal the intensity of emotional reactions experienced by a subject during the forensic interview and interrogation, facial expressions impart information about how he or she feels about the statements. The subject's eyes communicate acceptance and interest, and dilation of the pupils has been linked to deception. Studies of the general American population have shown that persons make less eye contact with

people they feel have more authority, disabled individuals, and strangers. Although it is often assumed that lack of eye contact suggests that a child is lying, only anecdotal evidences exists for this observation. There is a wide degree of cultural variation; some cultures, such as the traditional Navajo, consider it rude to make eye contact, while others consider lack of eye contact suggestive of insincerity.

Women tend to read gestures better than men and some cultures are more demonstrative than others. In addition, a gesture in one culture may have no meaning or an entirely different meaning in another. For example, some traditional Navajo speakers will gesture with their lips and chin to the general direction of the object or person rather than using their fingers to point. Kinetics is the study of body movements during communication and includes the analysis of expressive and receptive gestures. There are two general types of gestures: descriptive and reinforcing.

Descriptive gestures describe an action or an event, and are used when giving directions. Using the fingers, hands, arms, face, and head, the speaker physically describes what he or she is saying. A subject may show a sequence of events, spatial positions, and time relationships using his or her body to help explain details surrounding a crime. When a speaker uses descriptive gestures when giving directions, the listener may also perform similar gestures to clarify what has been said, and to show an understanding of the information.

Reinforcing gestures accentuate and emphasize verbal statements. They can be subtle or conspicuous. A fidgety subject may show indifference by restlessness, and an involved interviewee may hit a table with his or her fist expressing extreme emotional involvement with what is being discussed. A subject with his or her arms crossed may be expressing general disapproval, while one with an expansive posture may show openness with the content of the discussion. Reinforcing gestures include crossed legs, drumming fingers, leaning in or out, touch, pointing, and general body position changes during speech communication.

Proxemics is the speaker and listener's physical relationships to each other in space and time, and can profoundly affect the quality and quantity of information exchange during the forensic interview and interrogation. Consciously or subconsciously, proxemics influences all parties during communication. Proxemics involves both territory and personal space.

Territory is a physical zone a person stakes out as his or her own. During a forensic interview and interrogation, a subject may stake out a particular chair or position at an interview table as his or her own symbolic territory. He or she will likely be threatened and uncomfortable when deprived of his or her territory, symbolic and temporary though it may be. Whereas territory involves a fixed physical zone, personal space is moveable and surrounds a person wherever he or she goes. Authorities on nonverbal communication recognize four personal space zones of communication: public, social, personal, and intimate.

The farthest distance between speaker and listener is the public zone. It extends beyond 12 feet and is the distance for public lectures such as occurs in college classrooms, and police officers hailing suspects. Social distance extends from about 4 to 12 feet and is reserved for formal types of small group and two-person communication. Personal and intimate zones of communication have special relevance to the forensic interview and interrogation.

The personal zone of communication is reserved for casual conversations and discussion of topics where the discourse can be overheard. This distance extends to about 4 feet. With regard to personal zones, people stand closer to friends than enemies, farther away from strangers, authority figures, people from higher status, and individuals from different racial groups (Adler and Towne, 1978). Larger people demand and get greater amounts of personal space, and women show the least discomfort when the space around them is small. In this personal zone of communication, the subject is likely to feel comfortable discussing general information that is common knowledge. The intimate space of communication, which extends from the body to about 18 inches, is reserved for private, confidential types of information exchange.

When the subject and interviewer or interrogator voluntarily communicate in the intimate zone of personal space, they do not feel discomfort and there is a sense of trust. Freely talking in the intimate zone of personal space allows both parties to impart and receive information in a nonthreatening environment. If the interviewer or interrogator enters the subject's intimate zone of communication without some kind of consent, both parties are likely to feel discomfort and to be guarded. An example of this type of discomfort occurs when intimate space is violated in crowded elevators. Most people get quiet and simply watch the numbers change as the elevator descends or ascends. Interestingly, when a person tries to make small talk during such violations of intimate space, it only increases the discomfort of the elevator riders.

Unwanted violations of the subject's intimate zone of personal communication, "getting into his or her face," can be a productive method of extorting information, but is not conducive to obtaining information voluntarily. It is likely that information received during voluntary communication is more truthful than that received during forced violation of the subject's intimate communication zone.

21.14 Other Nonverbal Communication Cues

Ruthrof (2000) reports that mental images (icons) are essential to meaningful communication. Clothing and other accessories provide credible icons about the speaker during the act of communication. The mental images people project include clothing and accessories such as hair color, jewelry, cosmetics, ties, tattoos, piercings, religious symbols, and other adornments. They are used to express a variety of personal, political, religious, and social statements. Besides poor eye contact discussed above, gang members may show their affiliation using graffiti, certain colors and styles of clothing, quiet action, being secretive, and gesturing (Mosheim, 2005). The clothing people wear also project information about profession or occupation, income, and socioeconomic status. They also give information about the speaker's credibility. Verbal messages from speakers wearing medical white coats, power ties, police uniforms, military decorations, or baggy, low-hung pants, and other adornments give or take away from their credibility.

The senses of touch and smell also influence verbal communication. A hand-push or pat on the back can show the interviewer or interrogator's approval, affection, or repugnance about what the speaker is saying. A firm handshake can show strength and determination, whereas a lax one can suggest timidity and weakness. Lack of physical contact during communication can show disinterest and emotional detachment from what is being said. Offensive odors in an interview and interrogation room can decrease communication while pleasing smells and fragrances can have the opposite effect. Odors and other smells can also prompt recall of memories, much like hearing a song or tune can prompt memories of days-gone-by. Table 21.5 shows nonverbal cues and their effects during the forensic interview and interrogation.

Table 21.5
Speaker Profiling Nonverbal Cues

Profiling Nonverbal Cues	Nonverbal Effect
Facial expression	Attention and receptiveness to communicative act
Gestures	Accentuate verbal statements Describe actions and events
Proxemics	Physical comfort zone Movable bubble of space for appropriate communication
Clothing and accessories Touch, and smell	Socioeconomic status Credibility, communication ambience

21.15 Speaker Profiling Conjecture: Nonverbal Communication Cues

When there is a conflict between the words spoken by a subject during a forensic interview and interrogation, and his or her nonverbal communication, the latter is more revealing and likely more factual and truthful. Nonverbal cues, i.e., facial expressions, gestures, proxemics, and clothing, touch, and smell, can suggest not only how the speaker feels about what is spoken, but also give insight into his or her underlying agenda concerning the investigation. While there are cultural and gender variations in the use and reading of nonverbal communication, these cues can be invaluable sources of conjecture about subjects' attitudes, emotions, and behaviors during the forensic interview and interrogation.

The subject's eyes and lips are most revealing about the emotional involvement with the forensic interview and interrogation. Lack of eye contact shows that the subject is or wants to be disengaged from the interview and, with the exception of some gang members, recognizes the authority of the interviewer or interrogator. Although it is assumed that the subject cannot look the interviewer or interrogator directly in the eyes and lie, there is little scientific evidence for this observation. However, pupil dilation has been linked to making deceptive statements. A slight smile or frown can show the subject's true emotion linked to a statement even when the verbal and nonverbal communication is contradictory. For example, if a subject states: "I am unhappy at his death," the words suggest sadness, but when a slight smile accompanies the statement, it is likely that the subject's emotions are far from sad about his demise.

The gestures used by the subject, particularly reinforcing ones, can provide additional information about general emotional involvement and also the affect (emotional involvement) associated with a particular question or statement. A fidgety subject may be disengaged from the inter-

view and interrogation process or looking to escape the threatening situation. A subject with crossed arms and legs is likely less open and truthful than one sitting at the table with an open and expansive body posture.

The subject's and interviewer or interrogator's physical proximity can facilitate or obstruct truthful and factual information exchange. When the interviewer or interrogator is in the personal space of the subject, the quality and quantity of information obtained from him or her will be affected. If the subject willingly allows the interviewer or interrogator into this intimate zone of communication, he or she likely has a trusting relationship and will provide truthful and factual information. When this zone of communication is unwillingly entered, the subject feels threatened and violated, and will be less likely to be open and honest. However, some subjects may be threatened and provide information more readily when the interviewer or interrogator is aggressively violating his or her intimate zone of communication.

The subject's clothing and other adornments can express volumes about his or her underlying political, religious, social, and philosophical perspectives. The subject's hair color, jewelry, cosmetics, ties, tattoos, piercings, religious symbols, and so forth, should be looked upon as iconic representations reflecting his or her core beliefs, affiliations, and life perspectives. Physical contact between subject and the interviewer or interrogator can enhance communication or can hinder it. Odors, fragrances, and smells detract or contribute to the communication ambience.

21.16 Chapter Summary

General principles of profiling can be applied to the speaker's rate-of-speech, loudness, pitch, voice quality, and nasality, word choice and grammatical construction, and several nonverbal cues to get to the overall openness, truthfulness, and accuracy of statements during the forensic interview and interrogation. The forensic interviewer and interrogator can reach several conclusions and opinions based on speaker profiling information. Although speaker profiling conjecture is based on incomplete information, it provides the interviewer and interrogator with valuable additional information about the subject's veracity. Speaker profiling during the forensic interview and interrogation is a worthwhile skill to be learned and practiced by novice and experienced interviewers and interrogators alike.

Suggested Readings and Resources

Aronson, A. (1990). *Clinical Voice Disorders: An Interdisciplinary Approach*. New York: Thieme. This classic textbook address the psychology of the voice including psychogenic voice disorders.

Majeski, W. J. (2002). The art and sciences of communication during an investigation. In R. Montgomery and W. Majeski (Eds), *Corporate Investigations*. Tucson: Lawyers and Judges Publishing Company. This chapter, in an edited book, focuses on the important aspects of verbal and nonverbal communication in corporate investigations.

Tanner, D. (2006). *An Advanced Course in Communication Sciences and Disorders*. San Diego: Plural Publishing. This book provides an overview of the process of communication and Chapter 9 addresses accompanying nonverbal communication.

Walters, S. (2003). *Principles of Kinesic Interview and Interrogation* (2nd ed.). Boca Raton: CRC Press. This textbook provides a basic foundation to the forensic interview and interrogation.

References

Adler R. and Towne, N. (1978). *Looking out/Looking in: Interpersonal communication* (2nd ed.). New York: Holt, Rinehart and Winston.

Aronson, A. (1990). *Clinical voice disorders: An interdisciplinary approach*. New York: Thieme.

Boodstein, O. (1995). *A handbook on stuttering* (5th ed.). San Diego: Singular.

Brown, G. R. (2002). The statement as a crime scene: Low-tech tools for corporate investigations. In R. Montgomery and W. Majeski (Eds) *Corporate investigations*. Tucson: Lawyers and Judges Publishing Company.

Costanzo, F.S., Markel, N.N., and Costanzo, P.R. (1969). Voice quality profile and perceived emotions. *J. Counsel Psychol.*, 16:267-270.

Davidz. J.R. (1964). *The communication of emotional meaning*. New York: McGraw-Hill.

Davis, M., Connors, B., and Walters, S. (1999). Credibility analysis validity study: Nonverbal communication project final report. John Jay College of Criminal Justice.

Eldred, S.H. and Price, D.B. (1958). The linguistic evaluation of feeling states in psychotherapy. Psychiatry, 21:115-121.

Fairbanks, G. and Hoaglin, L.W. (1941). An experimental study of the durational characteristics of the voice during the expression of emotion. *Speech Monographs*, 8:85-90.

Fairbanks, G. And Pronovost, W. (1939). An experimental study of the pitch characteristics of the voice during the expression of emotion. *Speech Monographs*, 6:87-104.

Goldfarb, W., Brownstein, P., and Lorge, I. (1956). A study of speech patterns in a group of schizophrenic children. *American Journal of Orthopsychiatry*, 26: 544-555.

Huttar, G. L. (1968). Relations between prosodic variables and emotions in normal American English utterances. *Journal of Speech and hearing Research*, 11:481-487.

Kent, R. (1997). *Speech sciences*. San Diego: Singular Publishing Group.

Levin, H. and Lord, W. (1975). Speech pitch frequency as an emotional state indicator. *IEEE Trans. Sys. Man Cybernet.*, 2:259-272.

Majeski, W. J. (2002). The art and sciences of communication during an investigation. In R. Montgomery and W. Majeski (Eds) *Corporate investigations*. Tucson: Lawyers and Judges Publishing Company.

Mallory, E. And Miller, V. (1958). A possible basis for the association of voice characteristics and personality traits. *Speech Monographs,* 25:255-260.

Markel, N.N, Bern, M.F., and Phillis, J.A. (1973). The relationship between words and tone-of-voice. *Lang. Speech,* 16:15-21.

Moore, W.E. (1939). Personality traits and voice quality deficiencies. *Journal of Speech and Hearing Disorders,* 4:33-36.

Moses, P.J. (1954). *The voice of neurosis.* New York: Grune & Stratton.

Mosheim, J. (2005, December). Gang culture: Awareness of communicative characteristics key to evaluating, treating youth. *Advance*: Vol 15, No. 49, pp. 6-9.

Newman, S.S. and Mather, V.G. (1938). Analysis of spoken language of patients with affective disorders. *American Journal of Psychiatry,* 94:912-942.

Ostwald, P.F. and Skolnikoff, A. (1966, July). Speech disturbances in a schizophrenic adolescent. *Postgrad. Med.,* 40-49.

Puts, D.A., Gaulin, S., and Verdolini, K. (2006). Dominance and the evolution of sexual dimorphism in human voice pitch. *Journal of Evolution and Human Behavior,* Volume 27, Issue 4, pp.283-296.

Rosenman, R.H., Friedman, M., Straus, R., Wurm, M., Kositchek, R., Hahn, W., and Werthessen, N.J., (1964). A predictive study of coronary heart disease: The Western Collaborative Group Study. *JAMA,* 189: 15-22.

Ruthrof, H. (2000). *The body in language.* London and New York: Cassell.

Sanger, D., Moore-Brown, B., Magnuson, G. and Svoboda, N. (2001). Prevalence of language problems among adolescent delinquents: A closer look. *Communication Disorders Quarterly,* 23(1), 17-25.

Scherer, K.R., London, H., and Wolf, J. (1973). The voice of confidence: Paralinguistic cues and audience evaluation. *J. Res. Personal.,* 7:31-44.

Sedlácek, K. and Sychra, A. (1973). Die melodie als faktor des emotionellen ausdruchs. *Folia Phoniatria,* 15:89-98.

Sheehan J.G. (1953). Theory and treatment of stuttering as an approach avoidance conflict. *Journal of Psychology* 56: 27-49.

Skinner, E.R. (1935). A calibrated recording and analysis of the pitch, force and quality of vocal tones expressing happiness and sadness, and a determination of the pitch and force of the subjective concepts of ordinary, soft, and loud tones. *Speech Monographs,* 2:81-137.

Tanner, D. (2006). *An advanced course in communication sciences and disorders.* San Diego: Plural Publishing.

Tanner, D., Culbertson, B, and Secord, W. (2001). Cheers and jeers: Hollywood and the motion picture industry. An extended seminar presented to the annual convention of the American Speech-Language-Hearing Association, New Orleans.

Tanner, D. (2001, April 3). Hooray for Hollywood: Communication disorders and the motion picture industry. *ASHA Leader,* 6(6).

Walters, S. (2003). *Principles of kinesic interview and interrogation* (2nd ed.). Boca Raton: CRC Press.

Williams, C.E. and Stevens, K.N. (1969). Emotions and speech: Some acoustical correlates. *Journal of the Acoustical Society of America,* 52:1238-1250.

Yeschke, C. (1993). *Interviewing: A forensic guide to interrogation* (2nd ed.). Springfield, Ill.: Charles C. Thomas.

Zuberbier, E. (1957). Zur schreib-und sprechmotorik der depression. *Psychother, Med. Psychol,* 7:239-249.

Chapter 22

Speaker Profiling, Instrumental Voice Stress Analysis and Lie Detection

22.1 Chapter Preview

This chapter explores the use of speech patterns, particularly fluctuations of voice fundamental frequency, to detect speaker stress as a method of lie detection. There is a review of the history of lie detection instrumentation with a focus on polygraph and voice stress analysis technology and procedures. Types of voice stress instrumentation are reviewed for their validity and reliability in detecting speaker fear and anxiety, and for their use for lie detection. Instrumental voice stress analysis, while lacking the validity and reliability of the polygraph, can be used by law enforcement personnel to prompt confessions and as a forensic interview and interrogation tool.

22.2 History of the Polygraph and Voice Stress Analysis

There is no shortage of forensic applications for using the voice to detect stress and deception. Instrumental speaker profiling using voice stress levels can provide information about a person's intent to engage in a criminal act. For example, some airports are using voice evaluators for detecting air passenger stress levels. A provision in a federal aviation law enacted after September 11, 2001 allows for "voice stress analysis" as one of many technologies to prevent terrorists from boarding airplanes (Rubinkam, 2003). The goal

is to screen passengers at ticket counters and security checkpoints for abnormal anxiety and tension as measured by the voice. Voice stress analysis is used by federal and state law enforcement personnel to investigate a variety of criminal acts including corporate crimes (Palmatier, 2002). Local police agencies also use the voice for investigative purposes. For example, Upper Merion Township Police Department in suburban Philadelphia report they have successfully used voice stress analysis for crimes involving child abuse, employee theft, stolen credit cards, and other crimes (Rubinkam, 2003). Large corporate employers have used voice stress analysis for pre-hiring screening. There is strong appeal to surreptitiously use an instrument to analyze a person's voice for stress and deception. Unlike the polygraph, voice stress analysis can be used without a person's permission, without him or her being physically present, and the samples can be taken from commercial television, radio, websites, emails, and other audio broadcasts.

Instrumental assessment of a person's physiological responses for lie detection was first experimented with in 1895 when blood pressure changes and pulse rate were monitored (Majeski, 2002). The "Ink Polygraph" was invented by Dr. James MacKensie (Clede, 1998). According to Clede (1998), the original "lie detector" was the Larson Polygraph built in 1921 and took a half-hour to set up. Since the development of the polygraph, millions of tests have been conducted, and it is generally accepted that the polygraph is a valid and reliable method of determining deception. Most authorities conclude that when the polygraph examination is conducted properly, it is at least 95 percent accurate in lie detection. "Over the last ten years or so, the amount of polygraph examinations conducted has grown dramatically. Does the polygraph work? As an investigative tool, absolutely. Should it be used by corporations? Absolutely, given the proper circumstances and conditions" (Majeski, 2002, p. 275).

The psychological stress evaluator was invented in the 1970s by Army intelligence officers Allan D. Bell Jr. and Charles R. McQuiston (Clede, 1998). As will be discussed in detail below, the psychological stress evaluator (PSE) measures changes in laryngeal microtremors in response to emotional stress. These changes in the voice are largely imperceptible to the human ear and the device was marketed as a lie detector. The PSE-2000 is the third generation design of the instrument and patents have been issued in the United States, Canada, Great Britain, and Japan (Clede, 1998). Federal research into voice stress analysis is currently primarily the responsibility of the United States Department of Defense Polygraph Institute (DoDPI) (Krapohl, Ryan, and Schull, 2002). "Voice stress is currently one of the hot topics, and DoDPI has conducted or collaborated in several studies on voice stress devices that can provide answers to agencies and departments weighing the potential costs and benefits of fielding them" (Krapohl, Ryan, and Schull, 2002, p. 2).

22.3 Polygraph Procedures

Research on the accuracy of the voice to detect deception often compares voice stress devices with the polygraph. Whereas polygraph tests are highly controlled and the test procedures standardized, voice stress analysis typically lacks these controls, proving to be a forensic blessing and curse. The blessing is that voice stress analysis is more cost efficient, less time-consuming and has more utility. The curse is that accuracy of the procedure to detect deception is far less than that of standard polygraph tests.

According to Majeski (2002, pp. 271-272) modern polygraph tests are capable of simultaneously recording at least three physiological responses:

The cardiovascular measurement utilizes a standard blood pressure cuff by which it measures increases in the blood pressure changes in the heart rate.

The respiration component utilizes two pneumonic tubes, which are placed on the upper chest or thoracic region and the other on the abdominal region. These low-pressure tubes measure the depth and rate of the inhalation/exhalation cycles.

The third essential form of measurement is the GSR or galvanic skin reflex. This component utilizes two metal plates, which are placed on two fingers of the subject's hand, and they measure the conductivity of electricity across the surface of the skin.

Majeski (2002) summarizes three phases of the standard polygraph test. During the pretest interview, the examiner asks questions about the subjects' personal background, discusses the issue, event, or crime requiring the polygraph, and reviews the question formulation with the subject. The second phase is the explanation of the attachments and the actual testing of the subject. The third phase is the post-test interrogation or interview. The nature and extent of the post-test phase is determined on whether deception was indicated.

22.4 Lie Detection and the Fight-Flight Response

According to the Department of Defense Polygraph Institute (1996), the polygraph measures predictable changes in a person's body associated with deception. These physiological responses, alterations in heart rate, breathing, and electrodermal activity were chosen in the 1920s and 1930s because they were simple to record, sensitive to even minor changes in stress levels, and accurate. The DoDPI notes that other physiological changes also occur during deception such as pupil dilation, slowing of digestion, blood supply being redistributed away from the skin and gastrointestinal regions and toward the muscles, and so forth.

The idea behind both polygraph and voice stress testing is that during deception, normal people have predictable physiological changes to questions about their veracity. The physiological changes are in response to fear and anxiety. Anxiety and fear are related, but not identical physiologically. Walker (1981) and others consider fear to be a response to an external threat while anxiety is a disturbing reaction to an internal conflict. The human reaction to these threats is called the fight-flight response. The fight-flight response is a remnant of human evolution where a person experiencing threatening conditions could flee from the danger or fight it. When the person is confronted with a significant external (or internal conflict), the body prepares to flee or fight. Walker (1981, pp. 67-68) describes the physiological response:

The hypothalamus first relays the altering message through the reticular formation and spinal cord to the autonomic nervous system. It then activates the pituitary to release thyrotropic hormone and adrenocorticotropic hormone. Increased sympathetic tone results in a rise in respiratory rate, blood pressure, and pulse rate, and a transference of blood from the intestinal tract to muscles, heart and brain. Activation of the thyroid and adrenals produces gluconeogenesis, protein and fat mobilization, and an increase in metabolic rate. Stimulation of the parasympathetic nervous system and release of norepinephrine from the adrenals causes increase micturition and peristalsis.

Many researchers believe anxiety states can be differentiated from episodes of acute fear (Tanner, 1996). However, in detecting lies, these distinctions are not necessary because the subject experiences both fear from law enforcement personnel conducting the examination (external threat) and also anxiety occurring due to psychological conflicts associated with lying (internal conflict). These reactions happen in normal people when undergoing lie detection procedures. However, they will not be present in individuals who have little or no fear of the lie being detected and those who have convinced themselves that they are uttering truthful statements. In addition, those who confabulate, chronically remark about events without regard to the accuracy or truthfulness of the statements, will not show physiological responses to lying. Several psychiatric conditions can result in pathological lying.

The United States Army began researching the association of voice stress and the psychological and physiological states of the speaker in the 1960s (Palmatier, 2002). However, clinical research into the role of speaker psychological and physiological states and voice production began in the 1930s. By the 1960s, it was an established clinical concept that there were measurable and perceptual voice changes when the speaker was under emotional stress and that laryngeal tension was one of several etiological agents in voice disorders. (See Chapter 21 for a comprehensive review of voice parameters and their psychological correlates.) Aronson (1990, p. 119) describes the phylogeny to the respiratory and phonatory disintegration:

Clinical and instrumental studies prove that otherwise normal voice perceptibly and measurably changes under emotional stress. A smooth, well-modulated voice signifies cortical control over the emotionally primitive, phylogenetically older nervous system. During subcortical emotional release, phonatory and respiratory control disintegrates. Massive automatic fight-or-flight reactions prepare the organism for increased physical work--fixing the upper extremities to the thoracic cage

for combat, requiring firm adduction of the vocal folds and wide abduction to facilitate an increased volume and flow of oxygen in order to meet the body's increased metabolic demands. Such emergency physiologic states are incompatible with fine voice pitch, loudness, and quality control.

22.5 Physiological Dynamics Associated with Voice Stress

To understand the role of stress on voice production, it is necessary to address respiratory and laryngeal musculature, voice output, feedback, muscular compensation, and the self-concept evaluator (Tanner, 2006; Tanner, 2003). Figure 22.1 provides a schematic of the interrelated aspects of voice production as an overlaid biological function. Speech, including voice production, is secondary to the primary biological functions of respiration and digestion for life-sustainment.

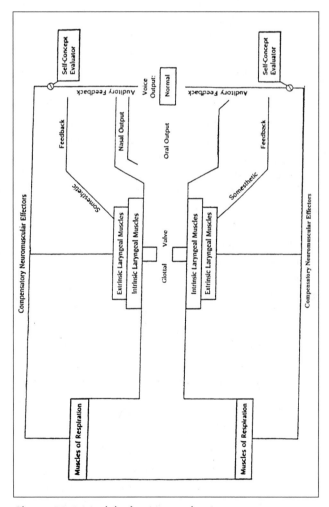

Figure 22.1 *Model of voice production*

Voice production is a result of muscular and aerodynamic forces. Respiration provides the driving energy and air supply for vocal cord vibration. Muscular forces compress air in the lungs and propel it through the tubes and cavities of the speech mechanism. Air movement is accomplished by increasing or decreasing the air pressure in the lungs relative to the atmospheric pressure. When the air pressure in the lungs is greater than the atmospheric pressure, muscular forces and air momentum in the speech tract are overcome, and there is an outward flow of the air to use for speech production. When the atmospheric pressure equals the pressure within the lungs, air movement ceases.

The respiratory muscular support necessary to vibrate the vocal folds is a small percentage of the total respiratory muscular potential. Humans are capable of using the muscles of respiration to create much greater subglottal air pressures (pressure below the vocal cords) and airflows through the glottis than are necessary for phonation. During normal phonation, some sounds are voiced while others do not have vocal cord vibration as part of their distinctive features. The voiced sounds create more impedance (resistance) in the vocal tract, and the respiratory support is adjusted appropriately. When less impedance exists in the tract, the respiratory muscles reduce their force. The respiratory-phonatory feedback and adjustment are highly coordinated and harmonious. Without this respiratory-phonatory feedback and adjustment, some speech sounds would be inappropriately loud and others too soft.

The outward flow of air through the glottis blows the vocal cords apart. The vocal cords would stay apart if not for elasticity and aerodynamic forces. Elasticity results in the muscles and tissues of phonation regaining their original shape after being stretched and distended. The aerodynamic force is the Bernoulli principle. The Bernoulli principle helps close the glottis during phonation by lowering air pressure on the vocal fold surfaces and drawing them toward the midline. The suction effect of the Bernoulli principle and the elasticity of the muscles and tissues in the larynx allows the vocal folds to vibrate very rapidly. This myoelastic-aerodynamic principle of vocal fold vibration accounts for the ability of the vocal cords to vibrate rapidly and not to fatigue over time. These forces are extremely susceptible to increased musculoskeletal tension.

As Figure 22.2 shows, air from the lungs is forced through the glottal valve. When the airflow and pressure reach a required threshold, the vocal cords are set into vibration. Pulses of air caused by the periodic valving of the vocal cords flow from the glottis through the speech mechanism. When the vocal cords close, they also create an acoustic shock wave, traveling at the speed of sound (1130 feet/

second) that radiates through the resonating chambers of the speech mechanism. The acoustic shock waves and pulses of air are valved by the velum (soft palate) approximating the posterior pharyngeal wall allowing more or less air and energy to pass through the velopharyngeal port for nasalization. The result of this aerodynamic event is a person's voice having distinctive qualities.

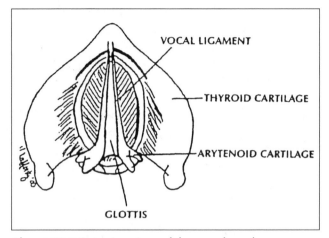

Figure 22.2 Superior view of the vocal cords

The hearing mechanism provides the first source of feedback a person receives about his or her voice. Air conduction auditory feedback occurs when the ears detect air pressure changes. The air pressure changes cause the tympanic membrane (eardrum) to vibrate in response to the frequency and amplitude pressure fluctuations of the sound waves. The ossicles, bones of the middle ear, vibrate in response to the movement of the tympanic membrane, which in turn, causes disruptions in the fluid-filled cochlea. Neurological impulses are transmitted from the cochlea through Cranial Nerve VIII to the brainstem. From the brainstem, the impulses are sent to higher centers of the brain.

Auditory feedback also occurs through bone conduction. In bone conduction feedback, the above process occurs but bypasses the external and middle ear. The energy produced by the vocal cords and other speech structures directly sets the cochlea into vibration. These two types of auditory feedback account for the observation that a person's voice "sounds differently" when heard on a recording. When talking, a person receives speech auditory feedback both through air and bone conduction, but when listening to his or her recorded speech, the feedback occurs only through air conduction.

Somesthetic feedback is the bodily sensation about voice production: tactition, kinesthesia, and proprioception. Tactition is the sense of touch, kinesthesia the sense of motion or movement, and proprioception is knowing body position in space. Somesthetic feedback occurs primarily at the level of the glottis and involves the extrinsic and intrinsic laryngeal musculature. Extrinsic laryngeal muscles are those with their origin outside the larynx. Intrinsic laryngeal muscles have both their origin and attachment within the larynx. Somesthetic feedback includes foreign body sensations on the vocal cords and excessive muscular tension in the throat.

The self-concept evaluator, a hypothetical construct of the personality, evaluates the auditory and somesthetic feedback about voice production. It judges the normalcy of the voice and activates the compensatory neuromuscular effectors when the abnormality exceeds a particular threshold of acceptability. Individuals have varying degrees of acceptance of abnormality in their voices. Some people accept major voice quality and somesthetic changes and others react to minimal alterations. When the self-concept evaluator senses unacceptable variations in the voice, it activates the compensatory neuromuscular effectors that increase the muscular forces involved in vocal cord vibration. The natural tendency for a person is to increase the muscular forces involved in voicing when there is significant abnormality. Clinically, this overcompensation contributes the development of voice pathologies such as vocal nodules, polyps, and contact ulcers (Tanner, 2003; Tanner, 1990).

As discussed previously, several factors related to the flight or fight response cause increased musculoskeletal tension. Minor musculoskeletal tension can be subconscious and the person is not aware of its effects on his or her voice. When there are perceptible abnormalities in voice production exceeding a person's tolerance levels, he or she may consciously produce voice with more force. As Figure 22.1 shows, voice production is a closed-loop system involving feedback and compensatory behaviors.

22.6 Vocal Microtremors, Pitch Instability, and Stress

Manufacturers of voice psychological stress evaluators propose that there are inaudible frequency modulations caused by microtremors of the laryngeal musculature. These frequency modulations occur between eight and twelve cycles-per-second. Like the above physiological reactions measured by the polygraph, these muscular ossicilations are altered in response to stress. Eight to twelve frequency modulations occur in normal speakers when they are relaxed and calm. Figure 22.3 shows a complex speech sound wave. Amplitude is displayed vertically and time horizontally.

As noted in Chapter 16, there are two measures of voice instability: shimmer and jitter. Shimmer is amplitude perturbation and a measure of loudness variation. Jitter, frequency perturbation, is a measure of fundamental frequency period-to-period variation. There is evidence that excessive jitter creates audible indications of voice abnormality.

The human larynx is not a perfect machine, and so we would expect some instability in a person's pitch, even when he or she was trying to produce a steady tone. However, extensive research on normal subjects and patients with voice disorders has shown that voices that are heard as normal do not manifest pitch instability, or jitter, that exceed 1 percent of the person's fundamental frequency. That is, we would not expect moment-to-moment changes in fundamental frequency to exceed an average of 1 Hz in a male subject with a 100 Hz fundamental or 2 Hz in a female subject with a 200 Hz fundamental. Jitter values exceeding about 1 percent are associated with voices that are judged to be hoarse (Dalston, 2000, p. 306).

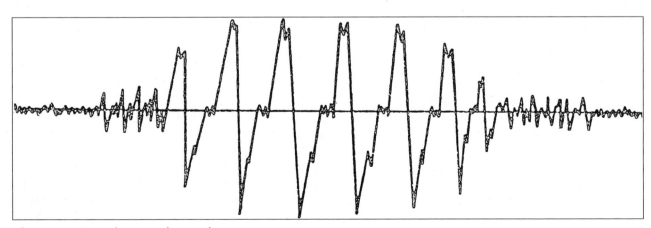

Figure 22.3 Complex speech sound wave

As reported in Chapter 21, clinical research suggests that a hoarse voice is associated with self-consciousness. Most marketers of voice stress evaluators suggest that laryngeal microtremors and related modulation in fundamental frequency are inaudible. Dalston (2002) suggests that jitter values in excess of 2 Hz create perceptible voice quality alterations even when the subject is trying to reduce the fundamental frequency instability.

Current voice stress technology that measures pitch instability is theoretically capable of detecting these variations in speaker stress levels. Although there are several voice parameters appearing to be responsive to physiological fluctuations related to the flight or fight response, such as loudness instability and variations in spectral energy distribution (time, frequency, energy variations), fundamental frequency variations are primary markers of laryngeal muscular hypertension.

22.7 Verbal Jeopardy and Confessions

The role verbal jeopardy plays in lie detection is an important variable in the accuracy of voice stress evaluators. The levels of verbal jeopardy and the accuracy of voice stress tests of deception were linked by Timm (1983). Perceived verbal jeopardy is the suspect's belief that law enforcement personnel and scientific instruments are testing his or her veracity. Voice samples taken during a formal interrogation and with a voice stress instrument in sight of the suspect creates greater verbal jeopardy than a sample taken surreptitiously. Because of the increased verbal jeopardy, the suspect is likely to display greater physiological responses when deceptively answering questions. Polygraphs create increased verbal jeopardy by the formality of the testing. The reliability of lie detection using voice stress analyzer is greater when subjects are experiencing verbal jeopardy during formal interrogation.

The commercial literature on voice stress analysis reports cases solved using voice stress analysis and a valuable use of voice stress devices is to prompt confessions from suspects. There are several cases where suspects confessed to crimes when shown graphics of their voice stress. Suspects' belief that voice stress analysis is an infallible method of lie detection can prompt confession. When used to prompt a confession, voice stress devices can be valuable regardless of their validity and reliability.

22.8 Voice Stress Instrumentation Propaganda

Given that certain voice stress parameters, especially pitch instability, are indicative of increased speaker stress, can voice stress analyzers be used as valid and reliable lie detec-

tors? The National Institute for Truth Verification (2006) there are six voice stress devices currently being marketed as lie detectors and provides validation studies. Most of these devices are based on the original Psychological Stress Evaluator technology developed in the 1970s, but have evolved from analog to digital systems. Some newer generation instruments have advanced filters and graphics for data analysis and presentation, and some analyze additional voice parameters.

Unfortunately, there is ambiguity in the analysis of microtremors for lie detection. Some reports, based on interviews from manufacturers and law enforcement personnel, say that there is an increase in the small frequency modulations occurring during deception. The National Institute for Truth Verification's home page reports that microtremors and the consequent frequency modulations "increase" during stress. According to Dennis (2006, p. 2), "In moments of stress, like when you tell a lie that you dare not get caught at, the body prepares for fight or flight by increasing the readiness of its muscles to spring into action. Their vibration increases from the relaxed 8 to 9 Hz, to the stressful 11 to 12 Hz range." These statements may refer to fear and anger being associated with increased frequency variation, and that newer generation devices examine selected parameters such as upper and lower side bands. In contrast, some reports suggest that the microtremors and consequent frequency modulations decrease in response to stress associated with lying. Due to increased muscular tension, the frequency modulations flatten out and disappear. When used for lie detection, the absence of these microtremors signals that the speaker is uncomfortable with what he or she is saying (Krapohl, Ryan, and Schull, 2002). As a lie detector, voice stress analysis operates in a similar manner to the polygraph with the exception that only one physiological measure is monitored. The manufacturers of the devices also claim voice stress analyzers are extremely reliable and valid for detecting lies when used by properly trained examiners. Most reports from the United States Department of Defense Polygraph Institute, and others, suggest that the psychological stress evaluator has serious flaws with regard to its military uses, and that currently, its validity and reliability are questionable.

It is rarely contested that vocal microtremors fluctuate in response to stress. As reported above, there are differing reports about whether they increase or decrease in amplitude and frequency. One possible explanation for the differing reports may have to do with verbal jeopardy. When a person is verbally deceptive without jeopardy, that is, he or she does not believe the veracity of the statements are being called into question, a case could be made that microtremors increase in amplitude and frequency. This would be due to the emotionality associated with the statements. However, when the veracity of verbal statements are being questioned, such as occurs in a formal voice stress analysis with the instrument in sight, it is possible that because of closed-loop feedback, the subject compensates with more muscular tension as shown in Figure 22.1. The increased muscular tension consequently reduces amplitude and frequency of the laryngeal microtremors.

22.9 Voice Stress Instrumentation for Lie Detection: Validity and Reliability Circa 2007

Validity is the extent to which voice stress devices do what they purport to do. Reliability is the dependability of the instruments and procedures, and the consistency of the results over repeated tests. Review of the research on the use of voice stress instrumentation suggests that the devices have the potential for accurately detecting deception. Over the past forty years, the studies conducted on voice stress and the detection of deception, with some exceptions, have shown a general increase in the validity and reliability of the devices. Since the discovery of vocal microtremors and the development of the first voice psychological stress evaluator, the instruments and the procedures for lie detection using voice stress have improved marginally. The following are factors to consider when using voice stress instruments as lie detectors.

1. The validity and reliability claims made by the manufacturers of voice stress instrumentation, although often appearing to be conclusions scientifically drawn from the available research, are excessive, extreme, and often unreasonable. They do not reflect the conclusions drawn from scientifically controlled studies. Some manufacturers claim voice stress evaluators are nearly infallible as lie detectors. These excessive claims about the validity and reliability of voice stress evaluators as lie detectors cloud their forensic applications.

2. Laryngeal microtremors and fundamental frequency instability are physiological and acoustic factors sensitive to deception-induced stress.

3. Current voice stress instrumentation and procedures are not as valid and reliable as polygraph instrumentation and procedures for detecting deception.

4. Voice stress instrumentation can theoretically approach the validity and reliability of the polygraph when the speaker is experiencing significant verbal jeopardy and the procedures used are similar to standard polygraph procedures.

5. The use of voice stress instruments during interrogations can be effective in obtaining confession because of the subjects' belief they are infallible in detecting lies.

6. Voice stress analysis for lie detection is not accurate beyond chance when the speech sample is taken surreptitiously and the subject is not experiencing verbal jeopardy. Additionally, there are "degrees of lies," and like the polygraph, voice stress evaluators are more accurate in detecting those with the most emotional significance to the subject.

7. The voice stress instruments analyzing additional aspects of the speech signal and using more complex algorithms are generally more accurate than those simply using fundamental frequency instability.

8. Voice stress analysis for lie detection is an evolving technology. The principle of detecting lies by monitoring changes in the human voice is theoretically sound. Future research should address lie detection procedures and applications of voice stress analysis, and experiment with using all voice parameters for testing the veracity of subjects.

22.10 Summary

During the past four decades, voice stress analysis technology has improved significantly. The major improvements involve digital rather than analog technology, sensitivity of the devices, analysis of additional aspects of the speech signal, and graphics. The scientific basis for using the voice for stress and lie detections is theoretically sound. Presently, voice stress analyzers can detect high levels of stress in subjects, and are marginally capable of lie detection beyond chance when the subject is experience significant verbal jeopardy and procedures used are similar to those for the polygraph.

Suggest Reading and Resources

Department of Defense Polygraph Institute Research Division (2006). http://www.dodpi.army.mil/div_RES.asp This website contains several studies addressing the validity and reliability of voice stress analysis.

Majeski, W. J. (2002). The art and sciences of communication during an investigation. In R. Montgomery and W. Majeski (Eds) *Corporate investigations*. Tucson: Lawyers and Judges Publishing Company. This chapter provides an overview of factors related to investigative procedures.

Palmatier, J. J. (2002). Assessing credibility: ADVA technology, voice and voice stress analysis. In R. Montgomery and W. Majeski (Eds) *Corporate investigations*. Tucson: Lawyers and Judges Publishing Company. This chapter explores voice stress analysis relative to corporate investigation.

References

Aronson, A. (1990). *Clinical voice disorders: An interdisciplinary approach*. New York: Thieme.

Clede, B. (1998). Technology, it helps find the truth. Retrieved July 2, 2003 from the World Wide Web: http://www.clede.com/articles/Police/truth.htm. (First published in *Law and Order*, July, 1998).

Dalston, R.M. (2000). Voice disorders. In R. Gillam, T. Marquardt, and F. Martin (Eds) *Communication sciences and disorders*. San Diego: Singular.

Dennis, P. (2006). Voice Stress Analysis. Retrieved September 27, 2006 from the World Wide Web: http://www.whatreallyhappened.com/RANCHO/POLITICS/VSA/truthvsa.html

Department of Defense Polygraph Institute (1996). Voice stress analysis position statement. Retrieved July 4, 2003 from the World Wide Web: http://www.polygraph.org//voice.htm. (Author).

Krapohl, D.J., Ryan, A. H., and Shull, K. W. (2002). Voice stress devices and the detection of lies. Retrieved July 3, 2003 from the World Wide Web: http://www.scpolygraph.org/pages/articles/voice_stress_devices. (Published 2002 in *Policy Review*, the official publication of the International Association of Chiefs of Police, National Law Enforcement Policy Center).

Majeski, W. J. (2002). The art and sciences of communication during an investigation. In R. Montgomery and W. Majeski (Eds) *Corporate investigations*. Tucson: Lawyers and Judges Publishing Company.

National Institute for Truth Verification (2006). Voice stress analyzer comparisons. Retrieved July 10, 2003 from the World Wide Web: http://www.cvsal.com/pricing.php. (Author).

Palmatier, J. J. (2002). Assessing credibility: ADVA technology, voice and voice stress analysis. In R. Montgomery and W. Majeski (Eds) *Corporate investigations*. Tucson: Lawyers and Judges Publishing Company.

Rubinkam, M. (2003). Police using voice stress analysis to detect lies. Retrieved June 30, 2003 from the World Wide Web: http://www.rss.com.np/latest/voice.html.

Tanner, D. (1990). *Tanner muscular relaxation program for voice disorders*. Oceanside, C.A.: Academic Communication Associates.

Tanner, D. (1996). *An introduction to the psychology of aphasia*. Kendall-Hunt Publishers, Dubuque, Iowa.

Tanner, D. (2001, December). The brave new world of the cyber speech and hearing clinic. *ASHA Leader*, 6(22).

Tanner, D. (2003). Exploring communication disorders: *A 21st century introduction through literature and media*. Boston: Pearson, Allyn & Bacon.

Tanner, D. (2006). *An advanced course in communication sciences and disorders*. San Diego: Plural Publishing.

Tanner, D., Culbertson, B, and Secord, W. (2001). Cheers and jeers: Hollywood and the motion picture industry. An extended seminar presented to the annual convention of the American Speech-Language-Hearing Association, New Orleans.

Timm, H.W. (1983). The efficacy of the Psychological Stress Evaluator in detecting deception. *Journal of Police Science and Administration*, 11: 62-68.

Walker, J. (1981). *Clinical psychiatry in primary care*. Menlo Park, CA.: Addison-Wesley.

Chapter 23

Speaker Profiling and Communication Disorders

23.1 Chapter Preview

This chapter examines speaker profiling and the large, heterogeneous communication-disordered population. There is a review of cognitive dissonance and the effects of negative stereotypes and prejudices on the general population of communication disabled. Speaker profiling conjecture is addressed as it pertains to the Deaf Community, persons with immature and regressive speech, adolescent and adult stuttering, psychogenic voice disorders, and neurogenic communication disorders.

23.2 Application of Speaker Profiling to the Communication Disordered Population

A large percentage of the population of the United States has a communication disorder. The type and severity of a communication disorder can be an important consideration when speaker profiling, and people with communication disorders have certain traits and characteristics that can provide valuable forensic information. According to Rubin (2000), in industrialized countries, the percent of people with communication disorders ranges between 5 percent and 10 percent. In non-industrialized countries, the incidence and prevalence of communication disorders vary greatly because of vague and imprecise definitions of what constitutes a communication disorder. In many underprivileged countries, epidemiological research is underfunded or nonexistent. Because the United States has modern and effective screening, diagnostics, and reporting of disabilities, the percent of the population with identified communication disorders is likely higher than what is reported by many other countries. With the population of the United States at approximately 300 million, a low estimate suggests that 30 million Americans have a communication disorder. Bello (1995) reports that roughly one in six Americans have a communication disorder, yielding about 50 million persons with speech, voice, language, and hearing disorders.

The reasons for a wide range of reported communication disorders are threefold. First, some communication disorders exist for a brief time. For example, some children have typical childhood articulation disorders such as substituting the "w" for the "r" speech sound in the word "wabbit." With maturation or because of therapy, most children outgrow or overcome the speech disorder. Consequently, there is a higher incidence of communication disorders in children; about 10-15 percent of school-aged children have speech, voice, language, or hearing disorders. Second, some communication disorders appear gradually and pinpointing precisely when people suffer from them is

273

difficult. Hearing loss, for example, is often gradual in onset in the elderly with about 33 percent of the people over the age of sixty-five years experiencing problems hearing (National Center for Health Statistics, 1988). Third, the actual percent of Americans with communication disorders is changing. Today, more at-risk babies are surviving due to medical advances, and many have complications with resulting communication disorders. Advances in medical sciences and emergency transportation services also have resulted in more adults surviving traumatic brain injuries and catastrophic illnesses, but they often do so with communication disorders.

23.3 General Social Characteristics of the Communication Disordered Population

When considering the social characteristics of the communication-disordered population, there are two categories of people with speech, voice, language, or hearing disorders. First, there are those individuals with cosmetic communication disorders. Persons with a cosmetic communication disorder have functional abilities to communicate, that is, they can exchange meaning with others, but their speech stands out as obtrusive. For example, a person who lisps can communicate effectively; even while lisping, the listener knows what he or she is saying. The lisper's speech is simply obtrusive; it is abnormal, draws attention to itself, and stands out as defective. Other examples of cosmetic communication disorders include speakers with the hypernasality of cleft palate, voice quality irregularities, and mild-to-moderate stuttering.

The second category of communication disorders involves loss of speech intelligibility, severe hearing loss and deafness, aphonia (loss of voice), and language delay or disorders that functionally limit the use of language. (Language disorders can affect thought, and prevent or significantly impair the expression and reception of information through any of the language modalities: speaking, auditory comprehension, reading, writing, and gestures.) People with these types of communication disorders have obstacles to happy, productive lives because of their disabilities. Examples of communication disorders reducing speech intelligibility, severe hearing loss and deafness, aphonia, and loss of speech and language due to strokes, laryngectomies, Parkinson's disease, and traumatic brain injuries. Many individuals with communication disorders have unique interpersonal and social challenges not experienced by other disabled persons.

The communication-disordered population is large, heterogeneous, and can be broken down into subcategories such as stuttering, stroke-related aphasia, autism, Down syndrome, multiple sclerosis, and so forth. The largest number of communication-disabled persons is those with hearing loss or deafness, and the smallest group is speech, voice, language, and hearing disorders associated with rare diseases and birth defects. The effects of communication disorders on quality of life range from a minor nuisance to the complete inability to communicate. For example, mild stuttering is a modest nuisance for the person who only has occasional breakdowns in speech fluency whereas global aphasia resulting from a stroke renders the patient unable to speak, read, write, and understand the speech and writing of others.

The age range for people with communication disorders is skewed to the young and old. Although persons in their middle years can suffer communication disorders such as noise-induced hearing loss, traumatic brain injury and aphasia, vocal nodules, etc., most communication disorders occur in children and elderly persons. Some persons with communication-disorders are normal cognitively while others are mentally retarded, autistic, or learning disabled. More males suffer from communication disorders than females, and in the case of stuttering, roughly four times more males than females stutter. With the exception of age-related hearing loss in the elderly, as a group, communication disordered persons are at an economic disadvantage; they tend be dependent children or adults and have less money and power. Not all communication disorders are continuously visually apparent. Some communication disorders are obvious such as cleft lip, laryngectomy, or Down syndrome. Other persons only show their disability when speaking such as stuttering and lisping. Most people with communication disorders have been or are in special education or rehabilitation programs. They are playing catchup with the normal population in an attempt to be like the social mainstream.

23.4 Self-Concept and Cognitive Dissonance

To effectively profile persons with communication disorders as a group, and get to their underlying psychological, personality, and emotional states and characteristics, it is necessary to address the notion of cognitive dissonance. The psychological concept of cognitive dissonance was initially advanced in the 1950s and explains how a person's mind modifies existing emotions, beliefs, and behaviors when confronted with incompatible cognitions (thoughts). Both people with communication disorders and the general public often have incompatible thoughts about communication disorders and the individuals who suffer from them. Negative stereotypes abound about these disabled individuals and many are inappropriately applied to individual communication-disabled persons or wrongly generalized to the group as a whole. Perhaps the best example of incorrect negative stereotypes about communication-disordered persons involves the renowned theoretical physicist Stephen William Hawking. Conventional wisdom suggests that a person in a wheelchair, unable to talk, and who drools is profoundly mentally retarded. The reality is that Dr. Hawking suffers from a pure motor speech disorder secondary to amyotrophic lateral sclerosis (ALS) and is far from mentally retarded. In fact, he is one of the most intelligent persons to have ever lived.

Historically, the communication-disordered population has been negatively stereotyped. Past attitudes and treatment of persons with communication disorders have been bigoted and often brutal. Primitive societies tolerated no weaknesses in their members as they struggled for survival, and disabled persons were buried alive, sacrificed to the gods, hurled from cliffs, and thrown into rivers (Van Riper and Erickson, 1996). As recently as the mid-1900s, the Nazi's in Germany engaged in systematic extermination of large numbers of disabled persons including those with communication disorders. And the word "handicapped" may have originated from the practice of disabled persons begging for food and money on street corners with cap in hand. Even today, movies and literature often portray communication-disordered persons as dim-witted, befuddled, and laughable (Tanner, 2001). Many persons with a communication disorder suffer from these negative stereotypes causing conflicts in their identity and reduced self-esteem.

Cognitive dissonance is defined here as the discrepancy between a person's perception of a stereotype and the actualization of a person who is labeled by the stereotype but does into fit the stereotyped perception. A person with a communication disorder can have many reactions and responses when confronted with public perceptions that are in conflict with the reality of [his or] her communication disorder. The most apparent reaction is an identity conflict. An identity conflict can occur when the person's concept of self with regard to the communication disorder is in conflict society's beliefs about people with communication disorder (Tanner, 2003a, p. 21).

Of course, some stereotypes are appropriate and accurate. Nevertheless, for many individuals with communication disorders, there is a conflict between their self-identity and society's perception. To add to the stigma associated with communication disorders, society reacts in a negative way to people with communication disorders by being impatient with their disabilities and with overt and covert rejection, ridicule, and pity. These societal reactions play a powerful role in not only the communication-disabled identities, but they also resultantly affect their behaviors.

Although generalizing to the heterogeneous group of people with communication disorders is difficult, as a rule, listeners treat most individuals with communication disorders discourteously. Because many communication-disabled persons take longer to express themselves, listeners may walk away midsentence or interrupt them. They are also subjected to overt rejection and outright ridicule, where listeners comment negatively about their communication disorders. Overt rejection and ridicule are common on playgrounds and can be devastating to the self-esteem and identity of a child with a communication disorder. Covert rejection is hidden and subtle, but powerful in creating a negative mind set for the disabled person. Covert rejection may occur when a hurried boss ignores what a communication-disordered person is saying, lacks eye contact, or frowns at his or her speech production. In many ways, covert rejection can be more disparaging than overt rejection because there is no avenue for the person to confront it. Pity is often a double-edged sword for the communication-disordered. The person expressing pity has a false sense of superiority, albeit with good intentions, while solidifying feelings of inferiority in the recipient. Combined, the above negative reactions of society to the communication-disordered population can have major effects on their psychology, emotions, self-esteem, and identity.

23.5 Speaker Profiling and the Deaf Community

Total deafness, the complete loss of hearing in both ears, is rare. Most individuals have some residual hearing and can sense air vibration. In the discussion that follows, profound hard-of-hearing and deafness are used interchangeably because both disorders similarly affect speech and language development. In the deaf community, there are two social and political philosophies concerning the stigma associated with deafness and treatment options. One group of deaf persons, the "oralists," believes that deafness is a disability that limits social interaction and vocational opportunities. According to oralists, deafness interferes with parent-child interaction, socialization with others, and educational and vocational opportunities. When the disorder is detected and evaluated, parents ascribing to this philosophy place their children in special education programs and classrooms, and take advantage of all resources available to minimize the social, educational, and psychological effects of the communication disorder. Children are prescribed hearing aids, and where medically indicated, they receive cochlear implants (see Chapter 14). They are also taught speech reading (lip reading) and given intensive speech therapy to learn how to talk. When all available resources are used to treat the deafness, most deaf persons learn to function well in the hearing-world and minimize the social and psychological effects of the disorder. Deaf individuals ascribing to the oralists philosophy seek full integration into society and view deafness as a treatable disability.

In contrast to the oralists philosophy, "manualists" do not want communication inclusion with the hearing-world; they take a contrary position about deafness being a disability. They believe manual communication, finger spelling and sign language, is the natural way for deaf persons to communicate. They are content with being members of the Deaf Community and take pride in their deafness; they do not feel stigmatized. They embrace sign language, which is a true language in that it meets all of the definitions of a standard language; it has rule-governed grammar and syntax, and an agreed-upon semantics. Central to the manualists philosophy is that sign language plays an important role in thought processes and the maintenance of the deaf culture. Manualists believe that deaf persons are a repressed linguistic minority, similar to other repressed social groups, and many are active politically and socially. There is also a subgroup of the deaf population ascribing to the "total communication" school of thought that embraces all forms of communication and integrates the manualist and oralist philosophies.

The social and psychological effects of deafness on a person depend, in large part, on when the deafness occurred. Hearing plays a critical role in speech and language acquisition, and when deafness occurs before they are fully developed, the person will not naturally learn to talk. Prelingual deafness is deafness before the development of speech and language. Perilingual deafness occurs during the speech and language development period. Postlingual deafness is when the loss of hearing occurs in children approximately eight years of age or older, and after the development of speech and language. The communicative, social, and psychological effects of postlingual deafness are less significant because speech and language are already basically learned. By about eight years of age, the grammatic structure and communicative functions of speech and language are established in most children, although people learn the meanings of new words throughout their lives. Although in postlingual deafness, there is deterioration of speech and language abilities overtime, the

speech distortion is not as severe as what occurs when a child is born deaf or loses his or her hearing during the primary communication developmental period.

The thought processes of individuals deprived of language from birth has been an impassioned psychological and philosophical topic of debate for decades. Obviously, because the prelingually deaf person has never heard speech, he or she does not have the same type of internal monologues, self-talk, occurring in people with normal hearing. For example, if one has never heard the word "truthfulness," he or she will not process the word during internal monologues. The noted author and neurologist Oliver Sacks (1990) addresses the dissimilar thought processes occurring in hearing and deaf persons. He notes that prelingually deaf persons using sign language have a fundamentally different way of representing reality during thought. Sign language, unlike speech, has four dimensions, three for space and one for time, giving it more capabilities to carry information. Although the nature of thought in hearing and prelingually deaf persons is far from understood, most authorities recognize that hearing and prelingually deaf persons process reality with fundamentally different units of thought.

23.6 Speaker Profiling Conjecture and Deaf Persons

When speaker profiling deaf individuals, a distinction must be made about deaf persons with postlingual and prelingual onset, and whether they ascribe to the oralists, manualists, or total communication philosophies. Those persons with a postlingual onset of deafness are likely to have the same social and psychological makeup as others with major communication disorders. Because of their communication disorder, people with postlingual deafness are likely to feel inferior to the normal population regarding their disability, suffer similar negative reactions by society, and experience frustration at their difficulties communicating. However, it is unlikely that these individuals will identify strongly with the larger group of deaf persons, particularly those ascribing to the manualist philosophy and those born deaf. What is most important, persons with postlingual deafness will think and process reality in the same manner as those with normal hearing; they will have basically the same types of internal monologues (verbal thoughts).

Speaker profiles about persons with prelingual and perilingual deafness should address "when" the onset occurred relative to the development of speech and language. If the speaker is born deaf, or if it occurred shortly thereafter, the effects of the disorder on speech and language development will be all-inclusive. Because no speech sounds will have ever been heard by prelingually deaf persons, their speech attempts will be profoundly distorted. Congenitally deaf speakers, if they have speech at all, will have the speech sound production typical of congenitally deaf persons; it will be nasal, monopitch, and distorted. If the deafness occurs between birth and about eight years of age, the exact date or period of time the deafness occurred influences the nature and level of the person's speech and language development. In speech development, there is a predicable sequence of speech sound acquisition. For example, most normal, hearing children acquire the speech sounds /m/, /h/, /w/, /n/, "ng," /f/, /p/, and /b/ by about three years, six months of age (Tanner, Culbertson, and Secord, 1997). As a general rule, if the onset of the deafness occurs after this age, these speech sounds will have been heard, perceived, distinguished, and motorically learned, and consequently, they will be produced more articulately than subsequently learned phonemes. After about eight years of age, the older is the person when the deafness occurs, the more precise is his or her speech sound production.

Language development in both hearing and deaf children is initially parallel. Both hearing and deaf babies produce the birth cry, engage in undifferentiated and differentiated crying, coo, and begin the babbling stage. The birth cry is the vocalization most children make immediately after delivery. Undifferentiated crying is the type of crying that has no different meanings to the mother; she cannot discern the baby's needs based on the way he or she cries. Differentiated crying emerges during the second month of life, and is the first true form of reciprocal communication between mother and child. The mother can typically distinguish as many as seven different types of cries reflecting the needs of the child. Cooing is the production and repetition of vowel sounds. Primarily because of tactile stimulation, the child randomly produces vowels, and both hearing and deaf children coo in the same ways. In addition, both hearing and deaf children enter the initial stage of babbling, which is the production and repetition of consonants. Babbling, like cooing, is initially done because of the tactile stimulation, but later it evolves into more complex utterance because of auditory stimulation. At this stage of language development, hearing and deaf children part ways. Without cochlear implants, speech and language therapy, aural habilitation, and special education, the deaf child will not progress beyond this stage of traditional language development.

Most speakers with prelingual deafness, and some with perilingual deafness which had its onset early in the speech and language development period, will identify with the Deaf Culture more than with the hearing population. The speakers' parents will have been pivotal to their child's Deaf Culture identities. As a rule, deaf parents who are manualists rear their children in the Deaf Culture, while many hearing parents prefer the oralist or total communication philosophies. Speakers who are manualist and identify with the Deaf Culture are likely to share many of the beliefs, attitudes, and behaviors of other alleged repressed social groups. They tend to seek out their mates and friendships within their own social milieu, resent outside social, political, and educational intrusion, lack trust in outsiders, and suspect the motives of many persons in the hearing world.

During the forensic interview and interrogation (see Chapter 21), deaf persons using sign language must be provided with interpreters. It should be noted that the translation of sign language into English carries the same, if not more, potential of inaccuracies and possible misinterpretations as does the translation into English of a foreign language, e.g., Arabic, French, Spanish. There are also several dialects of sign language, and individual signing fluency variations. Even written statements made by prelingually deaf persons may be inaccurate due to the special auditory representations and thought processes of persons deprived of hearing before the normal speech and language developmental period. To minimize the potential for misinterpretation and inaccuracy of translation, interviewers and interrogators should reword and repeat questions, and allow for the subject to have multiple responses to pivotal issues.

23.7 Speaker Profiling, Immature and Regressive Speech

The most common types of immature speech are "lisping," substituting the "th" for the /s/ speech sound such as occurs in "thee" for "see," and "lalling," substituting the /w/ for /r/ speech sound such as occurs in "wabbit" for "rabbit." The /r/ and /s/ speech sounds are also the most common articulation errors seen by therapists in schools. Developmentally, 75 percent of children have mastered correct production of /r/ and /s/ speech sounds in the initial, medial, and final positions of words by four years, six months, and four years, nine months respectively. Ninety percent of children have mastered these speech sounds in two of three positions of words by six years of age (Tanner, Culbertson, and Secord, 1997).

Lisping in adolescent and adult males has been associated with effeminate homosexuality. The motion picture industry often uses speech stereotypes to develop characters and to advance plots and storylines (Tanner, 2001). Hollywood continues to propagate the stereotype of the effeminate male homosexual as one with the immature speech pattern of a lisp. Certainly other characteristics are used by screenwriters to portray effeminate male homosexuality such as expansive gestures, softly spoken speech, exaggerated articulation precision, clothing, and so forth, but lisping is often a primary feature used for character development. Notwithstanding general public perceptions, it should be noted that there are no valid and reliable scientific studies showing a link between lisping and male homosexuality. There is no scientific evidence that males who are homosexuals lisp more frequently than the general population, lisp more than heterosexuals, nor is lisping in a male child suggestive of homosexual tendencies. There may be a lisping and male homosexual link, and the general public and Hollywood are accurately portraying the speech pattern, but to date, there are no valid and reliable scientific studies addressing the relationship. With regard to lalling, cartoons, movies, and televison sometimes use the /w/ for /r/ substitution for its humor value and to portray a character as being chronically befuddled, e.g., Warner Bros.' cartoon character, Elmer Fudd. As with the lack of scientific evidence about lisping, there is no evidence showing adults who substitute the /w/ for /r/ speech sound have lower intelligence nor are they more addlebrained than adults with normal articulation.

There are three reasons why an adult may talk with some of the speech characteristics of a child. First, he or she may have developed the speech disorder as a child and it was never discovered. In the United States, most children are screened for speech, voice, language, and hearing disorders when they are young, and the great majority of those with communication disorders are identified. Today, most newborns receive reflexive hearing screening tests when they are hours old and many school districts screen all preschoolers, kindergartners, and first graders. Nevertheless, some schools do not screen for communication disorders effectively, or at all, and some children are not tested for a variety of reasons including home schooling, chronic illnesses, failure to enroll in school, and so forth. Although rare, some children with speech, voice, language, and hearing disorders slip through the system and become adults with communication disorders. Second, some children have their communication disorder identified and evaluated. Even so, the treatment is completely or partially unsuccessful. Not all communication disorders are amenable to successful treatment, and some children do not respond to therapies. Third, because of the psychological defense mechanism and coping style of regression, some adults revert to childlike speech, or for social reasons, they prefer to talk abnormally. They have the ability to talk normally, but consciously or subconsciously engage in childlike speech.

Regression is a retreat to a more secure and comfortable level of adjustment (Stuart, 1998). This psychological defense and coping style reduces anxiety by allowing the person to become more dependent, and to return to thoughts, attitudes, and behaviors that he or she has outgrown. People utilizing the psychological defense and coping style of regression seek and find comfort in dependent relationships. Regression to more secure and comfortable thoughts, attitudes, and behaviors may include changes from adult to childlike speech patterns. Speaker profiling of adults with childlike speech patterns involves addressing possible reasons for their regression and immature speech production. Aronson (1990) notes that regressive speech patterns can involve phonatory and resonatory systems and include aberrant articulation with reduced mouth opening. "Regressive speech serves the purpose of relieving the person from the responsibility of relating to others on an adult plane. It says, in effect, that the person does not wish to be regarded as an adult with the responsibilities for mutual interaction that an adult relationship entails" (Aronson, 1990, p. 139).

23.8 Speaker Profiling Conjecture: Immature and Regressive Speech

Adult and adolescent speakers with longstanding articulation errors such as lisping and lalling will have likely spent years in speech therapy as school children. As such, part of their identity and self-concept will be that of a communication-disordered individual. However, in these cases, the therapies will have been unsuccessful in significantly minimizing or removing the disorders. Accompanying the identity and self-concept of these adult communication-disordered persons will be the sense of inferiority in speaking situations shared by most persons with a history of speech, voice, language, and hearing disorders, but also at least some guilt for the negative therapy outcomes. Often, adults and adolescents with lisping and lalling will have had a long history of suffering negative social reactions to their immature speech patterns. Listeners, including parents, siblings, friends, and acquaintances, will have been impatient with their childlike speech, and some speakers will have suffered the debasing and demeaning reaction of pity. Covert and overt rejection as well as blatant ridicule, often disguised as humor and good-natured ribbing, is likely to have been commonplace.

Adult-onset of lisping and lalling are likely the result of the psychological defense and coping style of regression, or an attempt by the speaker to create a new identity. Typical childhood speech patterns of lisping and lalling rarely have an adult-onset due to neurological injury or disease. When a period of mutism accompanies or precedes the adult onset of lisping and lalling, and when associated with psychological trauma and shock, they are likely a manifestation of hysteria. A hysterical psychological disorder involves extreme, volatile emotions, and is often accompanied by attention-seeking behavior such as the adult-onset of lisping or lalling. In hysterical disorders, there is often symbolism to the symptoms. For example, some persons who see distressing and tragic events lose their vision; they develop hysterical blindness. Loss of hearing sometimes occurs because a person hears abusive and traumatic things; he or she develops hysterical deafness. Hysterical loss of voice occurs when a person loses the ability to speak normally and the symbolism involves disruption of interpersonal communication with some significant individual, usually a spouse or family member. Adult-onset of lisping and lalling can also be a result of a type of hysteria, and the speech disorder is symbolic of problems communicating.

Some individuals may speak with lisps for social reasons. While there is no demonstrated scientific link between lisping and male effeminate homosexuality, some male adolescents and adults may lisp because it is part of an acquired identity. Because of society and the motion picture industry's linking of lisping and effeminate male homosexuality, they may speak with a lisp to portray their sexual orientation, preference, and identity. Just as some people wear types of clothing to show affiliation with certain groups, a lisping male may be showing his association with the homosexual subpopulation by his speech patterns. In this sense, the lisp is a nonverbal form of communication showing a desire for social inclusion into the male homosexual subpopulation.

23.9 Speaker Profiling, Adolescent and Adult Stuttering

Stuttering has afflicted speakers presumably since humans began to talk. There are hieroglyphic references to stuttering about 2,000 years before the birth of Christ and in the ancient records of the early Greek and Romans. Stuttering occurs in all languages, although it is more prevalent in some cultures than in others. Approximately 1-3 percent of the U.S. population currently stutters, and upwards of 5 percent of Americans report periods of their lives where they stuttered. Occurring mostly in males, stuttering ranges from mild inconveniences for some, and for others, devastating disabilities that have and continue to mold their lives. "I am a stutterer. I am not like other people. I must think differently, act differently, live differently–because I stutter. Like other stutterers, like other exiles, I have known all my life a great sorrow and a great hope together, and they have made

me the kind of a person I am. An awkward tongue has molded my life" (Johnson, 1930, p. 1). Analysis of this universal and age-old speech disorder can provide valuable insight into the personality of the speaker, and contribute substantially to his or her profile.

Because everyone has disfluent speech, i.e., occasional repetitions, prolongations, and hesitations in their ongoing speech, clearly defining and describing true stuttering is important. True stuttering, the type of aberrant speech seen in stuttering adolescents and adults is a combination of defective speech production and the stutterer's reaction to the disorder. Generally, stuttering consists of too many sound, word, and phrase repetitions, prolonging or stretching-out utterances, blocks in the smooth flow of speech, and the speaker's reactions to them. The reactions include visible avoidance and escape behaviors as the speaker tries to force his or her speech mechanism into functioning and to get out of the stuttering moment. Most confirmed stutterers report anxiety and associated negative emotions before, during, and after the moment of stuttering. For many, particularly those with long-standing and severe stuttering, the disorder affects their personalities, vocational choices, self-concepts, socialization, and self-esteem. "Stuttering affects a person in many ways, but one of the most critical social activities an adult individual undertakes is that of finding a partner and maintaining an intimate relationship" (Linn and Caruso, 1998, p. 12).

Besides the visible, eye-squints, hand slaps, jaw tremors, etc., and the audible repetitions, prolongations, and blocks, the frequent bouts of anxiety and associated negative emotions experienced by the stutterer are pivotal to their psychological reactions to speaking. Fear, dread, guilt, and apprehension are common associated negative emotions to speaking, be they speeches to large audiences or one-to-one acts of communication. Although stuttering authorities differ on whether there is a clinically definable "stuttering personality," most agree that stuttering is aversive and negatively affects the person suffering from it. Studies of large samples of stutterers compared to normal-speaking subjects have found that, as a group, people who stutter are not dramatically affected psychologically by the disorder. However, research using the Minnesota Multiphastic Personality Inventory (MMPI) shows that stutterers fall within the range of normal and resemble troubled persons seeking counseling.

Today, no one knows the cause or causes of stuttering. Although this communication disorder has been scientifically studied since the 1930s, no clear single etiology has emerged to account for the onset of stuttering in all people. However, there are certain generalities that can be drawn from the decades of research and speculation about stuttering. First, it is likely that there are multiple types of stuttering and several etiological factors. Most stuttering begins in children between two and seven years of age. Although these children may have an organic predisposition to stutter, physical and neurological irregularities do not directly "cause" stuttering; they only create conditions ripe for its development. Second, adult-onset stuttering is usually hysterically-based. A hysterically-based stutter is the type of fluency disruption seen in soldiers suffering from combat fatigue, shell shock, and by others who begin to stutter late in life due to stress. In the majority of these cases, stress and psychic trauma cause the stuttering, and the speech disorder is a conversion reaction and the turning of psychological turmoil into a physical manifestation. Third, learning and audience reactions to impaired speech play important roles in the maintenance and perpetuation of stuttering. The struggle to speak seen in so many people who stutter is a result of their adopting the belief that their speech disfluencies are abnormal and attempts to create perfect speech. Combined, anxiety and attempts to force normal speech actually contribute to stuttering, and a negative spiral of disrupted speech and forced compensation is set into motion. Fourth, audience rewards increase the likelihood of stuttering self-perpetuation. Especially for children, there are rewards for being a stutterer. Because of their stutter, some children are rewarded by non-interruption, more attention by parents and teachers, ready-made excuses for failure, exclusion from verbal class assignments, etc. In addition, the relief felt by the stutterer when the stuttering moment ends contributes to its maintenance and perpetuation. In the majority of stuttering, there are multiple etiological factors at work: organic predisposition, struggle-

compensation, the results of fluency disrupting anxiety, audience reactions, and relief rewards.

23.10 Speaker Profiling Conjecture: Adolescent and Adult Stuttering

Speaker profiles about adolescent and adult stutterers must take into account the wide variability in the severity and the chronicity of the disorder. While some people who stutter are minimally affected socially and psychologically by the disorder, the majority of adolescent and adult stutterers have suffered from it for many years, and many times, several decades. Particularly in persons plagued by severe stuttering, the disorder will have been a constant companion in all types of speech communication from simply asking a stranger for the time, to important verbal questions such as proposing marriage. It is likely that the stutterer has a family history of the disorder; fifty percent of people who stutter report that they have a family member with the same problem (Owens, Metz, and Haas, 2000).

During forensic interviews and interrogations (see Chapter 21), the severity of the stuttering will increase as the stress levels increase. Stuttering is often a barometer of how much stress and anxiety the speaker is experiencing. As stress and anxiety increases during forensic interviews and interrogations, there will be consequent increases in the number of repetitions, duration of prolongations, and the length and severity of blocks. However, as Table 23.1 shows, several factors must be considered when gauging the degree of stress and anxiety experienced by the stutterer: fluency management techniques, rhythm and melody, audience threat, speech cues, noise, and miscellaneous factors such as illness, alcoholic intoxication, and fatigue.

Table 23.1
Factors Affecting Fluency Levels in Stutterers

Factors	Effects on Some People Who Stutter
Fluency Management Techniques	Relaxed, slow, singsong speech with easy, light articulatory contacts improves fluency
Rhythm and Melody	Speaking with melody and a smooth rhythm improves fluency
Audience Threat	Nonthreatening audiences improve fluency
Speech Cues	Fluency improves when speaking in unison or repeating what has been spoken
Noise	Ambient noise improves fluency
Miscellaneous Factors	Illness, alcoholic beverages, and fatigue may increase fluency in some persons

For many stutterers who have undergone extensive therapy, the treatment outcome is "control" of the dysfluencies rather than a complete "cure" for the disorder. Many adolescents and adults who stutter control their stuttering by being relaxed during speaking, having light, easy, articulatory contacts, and a slow, purposeful, singsong manner of talking. Additionally, for the majority of people who stutter, the more nonthreatening the audience, the more improved is their fluency. For example, most stutterers can talk fluently to pets, babies, and aloud to themselves while having more problems with police officers, lawyers, and interrogators. Simply repeating what has been spoken often results in normal fluency; it is likely that a person who stutters will be able to repeat a confession when stated by an interrogator. When speaking in unison with another subject, the stutterer is also likely to be fluent. Ambient noise such as a loud interview and interrogation room, or an office in a precinct with high background noise levels are likely to cause some stutterers to be more fluent. Miscellaneous factors such as illnesses, alcohol intoxication, and fatigue may also affect the fluency levels of some people who stutter (see Chapter 20).

Adolescent and adult stutterers are likely to suffer from reduced self-esteem, particularly in speaking situations. They are also likely to be socially awkward. Typically, adolescent and adult stutterers have had years of suffering the pangs of rejection and ridicule. They will have the self-concept of a stutterer and the accompanying reduced self-esteem about social interaction that accompanies it. The seeds for this learned inferiority will have been planted early in their lives on playgrounds and in classrooms, and propagated by family, friends, and society's reaction to stuttering in adulthood.

Because most people who stutter can only control the disorder, and with vastly differing levels of success, there is a movement among some persons to redefine stuttering as a "different" rather than a "disordered" way of speaking. Yeoman (1998) reports in *Psychology Today* that some stutterers believe they are better off viewing the fluency interruptions as different, and learning to accept them, rather than considering them disordered and completely trying to overcome stuttering, which is often futile. Like members of the Deaf Community discussed previously, there is a movement among some persons who stutter to remove the negative assessment and inferior status of people who stutter, and to move the communication irregularity into the realm of a "nonstandard" rather than "substandard" way of talking.

Although most persons who stutter are only able to control their dysfluent speech symptoms, some individuals are truly cured of the disorder. Either because of therapy, self-control, spontaneous elimination of the disorder, or other factors, a small percentage of individuals believe they are completely cured of stuttering. If the disorder began in childhood, they have memories of being a stutterer, but as adolescents or adults, they are no longer plagued by stuttering. In the not-so-distant past, some authorities believed that stuttering is a manifestation of a psychological disorder, and that to cure it without the benefit of psychotherapy could cause the patient to be a danger to self or others. It was thought that stuttering was a safe expression of a deep-rooted psychological disorder and if removed without a psychotherapist providing another alternative, the person who stuttered would resort to a dangerous alternative expression of his or her psychological distress. Although symptom substitution is a well-established psychiatric phenomenon, there are no scientific studies showing that it applies to stuttering. "The scientific literature has never reported a case where eliminating stuttering resulted, directly or indirectly, in injury to anyone. No incident has been reported in which a person was cured of stuttering and replaced it with a destructive or harmful psychological substitute" (Tanner, 2003a, p. 37). However, it should be noted that because this has not been reported in the stuttering scientific literature does not mean that it has never happened nor will it ever occur in the future.

23.11 Speaker Profiling and Psychogenic Voice Disorders

The voice production mechanism is highly sensitive to musculoskeletal tension. As a result, an increase in anxiety and consequent elevation in physical tension as a response to stress can affect a person's pitch, loudness, and voice quality. While psychological factors do not cause cleft lip and palate, vocal paralysis, and laryngeal cancers, many voice disorders are either completely or partially psychogenic in nature. Voice disorders, such as screamer nodules (noncancerous growths on the vocal cords) and chronic laryngitis (longstanding inflammation of the vocal cords) occur, at least in part, because of the effects of external or internal stressors and the person's attempts to deal with anxiety. For example, hysterical aphonia (see below), the complete loss of voice due to a conversion reaction is wholly psychogenic in nature, while voice disorders related to vocal strain and abuse, such as vocal contact ulcers, are partially psychogenic.

The primary voice disorders related to vocal strain and abuse are nodules, polyps, and contact ulcers. Vocal nodules can be on one or both sides of the vocal folds and are usually about the size of a peppercorn. Vocal nodules in adults are more common in females and associated with vocally abusive behaviors. However, there is usually a psychogenic component involving the speaker's reaction to stress. "They are talkative, socially aggressive, and tense, and have acute or chronic interpersonal problems that generate tension, anxiety, anger, or depression. Even when the nodule may be the sole result of abuse from singing or other strenuous vocal activity, it is often found that these were not the only factors responsible for the vocal abuse; these patients had also entered a period of their lives in which concomitant emotional stress had surfaced" (Aronson, 1990, pp. 125-126).

Vocal polyps are small, fluid-filled blisters on the vocal folds. Chronic vocal polyps may be precancerous. When polyps occur because of vocal strain, they often result from one-time abuse. They are also associated with asthma and allergies (Hall, Oyer, and Haas, 2001). Vocal contact ulcers are ulcerations, breaks in the tissue of the vocal folds, and are associated with pain and a foreign body sensation in the throat. Contact ulcers occur more frequently in males than females, possibly due to some males talking in an unnaturally lower pitch to appear more masculine and powerful. Chemical exposure, heavy smoking and alcohol consumption, and vocal abuse have been associated with contact ulcers. Approximately one-third of voice disorders can be traced to some degree of increase in musculoskeletal tension and voice abuse (Cooper, 1973).

As noted above, hysterical aphonia is the complete loss of voice not due to organic, physical factors. Most authorities on hysterical aphonia attribute it to the conversion of significant emotional distress into a physical symptom, i.e., the loss of voice. Hysterical aphonia usually manifests itself in the patient's remarkable ability to voice during laughing, humming, coughing, and throat clearing, and his or her reverting to whispering during speech. Symbolically, patients with hysterical aphonia present with loss of voice to represent problems in social interaction, usually involving family members and significant others in sexual relationships.

23.12 Speaker Profiling Conjecture: Psychogenic Voice Disorders

For speaker profiling purposes, persons with voice disorders resulting totally or partially from psychogenic factors can be divided into two groups: tension-based and hysteria-based. The tension-based group consists of individuals with increased musculoskeletal tension due to their attempts to deal with external or internal stressors. In this group of subjects, psychogenic factors partially contribute to the voice disorder; however, vocal strain and abuse are equally or more important to their development. Vocal nodules, polyps, and contact ulcers are the primary voice pathologies

occurring in this group of speakers. The voice qualities of hoarseness and intermittent breaks in the ability to produce voice are the usual perceptual features of tension-based voice disorders. Some individuals will also have voice fatigue, particularly late in the day.

Typically, the person with a vocal nodule is a talkative, socially aggressive, middle-aged female. According to Aronson (1990), she suffers from persistent interpersonal problems that generate musculoskeletal tension, anxiety, depression, or anger. It is likely that she is also a singer without formal training. The person suffering from a vocal polyp may be allergic, asthmatic, and have engaged in one-time extreme vocal abuse such as screaming, shouting, or yelling very loudly. The typical person with a vocal contact ulcer is a talkative, socially aggressive, middle-aged male. "The classic profile of the contact ulcer patient is a male in his forties who uses his voice intensively in his daily life and is either a lawyer, teacher, minister, actor, or salesman. In personality, he is tense and hard-driving, and is often under chronic stress" (Aronson, 1990, p. 128).

A hysteria-based psychogenic voice disorder is an explicit signal sent by the person to seek medical, psychological, and family support for an underlying psychological turmoil (see Chapter 11). Hysteria-based aphonia and dysphonia are the complete and partial loss of the voice, respectively. These voice disorders are nonorganic, nonphysical in etiology, and sometimes called functional voice disorders. In many individuals, there is an inner conflict, usually the need to express a thought, feeling, or attitude, and fear of doing so. Curiously, the person with hysteria-based aphonia often presents with "la belle indifference" which means "the beautiful indifference." Although these patients may have been impaired or completely without voice for days, weeks, and even months, they do not appear distressed by their disorder. In fact, many appear unconcerned, lighthearted, and even relieved about it.

23.13 Speaker Profiling and Neurogenic Communication Disorders

There is no shortage of research and speculation about the role of brain damage and neurological impairments in antisocial personalities, psychopaths, and criminal behavior. Smith and Kling (1976) review the association of dissocial behavior with brain function including the role of frontal and temporal lobe lesions in aggressive behavior, violence, and impulse disorders. Lykken (1995) discusses genes, evolution, and brain dysfunction in the development of the antisocial personality, psychopaths, and perpetrators of violence. Stoff, Breiling, and Maser (1997) provide a comprehensive overview of brain damage and neurological dysfunction in antisocial behavior.

Neurogenic communication disorders are a large group of speech, voice, and language disorders caused by brain damage and neuromuscular impairments. For speaker profiling purposes, there are three etiological categories of neurogenic communication disorders: traumatic brain injury, degenerative diseases, and stroke. As a general rule, traumatic brain injuries are more common in young persons, degenerative diseases occur in the middle-years, and strokes primarily afflict individuals in the sixth, seventh, and later decades of life.

A. Traumatic Brain Injury

Neuroscientists have identified two types of traumatic head injuries causing brain damage: open and closed. Open head injuries occur when a projectile or missile penetrates the skull and enters the brain, tearing and shearing brain tissue. The projectile or missile is usually a hard object such as bullet, nail, or shrapnel. Closed head injuries occur from the head hitting a hard surface, such as during an automobile accident, or by a blunt blow from a weapon, such as a baseball bat hitting the head. The force of the impact causes brain damage at the site of the injury, and also acceleration and deceleration forces which rotate, tear, and shear the brain tissue. Today, neuroscientists know that both types of high-impact head injuries produce coup and contra-coup effects. The coup injury is the damage occurring at the site of the impact and the contra-coup effect occurs on the opposite side of the brain because of its recoil inside the skull. Both high-impact open and closed head injuries create focalized and diffuse brain damage. According to Fuller and Goodman (2001), if the head is not immobilized when struck, most of the injury is a contra-coup effect.

Because both open and closed head injuries can cause focalized and diffuse brain and neurological damage, the diagnostic category of traumatic brain injuries virtually spans the spectrum of neurogenic communication disorders. The language disorder of aphasia and the motor speech disorders of apraxia of speech and the dysarthrias can also occur as separate or combined entities. (Chapters 9 and 10 discuss neurogenic communication disorders and traumatic brain injuries from a medical malpractice standpoint). Persons with traumatic brain injuries can also suffer brain and neurological disorders that do not result in aphasia, apraxia of speech, or the dysarthrias, but impairs or disrupts awareness, reality testing, memory, orientation, and communication.

B. Degenerative Diseases

Degenerative diseases are major causes of the dysarthrias. Neuromuscular disorders such as amyotrophic lateral scle-

rosis or "Lou Gehrig's Disease," multiple sclerosis, and Parkinson disease cause slow degeneration of the muscles that produce speech. The list of degenerative diseases that can afflict humans is large and there are many types of neurological damage and symptoms. Many degenerative diseases have a slow, insidious onset and persons suffering from them have more difficulty coming to terms with their limitations. Because of the slow, pernicious nature of many degenerative diseases, the stages of grief are interrupted and there is back-and-forth movement through them. Many progressive diseases are often accompanied by exacerbation and remission of symptoms which may occur naturally or because of medical treatments. Consequently, the progression through denial, anger, bargaining, depression, and acceptance may be interrupted during periods of remission and exacerbation of symptoms. Some individuals may become fixed in a stage such as denial or anger for long periods, and some persons may never reach acceptance. When progressive degenerative diseases affect the frontal or temporal lobes of the brain, patients may also have many of the psychological reactions discussed below.

C. Stroke

Stroke is the leading cause of apraxia of speech and aphasia. There are two types of strokes: occlusive and hemorrhagic. An occlusive stroke is when an obstruction or "plug" stops or impairs the flow of blood to a part of the brain. A hemorrhagic stroke is the bursting of a blood vessel which also stops or impairs the flow of blood to a part of the brain. Occlusive strokes are the most common type of strokes, and hemorrhages also occur in traumatic brain injuries. Although an oversimplification, the main neurogenic communication disorders arising from brain and neurological injury involves aphasia (amnesia for words), apraxia of speech (problems programming words) and the dysarthrias (the effects of paralysis on speech muscles).

D. Communication Disorders and Frontal Lobe Damage

With regard to communication disorders, damage to the frontal lobes of the brain results in apraxia of speech, spastic dysarthria, expressive aphasia, and/or the frontal lobe syndrome seen in some traumatic brain injuries. Apraxia of speech involves the person's inability or impaired ability to plan, sequence, and activate the neuromuscular movements necessary to produce voluntary speech. Apraxia of speech results from damage to Broca's area proper in the third convolution (ridge) of the left frontal lobe in most right-handed persons. However, other areas of the frontal lobe of the brain are involved in planning, sequencing, and activating neuromuscular speech functions including the lateral premotor cortex (Wise, Greene, Büchel, and Scott, 1999).

Apraxia of speech can affect the five basic motor speech processes of respiration, phonation, articulation, resonance, and prosody, but usually involves the voluntary, articulatory processes. While some automatic utterances may be produced easily and without errors, persons with a mild-moderate apraxia of speech speak with articulatory groping, complications, and struggle. Many patients with severe apraxia of speech cannot produce meaningful speech. In pure apraxia of speech, which is rare, there are no other neurogenic communication disorders. Apraxia of speech is very frustrating for the speaker and listener.

Spastic dysarthria is the result of bilateral upper motor neuron damage. However, Duffy (1995) has identified a type of dysarthria resulting from unilateral upper motor neuron damage. The motor strips in the frontal lobes of both hemispheres of the brain regulate and inhibit muscular contraction. When there is damage to the motor strips, speech muscles become spastic and in a state of partial or complete contraction. Speech muscles become sluggish and their range of motion is limited. A person with spastic dysarthria often has a harsh voice, hypernasality, and slowly produced, distorted speech sound production.

Expressive aphasia is an inaccurate term used as a convenience primarily by clinicians to separate language into expressive and receptive functions. Expressive aphasia is assumed to result from damage to the left frontal lobe, in and around Broca's area, in most right-handed persons. Other terms for adult expressive language disturbances are Broca's, nonfluent, motor, and anterior aphasias. Expressive aphasia is an inaccurate term because it suggests that pure expressive language disorders exist and that there is a clear distinction between expressive and receptive vocabularies. Brownell (2000), and others, notes that expressive and receptive vocabularies are similar but expression involves motor speech memory and production. It is accurate to label this type of aphasia as "predominantly" expressive aphasia because usually patients have disruptions in all language functions albeit to differing degrees.

Frontal lobe syndrome is primarily associated with traumatic brain injuries and there is a collection of symptoms that occur together. Frontal lobe syndrome occurs when there is damage to the frontal lobes of the brain, and the patient is reduced in overall awareness and there is a decrease in the ability to monitor and regulate his or her behavior. Patients with frontal lobe syndrome tend to be concrete in their thinking, have difficulty initiating behaviors, and are often delayed in response time to questions and other stimuli.

E. Communication Disorders and Temporal Lobe Damage

With regard to communication disorders, temporal lobe damage is associated with auditory perceptual impairments and receptive aphasia. Auditory information coming from the ears is routed to the superior temporal gyrus of the cortex. Technically, the auditory cortex extends into the parietal lobe of the left hemisphere, but the primary neurons are found in the temporal lobe especially for pure auditory information. Martin and Clark (2003) note that auditory discrimination occurs cortically and subcortically.

Auditory perceptual disorders go by several clinical labels, and affect the ability to attend to and process auditory information. Auditory perception involves sound detection, localization, categorization, and identification. Higher in the perceptual process are speech reception and discrimination. Auditory processing disorders include attentional deficits with and without hyperactivity and the agnosias. Clinically, auditory processing disorders are a collection of vaguely defined disorders that include several learning disabilities, attentional deficits, cognitive impairments, and specific language disorders primarily occurring in children. Agnosia, a term first coined by Sigmund Freud, is a processing disorder usually limited to one sense modality. Auditory agnosia, difficulty perceiving and attaching meaning to general environmental and speech sounds, is often an indistinguishable component of receptive aphasia. Other terms for receptive aphasia are Wernicke's, sensory, jargon, and posterior aphasias.

Receptive aphasia is assumed to be caused by focalized lesions to the primary and secondary auditory cortex of the brain, Wernicke's area, which is found in the left temporal lobe of most persons. However, some authorities include parts of the parietal lobe in receptive aphasia especially as it relates to reading deficits and denial of disability. Receptive aphasia, like expressive aphasia discussed above, is an inaccurate but a convenient diagnostic category. Although the auditory cortex is important for auditory comprehension, it is not the "center" for receptive language nor does damage to it exclusively cause all of symptoms typically associated with receptive aphasia (Tanner, 2007, 2006b). Describing this multimodality language disorder as "predominantly" receptive aphasia is more accurate and recognizes that perceptual functions are involved and that comprehension involves the totality of the brain. Like predominantly expressive aphasia, predominantly receptive aphasia cuts across all language modalities to differing degrees. The person with predominantly receptive aphasia suffers from the inability or impaired ability to communicate in all modalities with primary involvement of the receptive avenues of communication: auditory perception and comprehension, reading, and understanding gestures.

Some patients with predominantly receptive aphasia speak jargon. Aphasic jargon speech is the fluent uttering of words and phrases which are lacking in meaning, sometimes called "empty speech." Jargon aphasia is often associated with anosognosia, the denial of disability, and projection, the psychological process of attributing the disorder to someone else. Jargon aphasics often fluently produce meaningless speech and act as if they could be understood should listeners simply try harder.

23.14 Speaker Profiling Conjecture: Neurogenic Communication Disorders

Tempting though it may be, drawing conclusions about dissocial, aggressive, violent, impulsive, and other behaviors in a particular person exclusively from brain site of lesion is fraught with error. Certainly, broad generalizations can be made about the functions brain hemispheres, lobes, tracts, and neuronal bundles play in thoughts and behaviors in large groups of people. However, it should be recognized that significant numbers of individuals will be exceptions to any generalization. Brain and central nervous system functioning is very complex and varies significantly from person to person.

The localization movement in neurogenic communication disorders, the attempt to find and map parts of the brain responsible for specific speech and language functions and disorders has a long and checkered history. While motor and sensory tracts can be identified with some degree of accuracy, pinpointing a mass of brain cells responsible for many other aspects of communication in all persons is theoretically unsound. The brain works holistically and there are individual differences in the location of speech and language functions and manifestations of brain damage. No better example exists of this localization futility than the mapping of language functions and projecting them to disorders. For example, while it is true that the majority of right-handed persons have language functions represented in the left brain hemisphere, some persons have them located in the right-hemisphere. And what is most remarkable, many normal left-handed persons have language represented in their right hemispheres. A stroke for example, in the left hemisphere of the brain will not necessarily result in aphasia in all persons.

At the core of controversies regarding the localization movement is the "brain-mind leap." This scientific, philosophical, and religious issue is the projecting of the neurological activities in the brain to what occurs in a person's mind.

The magnitude of the brain-mind leap can be demonstrated by addressing semantic representations in the brain. Neurologically, the meaning of the word "truthfulness," for example, can be found in the atomic particles in neurons, and the chemical interactions of neurotransmitters at their synaptic junctions. The meaning of the word "truthfulness" is likely a composite of these changes to cellular chemistry and continuous action potentials in thousands of neurons and their dendrite-to-axon connections. These electrochemical reactions somehow create the continuous imagery and semantic associations necessary to sense the meaning of the word and to use it expressively. Interestingly, the neuronal impulses, their action potentials, and cellular chemical stores have continuity. They are consistent from one semantic retrieval to another, yet the meaning of the word evolves with life experience. Through this ongoing continuous nervous energy and chemical changes at the cellular level, a person is conscious of the meaning of "truthfulness," and in fact, the semantics of the word becomes part of his or her consciousness (Tanner, 2006b, pp. 162-163).

With the above qualifiers, valuable profiles can be drawn about dissocial, aggressive, violent, impulsive, and other behaviors based on the site or sites of lesion causing neurogenic communication disorders.

23.15 Speaker Profiling Conjecture and Traumatically Induced Neurogenic Communication Disorders

The majority of individuals with traumatic brain injuries have communication disorders either as a direct result of damage to the major speech and language centers, indirectly as a consequence of reduced or disordered awareness, or a combination of factors. Regardless of the specific manifestations of the brain damage, accurate profiles can be drawn for the typical adult person likely to suffer a traumatic brain injury. First, according to Hickey (1997), the presumptive causes of TBI are motor vehicle accidents (50 percent), followed by falls (21 percent), and assaults or other type of violence (12 percent). However, there is evidence that assaults and other types of violence, such as drive-by shootings, have increased in recent years. Kraus and Sorenson (1994) show that the age group of fifteen to twenty-four is at the highest risk for traumatic brain injury. All studies show that single males are at more risk for TBI than married persons or females. Males tend to be aggressive, chance-takers, and single ones are more likely to take greater sport and climbing risks, and drive vehicles fast and recklessly. Alcohol and drugs are involved in more than 50 percent of traumatic brain injuries. Typically, the traumatic brain injured person has a poor education and is employed, if at all, in a low-paying risky job. Although there are no studies showing traumatic brain injured persons have lower intelligence, they are likely learning disabled which has contributed to academic and other learning frustration throughout school. Perhaps because of their problems learning and profiting from experience, traumatic brain injury patients are likely to have been previously admitted to a hospital for a head injury.

A patient in a coma, stupor, delirium, or who has significant clouding of consciousness is likely to be institutionalized and consequently not of forensic or legal interest. When traumatic brain damage does not cause coma, stupor, delirium, or significant clouding of consciousness, psychological generalities can be made about patients with neurogenic communication disorders. As Table 23.2 shows, the patient with traumatic brain damage, regardless of whether the major speech and language centers have been impaired, can have problems with reality testing, memory, and orientation.

A patient with TBI-induced reality-testing problems has posttraumatic psychosis. Smeltzer, Nasrallah, and Miller (1994) note that psychosis in traumatic brain-injured persons is highly variable and ranges from 20-50 percent. The patient with posttraumatic psychosis has general prob-

lems with reality testing and suffers from minor and occasional delusions and hallucinations, or he or she may be plagued by frequent, or even constant, psychosis. The traumatic brain-injured person with functional communication abilities will communicate the occurrence and nature of these breaks with reality. It is important that when investigating delusions and hallucinations that the TBI patient's reports be confirmed by his or her actions. Persons with aphasia often use words with related meanings to the appropriate ones or association errors (see Chapter 10). Psychotic statements made by the patient may be misleading and indicate delusions and hallucinations, when in fact, the reports are simply a result of impaired language abilities (Tanner, 2006a). However, if psychotic actions accompany the reports, then it can be assumed that the patient is indeed suffering from posttraumatic psychosis.

A patient with TBI-induced amnesia may be suffering from memory loss for events occurring before the injury, retrograde amnesia, or have difficulty remembering new information, anterograde amnesia, or both. The person with retrograde amnesia may have selected memory deficits, including committing crimes and specific events related to them, or complete loss of memory for weeks, months, years, and even decades. The person with anterograde amnesia will have problems remembering events since the traumatic brain injury including forensic interviews and interrogations, statements made about a crime, and even meeting forensic interviewers and investigators. Reports from persons with posttraumatic amnesias must be considered suspect.

Table 23.2
Reality Testing, Memory, and Orientation Disorders in Traumatic Brain Injury

Function	Disorder	Description
Reality Testing	Posttraumatic psychosis	Break with one or more aspects of reality: delusions and hallucinations
Memory	Retrograde and anterograde amnesia	Memory loss of events before and/or after the TBI, problems learning
Orientation	Disorientation to time, place, person, and/or predicament	Confusion about time events and/or the passage of time, people (including self), place, and his or her predicament

The person with disorientation may be completely confused about time, place, person, and predicament, or partially disoriented to one or more of these facets of reality. Disorientation to time involves two factors: perception of the passage of time and remembering time events. The TBI person may have difficulty accurately perceiving the passage of time; he or she may believe ten minutes lasted one minute or an hour. Time disorientation includes problems remembering days of the week, months of the year, seasons, the correct year or decade, and so forth. Disorientation to place involves bewilderment about buildings, cities, states, and country of origin; the person is confused about specific or general locations. Disorientation to person involves mental confusion about relationships such as family members, past and current spouses, partners, and associates. On a fundamental level, a person with this type of disorientation may be confused about his or her self, gender, occupation, and other basic self-concept information. The TBI person disoriented to predicament may be confused about whether or not he or she has indeed suffered brain injury, and also events surrounding a crime or incident. A person mixed-up about predicament is not simply denying involvement with a crime or incident, but is actually mentally confused about his or her actual involvement in them. The memory deficits discussed above play important roles in orientation, for if a person could remember aspects related to time, place, person, and predicament, he or she would have basic orientation. This is not to say that all disorientation is a product of memory impairments, only that memory and orientation are fundamentally related.

Most persons with significant traumatic brain injuries have impaired "metacognition" or "thinking about thinking." According to Gillis (1996, p.111), they have difficulty recalling information, organizing, planning, and monitoring behaviors, and problems with inhibition:

> It is involved in the monitoring of cognitive processes (input and output). This monitoring includes knowing how and when to attend to and organize information; knowing how, when and what to remember; knowing when a problem exists and which solutions have worked or failed; and knowing the individual strengths and weaknesses of different processes and strategies.

Metacognition is sometimes referred to as mental executive functioning and has been linked to damage to the frontal and temporal lobes.

As can be surmised from the above discussion of neurogenic communication disorders related to traumatic brain injury, the subject's veracity about his or her involvement with a crime or incident, and information surrounding these events, is suspect. The speaker profile conjecture of a person with significant traumatic brain injury and functional communication abilities is a young unattached learning-disabled male earning low wages and working in a risky job with reality testing, memory, and orientation problems. He also is likely to be a risk-taker, engages in substance abuse, and has probably been repeatedly hospitalized for traumatic head injuries. While the traumatically brain-injured person may be consciously deceptive, it is also likely that he cannot accurately remember events related to a crime or incident.

23.16 Speaker Profiling Conjecture and Non-Traumatically Induced Neurogenic Communication Disorders Arising from Frontal Lobe Damage

The psychological reactions associated with non-traumatically induced neurogenic communication disorders has been studied extensively (Tanner (2003b), Gordon, et al. (1996), Tanner and Gerstenberger, (1996), Gainotti, (1989), Robinson, et al., (1988), Lipsey, et al., (1986), Robinson, (1986), Robinson, et al., (1985), Gordon, et al., (1985), Sackeim and Weber, (1982), Sackeim, et al, (1982), Robinson and Benson, (1981), Gasparini, et al., (1978), Black, (1975), Weinstein and Puig-Antich, (1974), Gainotti, (1972), Weinstein, et al., (1966), and others.) Neuroscientists have discovered that many of the psychological reactions caused by brain injury are similar to the psychological reactions seen in emotional disturbances not caused by brain damage. Consequently, many non-traumatically induced brain-injured speakers show many of the psychological reactions displayed by normal, psychologically disturbed persons.

There is no shortage of studies linking frontal lobe brain damage to dissocial, aggressive, violent, impulsive, and other behaviors. Many authors have tied damage to the frontal lobes of the brain with the propensity for violence, impulsivity, aggression, hostility, and many other potentially antisocial behaviors. Some have concluded that most violent offenders have frontal lobe irregularities or brain damage, and may have inherited the propensity for criminal behavior. However, regarding non-traumatically induced frontal lobe damage and cooccurring neurogenic communication disorders, there are four psychological concomitants: emotional lability, perseveration-echolalia, anxiety-depression, and catastrophic reactions. These reactions are likely to be part of a speaker profile for a person with apraxia of speech, spastic dysarthria, and/or expressive aphasia arising from non-traumatically induced frontal lobe damage.

A speaker with spastic dysarthria is probably emotionally labile. Emotional lability, sometimes called "pseudobulbar emotional lability" is usually seen as unwarranted and uncontrolled crying. Technically, emotional lability refers to wide swings in emotions and can include uncontrolled laughing and other emotional behaviors. However, because there is more to be sad about for many brain-injured persons, crying is the most common emotional reaction resulting from bilateral damage to the motor strips in the frontal lobes and associated corticobulbar tracts of the brain. A speaker with emotional lability usually does not have "inappropriate" emotions; his or her emotions are "exaggerated." However, in rare instances, a speaker may have emotional behaviors disconnected to true emotions. Three stimuli may prompt bouts of emotionally labile speakers: highly charged words, being placed in emotional situations, and certain thoughts. Once the emotional response is set into motion, it is often difficult to stop. A speaker with severe emotional lability may give the impression of being demented (Duffy, 1995), but it can also occur in persons with normal cognition. When a speaker has spastic dysarthria and is highly emotional, his or her emotions are likely to be partially or completely exaggerated as a result of the brain and neurological injury.

Perseveration is the tendency to continue an activity for a longer time than is warranted by the significance of the stimulus prompting it. Echolalia, a manifestation of perseveration, is the automatic repeating of what has been said. Both are associated with damage to the frontal lobes of the brain. Perseveration-echolalia can be likened to a song or tune that repeatedly goes through a person's mind, only in patients with neurogenic communication disorders, much more extreme. A subject with frontal lobe brain damage who cannot seem to break from a topic or automatically repeats what has been spoken is likely suffering from the effects of the brain and neurological damage, and is not necessarily being evasive, deceptive, or uncooperative for self-serving reasons.

When a subject has left frontal lobe brain damage and accompanying neurogenic communication disorders, he or she is more likely to suffer from anxiety-depressive disorders than a person who has had right hemisphere or temporal lobe damage. When a person has brain injury to the anterior (front) part of the left hemisphere, he or she is likely to endure anxiety-depression that will be long-lasting. How-

ever, if the brain damage is in the posterior part of the left hemisphere, the subject is likely to display indifference, lack of awareness of his or her disabilities, and even euphoria. It also appears that the smaller the brain lesion, the more likely the subject will be aware of his or her disorder, and suffer more anxiety, frustration, and depression. For some yet-to-be-determined reason, females have more strokes involving the anterior part of the brain, and males suffer more from strokes affecting the posterior region. Consequently, speakers with nonfluent, predominantly expressive aphasia are likely to be anxious-depressed women, while speakers with fluent, predominantly receptive aphasia are likely to be indifferent, unaware, and euphoric men.

A catastrophic reaction can be described as an anxiety attack, and the more nonfluent the speech output, the more likely the subject will suffer from it. A subject with nonfluent aphasia has trouble remembering words for expression and difficulty producing them. Speech is produced with hesitations, struggle, revisions, and complications, and because the understanding parts of the brain have not been damaged, the speaker is aware of the nonfluencies and errors. Consequently, nonfluent aphasia is frustrating, especially when an aphasic person is placed in a situation where important and critical speaking is required such as a forensic interview and interrogation. Some aphasic persons may suffer from one or more catastrophic reactions in these situations. When too much pressure builds, they may strike out physically and verbally. Most catastrophic reactions occur when stimuli overwhelm the speaker and rapid responses are required of him or her. The subject with expressive aphasia who strikes out when under pressure to respond verbally is doing so, at least partially, because of the brain and neurological damage.

23.17 Speaker Profiling Conjecture and Non-Traumatically Induced Neurogenic Communication Disorders Arising from Temporal Lobe Damage

Neuroscientists have linked temporal lobe brain damage to dissocial, aggressive, violent, impulsive, and other behaviors. Kling (1976) provides a review of animal and human behavioral changes, particularly aggression, in temporal lobe damage. Tardiff (1997), and others, have found organic brain disease affecting the temporal lobes to result in a propensity for violence. Temporal lobe epilepsy has been associated with purposeless violence as have brain infections, diseases, and strokes. Temporal lobe damage and many accompanying antisocial behaviors are well-accepted aspects of traumatic brain injury (see above). The amygdala, part of the reticular activating system which is deep in the temporal lobe, appears to play an important role in regulating violent, aggressive, and other antisocial behavior.

There are three non-traumatic induced temporal lobe damage and cooccurring neurogenic communication disorders psychological concomitants: denial of disability, projection, and jargon-confabulation. They are likely to be a part of the speaker profile for a person with predominantly receptive aphasia and auditory processing disorders.

When a subject produces aphasic jargon speech, he or she is likely to have damage to Wernicke's and adjacent areas of the left temporal-parietal lobes. Denial of disability, anosognosia, is also a frequent occurrence in many persons with this type of neurogenic communication disorder (Weinstein et al., 1966; Weinstein and Puig-Antich, 1974, Tanner, 2006b). Denial of disability and other aspects of the communication situation account for the persistent meaningless speech in many persons with aphasic jargon. If not for denial, persons with aphasic jargon would recognize that their communication acts are unsuccessful and would stop talking. When a subject, not employing denial, realizes that his or her requests and answers to questions are not understood, he or she will stop talking altogether and recognize the futility of the situation. However, when a jargon aphasic persists in his or her meaningless output, even when it is apparent that little if any functional communication occurs, denial prohibits the individual from appreciating the futility of the interaction. The subject with persistent partial or complete jargon output is engaging, at least in part, in the psychological coping style and defense of denial, and does not appreciate the significance of the communicative situation. Many denying persons with persistent jargon also engage in the coping style and psychological defense of projection.

Projection is the attributing of one's own intolerable thoughts and feelings to another person. Projection, in the extreme, plays an important role in the genesis of psychotic behaviors and delusions. Project and denial go together; one must deny negative emotions and psychological upheaval in himself or herself to project them to another. The denying, projecting subject with aphasic jargon speech denies that he or she is communicatively impaired, that communication is malfunctioning, and additionally, projects the problems onto the listener. Many subjects with aphasic jargon output utter nonsense and act as if the listeners would simply try harder, they would understand the perfectly normal attempts at communication. Because of the neurogenic communication disorder, denial, and projection, most if not all statements made by the subject are meaningless for legal and forensic purposes.

Confabulation is more than just lying; it is remarking about an event without consideration of the facts related to it, and in the extreme, disregard of the reality associated with an event. During forensic interviewing and interrogation, confabulation is the speaker giving answers to questions with little or no regard to their truthfulness. The subject engaging in confabulation makes up false stories, often to fill in unknown gaps in a real occurrence, and may or may not be self-serving. Confabulation is related to the coping style and psychological defense of fantasy and a form of psychological escape. It can also be reporting of excessive, wish-fulfilling daydreaming that has become so chronic that the speaker believes the events and confuses true and false memories. Confabulation is associated with frontal lobe injury, dementia, and widespread cortical and subcortical damage, but also with partial jargon aphasia and temporal-parietal lobe damage (Wernicke's encephalopathy). The subject with partial jargon aphasia may confabulate as part of denial-projection and disregard the facts surrounding an event. A confabulating subject may be reporting a false memory where he or she remembers an earlier traumatic experience that had been repressed. Regardless of the organic or functional causes of confabulation, by definition, the veracity and accuracy of a confabulating speaker's reports are suspect. Table 23.3 summarizes the communication processes, disorders, and important speaker profiling conjecture regarding communication disorders.

23.18 Chapter Summary

With approximately one-in-ten persons having a communication disorder, there is forensic value in examining speakers from this subpopulation. Although generalities are difficult to make about the heterogenous communication disordered population, many speakers suffer from reduced self-esteem, particularly in speaking situations. Some members of the Deaf Community consider themselves a repressed minority due to their adherence to sign language and rejection of other forms of communication. Some speakers engage in immature and regressive speech for identification purposes and to avoid having mature relationships. Speakers who stutter, especially those with adult-onset, may have underlying psychological reactions causing or contributing to the dysfluencies. Many voice disorders are psychogenic in origin. Speakers suffering from neurogenic communication disorders have predictable psychological reactions related to type of brain damage and sites of lesions.

Table 23.3
Speaker Profiling and Neurogenic Communication Disorders

Communication Process	Communication Disorder	Speaker Profile
Hearing	Deafness	May ascribe to the repressed minority viewpoint about deafness and the Deaf Community.
Articulation	Immature and regressive speech	Adults who lisp and lall may be using speech patterns to avoid mature, adult relationships.
Fluency	Stuttering	Adults who stutter may feel inferior to normal speakers, have repressed hostility, and experience reduced self-esteem in speaking situations.
Voice	Psychogenic voice disorders	Talkative, socially aggressive person with vocal nodules, polyps, and contact ulcers; inner conflicted person with hysterical aphonia.
Neurogenic Communication Disorders	Communication disorders associated with traumatic brain injury and/or focalized frontal and temporal lobe damage	TBI subjects have deficits with reality testing, memory, and disorientation; frontal lobe damage associated with depression, anxiety, emotional lability, perseveration-echolalia, and catastrophic reactions; temporal lobe damage associated with denial of disability, projection, and jargon-confabulation.

Suggested Readings and Films

Aronson, A. (1990). *Clinical Voice Disorders: An Interdisciplinary Approach.* New York: Thieme. This clinical textbook addresses many psychological issues associated with voice disorders.

Gillis, R., & Pierce, J. (1996). Mechanism of traumatic brain injury and the pathophysiologic consequences. In R. Gillis (Ed), *Traumatic Brain Injury Rehabilitation for Speech-language Pathologists.* Boston: Butterworth-Heinemann. This chapter reviews many of the cognitive and psychological issues in traumatic brain injury.

Tanner, D. (2003). *The Psychology of Neurogenic Communication Disorders: A Primer for Health Care Professionals.* Boston: Allyn & Bacon. This book provides an overview of the psychological issues associated with neurogenic communication disorders.

Yeoman, B. (1998, November/December). Wrestling with words. *Psychology Today,* 31(6): 42-47. This article addresses societal views of stuttering.

Two movies about posttraumatic amnesia accurately illustrate the crime-related issues. *The Bourne Identity* portrays retrograde amnesia and *Memento* illustrates the difficulty experienced by a person with anterograde amnesia.

References

Aronson, A. (1990). *Clinical voice disorders: An interdisciplinary approach.* New York: Thieme.

Bello, J. (1995). Hearing loss and hearing aid use in the United States. *Communication facts.* Rockville, MD: American Speech-Language-Hearing Association.

Black, F. (1975). Unilateral brain lesions and MMPI performance: A preliminary study. *Perceptual and Motor Skills*, 40: 87-93.

Brownell, R. (2000). *Expressive One-Word Picture Vocabulary Test* (3rd ed). Novato, C.A.: Academic Therapy Publications.

Cooper, M. (1973). *Modern techniques of vocal rehabilitation*. Springfield, Ill.: Charles C. Thomas.

Duffy, J. (1995). *Motor speech disorders*. St. Louis: Mosby.

Fuller, G. N. and Goodman, J.C. (2001). *Practical review of neuropathology*. Philadelphia: Lippincott, Williams, and Wilkins.

Gainotti, G. (1989). The meaning of emotional disturbances resulting from unilateral brain injury. In *Emotions and the dual brain,* G. Gainotti, and C. Caltagirone (Eds). New York: Springer-Verlag.

Gainotti, G. (1972). Emotional behavior and hemisphere side of the lesion. *Cortex*, 8: 41-55.

Gasparini, W., Satz, P., Heilman, K., and Coolidge, F. (1978). Hemispheric asymmetries of affective processing as determined by the Minnesota Multiphasic Personality Inventory. *Journal of Neurology, Neurosurgery and Psychiatry*, 41: 470-473.

Gillis, R., & Pierce, J. (1996). Mechanism of traumatic brain injury and the pathophysiologic consequences. In R. Gillis (Ed), *Traumatic brain injury rehabilitation for speech-language pathologists.* Boston: Butterworth-Heinemann.

Gordon, W., Hibbard, M., and Morganstein, S. (1996). Response to Tanner and Gerstenberger. In *Forums in Clinical Aphasiology*, C. Code (Ed). London, UK: Whurr Publishers.

Gordon, W., Hibbard, M., Egelko, S., and Diller, L. (1985). The multifaceted nature of the cognitive deficits following stroke: Unexpected findings. *Archives of Physical Medicine and Rehabilitation*, 66: 338.

Hall, B.J., Oyer, H.J., and Haas, W. H. (2001). *Speech , language, and hearing disorders: A guide for teachers.* Boston: Allyn & Bacon.

Herrmann, M. and Wallesch, C. (1989). Psychosocial changes and psychosocial adjustments with chronic and severe non-fluent aphasia. *Aphasiology,* 3(6): 513-526.

Herrmann, M., Barrels, C., and Wallesch, C. (1993). Depression in acute and chronic aphasia: symptoms, pathoanatomical-clinical correlations and functional implications. *Journal of Neurology, Neurosurgery, and Psychiatry,* 56(6): 672-678.

Hickey, J. (1997). Craniocerebral injuries: In J. Hickey (Ed), *The clinical practice of neurological and neurosurgical nursing* (4th ed.). Philadelphia: Lippincott.

Johnson, W. (1930). *Because I stutter*. New York: Appleton-Century-Crofts.

Kling, A. (1976). Frontal and temporal lobe lesions and aggressive Behavior. In W. Smith and A. Kling (Eds). *Issues in brain/behavior control* (pp. 11-22). New York: Spectrum Publications.

Kraus, J. and Sorenson, S. (1994). Epidemiology. In J. Silver, S. Yudofsky, and R. Hales (Eds) *Neuropsychiatry of traumatic brain injury.* Washington, DC: American Psychiatric Press.

Linn, G.W., & Caruso, A.J. (1998, July-September). Perspectives on the effects of stuttering on the formation and maintenance of intimate relationships. *Journal of Rehabilitation,* 64(3): 12-14.

Lipsey, J., Spencer, W., Rabins, P., and Robinson, R. (1986). Phenomenological comparison of poststroke depression and functional depression. *American Journal of Psychiatry*, 143:4.

Lykken, D.T. (1995). *The antisocial personality*. Hillsdale, N.J.: Lawrence Erlbaum Associates, Publishers.

Martin, F. and Clark, J. (2003). *Introduction to audiology* (8th ed.). Boston: Allyn & Bacon.

National Center for Health Statistics. (1988). Current estimates from the National Health Interview Survey, United States, 1988. *Vital and health statistics*, Series 10, No. 173 DHHS Publication No. (PHS) 89-1501.

Owens, R., Metz, D.E., & Haas, A. (2000). *Communication disorders: A life span perspective.* Boston: Allyn & Bacon.

Robinson, R., Lipsey, J., Bolla-Wilson, K, Bolduc, P., Pearlson, G, Rao, K., and Price, T. (1985). Mood disorders in left-handed stroke patients. *American Journal of Psychiatry* 142:12.

Robinson, R., Boston, J., Starkstein, S. and Price, T. (1988). Comparison of mania and depression after brain injury: causal factors. *American Journal of Psychiatry*, 145:2.

Robinson, R. (1986). Depression and stroke. *Psychiatric Annals*, 17(11): 731-740.

Robinson, R., and Benson, D. (1981). Depression in aphasic patients: frequency, severity, and clinical-pathological correlations. *Brain and Language*, 14: 282-291.

Ruben, R.J. (2000). Redefining the survival of the fittest: Communication disorders in the 21st century. *Laryngoscope, 110*: 241-245.

Sackeim, H., Greenberg, M., Weiman, A., Gur, R., Hungerbahler, J., and Geschwin, N. (1982). Hemispheric asymmetry in the expression of positive and negative emotions: neurological evidence. *Archives of Neurology,* 39: 210-218.

Sackeim, H. and Weber, S. (1982). Functional brain asymmetry in the regulation of emotion: Implications for bodily manifestations of stress. In *Handbook of Stress*, L. Goldberger and S. Breznitz (Eds). New York: Macmillan.

Sacks, O. (1990). *Seeing voices: A journey into the world of the deaf*. New York: Vintage Books.

Smeltzer, D., Nasrallah, H., and Miller, S. (1994). Psychotic disorders. In J. Silver, S. Yudofsky, and R. Hales (Eds) *Neuropsychiatry of traumatic brain injury*. Washington, DC: American Psychiatric Press.

Smith, W. L. and Kling, A. (1976). *Issues in brain/behavior control*. New York: Spectrum Publications.

Stoff, D.M., Breiling, J., and Maser, J.D. *Handbook of antisocial behavior*. New York: John Wiley & Sons.

Stuart, G. (1998). Self-concept responses and dissociative disorders. In *Principles and practice of psychiatric nursing (6th ed.),* G. Stuart and M. Laraia (Eds). St. Louis: Mosby

Tanner, D. and Gerstenberger, D. (1996). Clinical Forum 9: The Grief Model in Aphasia. In *Forums in Clinical Aphasiology*, C. Code (Ed). London: Whurr Publishers

Tanner, D. (2001). Hooray for Hollywood: Communication disorders and the motion picture industry. *ASHA Leader*, 6(6): 10.

Tanner, D. (2003a). *Exploring communication disorders: A 21st century introduction through literature and media*. Boston: Allyn and Bacon.

Tanner, D. (2003b). Eclectic perspectives on the psychology of aphasia. *Journal of Allied Health*, 32, 256-260.

Tanner, D. (2006a). *Case studies in communication sciences and disorders*. Upper Saddle River, N.J.: Pearson Merrill Prentice Hall.

Tanner, D. (2006b). *An advanced course in communication sciences and disorder*. San Diego: Plural Publishing.

Tanner, D. (2007, In Press). Redefining Wernicke's area: receptive language and discourse semantics. *Journal of Allied Health*.

Tanner, D., Culbertson, W., and Secord, W. (1997). *The developmental articulation and phonology profile (DAPP)*. Oceanside, C.A.: Academic Communication Associates.

Tardiff, K. (1997). Evaluation and Treatment of Violent Patients. In D. Stoff, J. Breiling, and J.D. Maser (Eds). *Handbook of antisocial behavior* (pp. 445-453). New York: John Wiley & Sons.

Van Riper, C., & Erickson, R. (1996). *Speech correction* (9th ed). Boston: Allyn & Bacon.

Weinstein, E. and Puig-Antich, J. (1974). Jargon and its Analogues. *Cortex*, 10:75-83.

Weinstein, E., Lyerly, O., Cole, M., and Ozer, M. (1966). Meaning in Jargon Aphasia. *Cortex*, 2: 165-187.

Wise, R.J.S., Greene, J., Büchel, C., & Scott, S.K. (1999). Brain regions involved in articulation. *Lancet*, 353: 1057-61.

Yeoman, B. (1998, November/December). Wrestling with words. *Psychology Today,* 31(6): 42-47.

Glossary of Terms

A

AAA: American Academy of Audiology.

Abduction: In voice, the moving away from the midline of the two vocal folds; opening of the glottis.

Abductor: In voice, the muscle that performs abduction; posterior cricoarytenoid muscle.

ABLB: Alternate binaural loudness balance.

Abstract attitude: Ability to symbolize and categorize verbal and nonverbal information; generalized ability to understand relationships.

Abulia: The chronic inability to make decisions or to perform voluntary activities. Chronic procrastination.

Abusive voice: Phonatory action involving excessive force. This force usually results from excessive muscular tension during phonation and/or inefficient use of pulmonary airflow.

Acalculia: The inability to perform and understand simple mathematics.

Accent: A distinctive speech pattern associated with a particular geographical, cultural, socioeconomic, or a dialectical group; carryover of the traits of one language to another.

Accessory behaviors: Habituated avoidance and escape reactions to stuttering that vary from stutterer to stutterer.

Acoustic agnosia: Inability to perceive differences in speech signals, errors of speech sound discrimination, and the inability to perceive salient auditory linguistic features.

Acoustic gain: Difference between the intensity of an input signal and intensity of an output signal of a hearing aid or other electroacoustic device.

Acoustic impedance: Opposition to or resistance of sound energy through the middle ear.

Acoustic nerve: The cochlear branch of cranial nerve VIII; the vestibulocochlear nerve.

Acoustic neuroma: A tumor of the auditory nerve.

Acoustic reflex: Automatic contraction of the stapedius and tensor tympani muscles in response to a loud tone; also called the stapedial reflex.

Acoustic reflex threshold: Lowest intensity or loudness of a tone producing the acoustic reflex.

Acoustics: A branch of physics dealing with the audible displacement of air molecules.

Acquired hearing loss: Hearing loss that is not congenital. Hearing loss occurring after birth as a result of disease or injury.

Addition: In speech articulation, a sound placed in a word where there should not be one.

Adductors: In voice, the muscles that perform adduction. These include the lateral cricoarytenoid, transverse arytenoid, oblique arytenoid, and thyroarytenoid muscles.

ADL: Activities of daily living.

Adventitious deafness: Deafness occurring after birth because of disease or injury. Acquired deafness.

Affect: Emotion associated with a thought or statement.

Affricate: A speech sound that consists of a plosive and a brief fricative.

Agnosia: The inability to recognize and appreciate the significance of sensory stimuli; usually specific to one modality of communication.

Agrammatism: Loss of the ability to understand and use the grammar of a language. The omission of grammatical units of language. See Telegraphic Speech.

Agraphia: The inability to express oneself in writing. The inability to write secondary to central language deficits and not due to limb paralysis or weakness.

AIDS: Acquired immune deficiency syndrome.

Air conduction testing: Measurement of the auditory system by presenting tones of different frequencies and loudness levels.

Air-bone gap: In audiology, the difference, measured in decibels, that an air conduction threshold exceeds bone conduction threshold at any frequency.

Alexia: The inability to read secondary to a perceptual or language deficit; the inability to read not due to visual acuity deficits or blindness.

Alternate binaural loudness balance: An auditory test to measure loudness growth or recruitment in the impaired ear.

Alveolar: A phonetic place of articulation that refers to the ridge of tissue just behind the upper incisors: the anterior part of the superior (maxillary) dental alveolus, posterior to the incisors.

Amnesia: Partial or complete inability to recognize or recall past events; loss of memory.

Anomia: Loss of the ability to recall words; not limited to nouns.

Anoxia: Lack of oxygen to the brain.

Anterograde amnesia: Loss of the ability to form, store, and recall new memories.

Aperiodic: Without periodicity; irregular.

Aphasia: Multimodality inability to encode, decode and/or manipulate symbols for the purposes of verbal thought and/or communication. The loss of the ability to use language due to damage to the speech and language centers of the brain.

Aphonia: Loss of the ability to vibrate the vocal folds to produce voice. The complete lack of phonation; without voice.

Apraxia of speech: Loss of the ability to plan and sequence speech acts due to a neurological disorder.

Articulation: Shaping compressed air from the lungs into individual speech sounds. The act of moving the vocal tract structures in such a manner that speech sounds are produced.

Articulator: An organ of the speech mechanism that valves the compressed air coming from the lungs.

ASHA: The American Speech-Language-Hearing Association.

asp: Aspirate.

Aspiration: In phonetics, addition of the whispered glottal sound source to the normal sound of a phoneme. In dysphagia, ingestion of food or liquid into the respiratory system.

Association: The internalization of information and the process of making it personally relevant. Relating of experiences, perceptions, and thoughts.

Ataxic dysarthria: A subtype of dysarthria usually associated with damage to the cerebellum and the tracts leading to and from it. Speech is produced with improper timing, stress, and coordination.

Audiogram: Graph for recording air and bone conduction thresholds.

Audiology: Branch of science concerned with the study, diagnosis, and treatment of hearing disorders.

Audiometrist: An audiology technician working under the supervision of an audiologist or otologist.

Auditory acclimatization: The gradual process of becoming accustomed to the increased loudness of a sound.

Auditory-acoustic agnosia: Inability to perceive differences in speech and environmental signals. The inability to perceive salient auditory features.

Auditory agnosia: Inability to perceive differences in auditory stimuli, including environmental sounds.

Auditory cortex: Auditory area located in the superior temporal lobe of the cerebral cortex, also called Heschl's gyrus.

Auditory canal: External auditory meatus. The anatomical conduit between the pinna and the tympanic membrane; the ear canal.

Auditory closure: Process by which auditory stimuli are integrated into a perceptual whole.

Auditory discrimination: Ability to perceive differences in sounds.

Auditory evoked potentials: A passive test to predict hearing sensitivity and the functioning of cranial nerve VIII and auditory brainstem structures.

Auditory perception: The process of detecting salient features from the hearing mechanism. The mental awareness of a sound and organization of sensory data received from the ears.

Auditory training: Therapy provided to a patient with a hearing loss to maximize the use of residual hearing.

Aural rehabilitation: Therapies to improve a hearing-impaired person's ability to communicate and includes speech and language therapy, speech reading, manual communication, and amplification.

Auropalpebral reflex: Contraction of the muscles of the eyelids in response to an unexpected sound.

B

Bel: A unit of sound intensity measurement where ten decibels equal one Bel. A logarithmic unit named after Alexander Graham Bell.

Benign vocal nodule: A nonmalignant neoplasm on the vocal folds; a noncancerous vocal tumor.

Bernoulli principle: A fluid dynamics principle which describes the decrease in air pressure associated with increased airflow velocity. The Bernoulli principle helps close the glottis during phonation by lowering air pressure on the vocal fold surfaces and drawing them toward the midline.

Bifid uvula: Uvula divided into two sections. A cleft of the uvula.

Bilabial: Pertaining to two lips. Sounds produced with both lips, such as /b/ and /p/.

Binaural: Pertaining to both ears.

Bisyllable: A word with two syllables.

Blend: Two or more consonant sounds without a vowel separating them; also called a consonant cluster.

Blockages: In stuttering, the inability to get speech started. Obstruction of airflow below speech valves or the sensation that the ability to phonate is blocked.

Blom-Singer prosthesis: A surgical procedure in which a plastic tube in placed into the pharynx to serve as a voice source following laryngectomy.

Bone conduction: Acoustic stimulation of the inner ear and auditory structures medial to the inner ear through application of a sound transducer or vibrator to the mastoid process of the temporal bone, thus bypassing the air conduction mechanism.

Boyle's law: A principle of physics describing the inverse relationship of the volume of a fixed amount of gas to its pressure in a closed system at a constant temperature [Robert Boyle, 1662]. As it applies to respiration, increasing thoracic volume decreases the air pressure within and draws air into the lungs, and relaxing the thorax increases its internal air pressure, expelling air.

Brainstem: The upper part of the spinal cord located where the neck meets the skull.

Breathy: Voice quality created by excessive leakage of air when the vocal folds vibrate.

Broca's area: Motor speech and expressive language area in the frontal lobe in the dominant cerebral hemisphere named after the French neurologist Paul Broca. Cortical area associated with expressive language and motor speech production.

C

Calibrate: In audiology, to adjust the output on a hearing testing instrument to the standard level for audiometric zero.

CAT: Computerized axial tomography.

Catastrophic reaction: A psycho-biological breakdown [Eisenson] resulting from excessive stimulation, frustration, and anxiety. A sudden overwhelming feeling of anxiety and the reaction to it including irritability, withdrawal, fainting, or other nonadaptive behaviors; an anxiety attack.

CCC-A: Certificate of Clinical Competence in Audiology.

CCC-SLP: Certificate of Clinical Competence in Speech-Language Pathology

Central nervous system: The brain and spinal cord.

Central deafness: Loss of hearing resulting from damage to the central nervous system.

Cerebellum: The part of the brain responsible for muscle tone, balance and coordination lying posterior to the pons and medulla.

Cerebral cortex: Thin layer of gray matter surrounding the cerebral hemispheres.

Cerebral dominance: Tendency for one cerebral hemisphere to be dominant over the other for a particular function.

Cerebral hemispheres: The two sides of the cerebrum.

Cerebral vascular accident: A disruption of the flow of blood to the brain; a stroke.

Cerumen: Waxlike secretion in the auditory canal.

CFE: Clinical fellowship experience.

CFY: Clinical fellowship year.

CHI: Closed head injury.

Chink: The sound made during esophageal speech by air being forced into the esophagus.

Chord: Cord.

Circumlocution: The substitution of a word to avoid a feared one; rearranging or rephrasing the original thought. Using a substitute word for the one that cannot be remembered or spoken.

Clavicular breathing: A type of shallow breathing accomplished primarily with the upper thoracic muscles.

Cleft lip: A congenital cranio-facial malformation of the upper lip involving failure of fusion; may be unilateral or bilateral.

Cleft palate: A congenital cranio-facial deformity involving a failure of maxillary fusion resulting in a complete or incomplete fissure in the hard palate, velum and/or uvula; may be unilateral or bilateral.

Closed head injury: Cerebral trauma of the non-penetrating variety in which one or more cognitive functions are impaired or destroyed.

Cluttering: A thought-organization fluency disorder characterized by short attention span, excessive rate of speech, and transpositions and omissions of sounds and words.

Coarticulation: Overlapping articulatory influences during connected speech.

Cochlea: Sensory mechanism of hearing in the inner ear; the end organ of hearing.

Cochlear implant: An electronic device surgically implanted into the ear to augment cochlear function.

Cochlear nerve: Auditory or acoustic branch of cranial nerve VIII.

Cognates: In articulatory phonetics, consonants produced in the same manner and place and differing only by voicing.

Cognition: Higher mental functions that include reasoning and information processing. Mental processes of thinking, judgment, and abstraction.

Communicative stress: Anxiety and fear associated with speaking to authority figures, large groups, or under conditions of temporal urgency.

Complete cleft: Cleft extending from the lip through the velum; may be unilateral or bilateral.

Compliance: Ease of energy transfer through the outer or middle ear.

Compulsivity: Unwanted, recurring urges to perform an act.

Computerized axial tomography: Obtaining an image of a body structure by gathering anatomical information from a computer synthesis of X-ray transmission data. Image of a body part obtained from computed tomography.

Conduction: In audiology, transmission of sound pressure waves through the peripheral auditory system.

Confabulation: Giving answers to questions with no regard for their truthfulness; making up false stories.

Congenital deafness: Loss of hearing occurring before or during birth.

Consciousness: Awareness of the self and the environment.

Consonant: Speech sound produced with or without voicing by movements of the articulatory structures that modify the air stream.

Continuants: Speech sounds such as /s/ and /v/ that do not have interruptions of the airstream.

Conversion: Somatization of an emotional conflict and resulting disorder.

Conversion aphonia: Loss of voice resulting from psychic trauma; psychogenic aphonia.

COPD: Chronic obstructive pulmonary disease.

Conversion deafness: Deafness resulting from psychic trauma; psychogenic deafness.

Coprolalia: Unprovoked use of obscene or profane language; excessive swearing.

Cortex: The layer of gray matter covering the surface of the cerebral hemispheres. The thin outer layer of the brain, also known as the gray matter.

Covert reactions: In stuttering, the feelings, reactions, and attitudes occurring during a moment of stuttering.

CP: Cleft lip; cerebral palsy.

Cranial nerves: Twelve pairs of neuron bundles emerging from the cerebral hemispheres, thalamus, and brainstem.

Cross hearing: Phenomenon by which sound presented to one ear is heard in the other one.

Croup: An inflammatory laryngeal condition with hoarseness, barking cough, audible inhalation, and inhalatory stridor.

CT: Computed tomography.

CVA: Cerebral vascular accident; a stroke.

Cx-x: Cervical spine designation.

D

DAI: Diffuse axonal injury.

Damping: The decrease of energy amplitude in an acoustic system over time, distance, impedance, or opposing energy; also called dampening.

Deaf: Without the sense of hearing; hearing which is nonfunctional.

Deaf mute: Slang term for one who can neither speak nor hear.

Decibel: One-tenth of a Bel. A logarithmic unit for measuring acoustic energy amplitude.

Decode: The process of breaking down and analyzing a signal, such as speech and language, into its component parts.

Degenerative disease: A condition which results in inhibition or destruction of a tissue or organ's ability to function normally.

Delayed auditory feedback (DAF): Time delay in sensing and perceiving one's own speech. DAF is associated with increased dysfluency in normal speakers.

Dementia: Generalized cognitive deterioration including disorientation, impaired judgment, and memory defects; generalized intellectual impairment.

Denasality: Voice quality characterized by lack of nasal resonance on normally nasal phonemes; reduced nasality.

Dental phoneme: A speech sound made by approximating the lip or tongue with the upper incisors.

Developmental stuttering: During the developmental period, speech containing more frequent and severe dysfluencies than what would be considered normal; incipient stuttering.

Diagnosogenic Theory of Stuttering: See Semantic Theory of Stuttering.

Dialect: Phonological, semantic, and/or syntactic variation of spoken language associated with geographical, economic, or social factors.

Dichotic listening: Presentation of different signals to both ears at the same time.

Difference limen: Smallest difference than can be detected between two signals; minimal perceptual difference.

Diphthong: Phoneme produced by moving the structures of articulation from one vowel articulatory gesture to another.

Diplophonia: Vibration of the true vocal folds and the ventricular folds producing two tones simultaneously.

Direct laryngoscopy: A diagnostic procedure where a laryngoscope is guided downward to the view the vocal folds.

Discomfort level: In audiology, loudness level perceived to be uncomfortable.

Disguise reaction: When an individual attempts to minimize the stuttering moment by hiding or concealing the stuttering behaviors.

Disorientation: Inaccurate perceptions and judgments about time, place, person, and/or situation/predicament.

Distortion: In speech articulation, the indistinct production of a sound.

Doppler effect: In acoustics, change in pitch caused by movement toward or away from the source of a sound.

Dyne: The amount of force necessary to accelerate 1 gram a distance of 1 centimeter per second.

Dysarthrias: A group of neuromuscular speech disorders. Impaired speech due to neurological and/or muscular deficits.

Dyscalculia: In aphasia, the impaired ability to comprehend and perform simple arithmetic.

Dysfluency: A breakdown in the rhythm and flow of speech caused by repetitions, prolongations, blocks, and/or pauses.

Dysgraphia: Problems with writing not due to hand or arm paralysis.

Dyslexia: Impaired ability to read not due to visual acuity deficits or blindness.

Dysphagia: Impairment of the emotional, cognitive, sensory, and/or motor acts involved with transferring a substance from the mouth to stomach, resulting in failure to maintain hydration and nutrition and posing a risk of choking and aspiration.

Dysphonia: Impaired voice

E

Ear: External, middle, and inner aspects of the organ and structures of hearing.

Ear canal: External ear or external auditory meatus, not including the pinna.

ECC: Early childhood caries.

Echolalia: The repetition of that which has recently been spoken. Automatically repeating or "parroting" something which has been heard.

EENT: Eyes, ear, nose, throat.

Egocentric: Self-centered.

Electrolarynx: Electrical device used to produce voice in patient's with laryngectomies; an artificial larynx.

Endoscope: A device used to examine the inside of a body cavity including the cavity of the larynx.

Engram: A location or a physical representation of a memory.

ENT: Ear, nose, and throat.

Enunciate: To articulate speech sounds precisely.

Equal loudness contour: Sound pressure necessary to produce sensation of equal loudness across frequencies.

Escape behavior: In stuttering, an attempt by the stutterer to remove himself or herself from a stuttering moment.

Esophageal speech: A type of alaryngeal speech in which compressing air in the esophagus produces a pseudovoice by releasing it through a constriction; belch talking.

Esophagus: Muscular tube leading from the throat to the stomach.

Euphoria: Heightened sense of well-being.

Eustachian tube: Air passageway from nasopharynx to middle ear allowing equalizing of pressure.

Executive function: Cognitive skills involved in planning, organization, self-monitoring, and strategy formulation for complex behaviors; metacognition.

Expiration: During breathing, the process of removing air from the lungs; air moving from a high-pressure region in the lungs to an external region of lower pressure.

Expressive aphasia: A neurologically based loss of the expressive components of speech and language: speaking, writing, and gesturing.

Expressive language: Use of socially shared encoded symbols to communicate spoken, gestured, or written concepts, ideas, and emotions. Expression of the speaker's psychological state.

External auditory meatus: External part of the ear; tube extending from the auricle (pinna) to the tympanic membrane.

External ear: The most distal parts of the anatomical structure for receiving sound, including the pinna and the external auditory meatus.

Extrapyramidal system: Cell nuclei and nerve fibers involved in automatic, unconscious aspects of motor coordination, posture, and movement; other than those of the pyramidal system.

F

False positive: In dysphagia, test results indicating aspiration when, in fact, aspiration does not exists.

False negative: In dysphagia, test results indicating the absence of aspiration when, in fact, aspiration exists.

Falsetto: Highest voice register produced by vibration of only the medial part of the vocal folds.

FAPE: Free and appropriate public education.

Fiberscope: A flexible fiberoptic bundle with the tip providing its own light source and magnifying capacity.

Filler: An interruption of the flow of speech by sounds such as "uh,""um," and""er."

Fixations: In stuttering, when the flow of speech is disrupted by moments of static articulatory positioning.

Flaccid dysarthria: Neuromuscular speech disorder associated with lower motor neuron damage. Speech may produced with hypernasality, breathiness, and indistinct sound production.

Flat affect: Narrowed mood, emotions, and temperament; reduced subjective experience of emotion.

Fluent speech: The act of speaking smoothly and easily.

fMRI: Functional Magnetic Resonance Imaging.

fo: Fundamental frequency.

Foreign accent: Speech characteristics of nonnative speakers of a language.

Formant: On a spectrogram, a frequency band in which there is a relatively high degree of acoustic energy (resonance) for vowels and voiced consonants.

Fricatives: Speech sounds made by forcing air through a constricted area, resulting in turbulence and a continuous, aperiodic sound.

Functional communication: The ability to express and understand basic ideas, needs, and wants.

Fundamental frequency: In voice, average frequency of vibration of the vocal folds. In acoustics, the lowest frequency of a complex periodic sound wave.

G

Gag reflex: The automatic tendency to gag, retch, or heave when stimulated; also called the pharyngeal reflex.

Geriatrics: Medical science devoted to the study and treatment of long-lived individuals.

GII: Generalized intellectual impairment.

Glide: In speech articulation, a sound requiring movement of the articulators from one position to another.

Glossal: Pertaining to the tongue.

Glossectomy: Surgical removal of all or part of the tongue.

Glottal cycle: Cycle of vibration of the vocal folds during phonation.

Glottal fry: Low pitched, pulsating, creaking, or gravel type voice quality.

Glottal opening: The space between the vocal cords.

Glottal stop: A sound made by stopping and releasing the airstream at the level of the vocal folds.

Glottal tone: Sound produced by the vibrating vocal folds.

Grammar: Rules of the form and usage of a language.

Grapheme: Printed or written symbols.

Gravel voice quality: Glottal fry.

GSW: Gunshot wound.

Guttural: Produced in the throat; pertaining to the throat or voice.

H

Habilitation: Therapeutic intervention to build or develop a deficient function, such as communication.

Habitual pitch: The fundamental frequency most used by a person. A range of pitches used most often during spontaneous speech; also called modal pitch.

Hard contacts: Speech produced with excessive pressure or force.

Hard glottal attack: Forceful vocal fold initiation of phonation.

Hard of hearing: Reduced hearing sensitivity.

Harmonic: In acoustics, whole number multiples of the fundamental frequency of a complex sound wave.

Harshness: In voice, acoustic qualities associated with great medial compression force and hypertension of the vocal folds.

Hearing: The function of the ears, auditory nerves, and centers of the brain permitting detection, perception, and association of sound.

Hearing aid: Any device which amplifies sound and directs it to the ear.

Hearing conservation: Educational and screening programs designed to preserve the sense of hearing.

Hertz (Hz): Cycles per second.

Hippocampus: A structure located in the medial aspect of the temporal lobe which plays a role in learning and memory.

Hoarseness: Raspy voice quality; a combination of harsh and breathy voice qualities.

Hostility: Chronic antagonistic attitude or feeling.

Husky voice quality: Voice quality that is breathy or whispered resulting from incomplete glottal closure.

Hyper-: Prefix meaning "too much."

Hyperkinetic dysarthria: Neuromuscular speech disorder associated with damage to the extrapyramidal system. Speech may be impaired by quick or slow unwanted muscular and structural movement.

Hypernasality: Excessive perceived nasality; too much nasal resonance.

Hypo-: Prefix meaning "too little."

Hypokinetic dysarthria: Neuromuscular speech disorder associated with damage to the extrapyramidal system usually as a result of Parkinson's disease. Speech may be produced slowly with tremors and distorted sounds.

Hyponasality: Reduced perceived nasality; too little nasal resonance. Lack of nasal resonance on the three nasal consonants in English; also called denasality.

Hysterical aphonia: Loss of voice because of psychogenic factors.

Hysterical deafness: Deafness occurring because of psychogenic factors.

Hysterical stuttering: Typically late onset stuttering which usually results from extreme anxiety or from psychogenic causes.

I
IAES: Interim alternative educational setting.

IDEA: Individuals with Disabilities Education Act

Ideation: Creation of ideas into formal concepts.

Ideational apraxia: Disruption of the ability to conceptualize, program, and transmit a motor impulse.

Idiolect: An individual speaker's variation in phonology, semantic, or syntactic aspects of language.

IDPH: Impartial due process hearing

IEP: Individual education program (plan).

IICP: Increased intracranial pressure; increased cranial pressure (ICP).

Image: Mental representation of some aspect of reality.

Immittance: In audiology, measurements made of tympanic membrane compliance or impedance.

Impedance: Resistance to a flow of energy.

Impedance bridge: An instrument to measure tympanic resistance to acoustic energy.

Incidence of a communication disorder: The number of new cases that occur; the frequency of occurrence.

Incus: One of three bones in the ossicular chain; the anvil.

Indirect laryngoscopy: The technique of viewing the interior of the larynx indirectly with a mirror and a light source.

Infarct: The death of tissue because of a lack of blood supply.

Infraglottic: Those parts of the larynx below the vocal folds.

Inhalatory stridor: A glottic sound due to near approximation of the vocal folds during inhalation.

Inner ear: That part of the ear where mechanical energy is transformed into hydraulic and electrical-chemical (neural) energy.

Inspiration: During breathing, the process of taking air into the lungs; air moving from an external region of high pressure to the low pressure in the lungs.

Intelligence: The abilities to reason, abstract, problem solve, acquire, and retain knowledge.

Intelligibility: The ability to be understood by a listener, usually measured in percentages. The degree a person can be understood by others.

Intensity: In audiology, the power of a sound wave, usually measured in decibels.

Interdental: A consonant produced with the tongue approximating the upper teeth.

Internal monologue: Communicating with one's self; self-talk or inner speech.

Interrupter device: In stuttering, a sudden surge of tension, jerk, or other muscular movement used by the stutterer to terminate the stuttering moment.

Intrusive sound: An extraneous sound produced between other speech sounds.

Intubation: Insertion of a tube into the body. Placement of a tube into the trachea or larynx to keep it open and ensure air flow for respiration.

Ischemic: Inadequate flow of blood to a part of the body.

IV: Intravenous.

J
Jargon: Fluent but unintelligible speech; fluent speech that makes no sense.

Jargon aphasia: A type of aphasia where the patient utters fluent speech but it makes little or no sense.

Jitter: In voice, the cycle-to-cycle variation in the periods of glottal cycles. Rhythmic variations in the frequency of a sound; frequency instability.

K

Korsakoff's syndrome: Confusion, disorientation, apathy, and confabulation resulting from chronic alcoholism.

L

Labial: In phonetics, a sound produced by one or both lips.

Labiodental: A consonant produced by approximating the lower lip with the upper incisors.

Language: The multimodality ability to encode, decode, and manipulate symbols for the purposes of verbal thought and/or communication. Rule-governed, socially shared code for representing concepts through the use of symbols.

Larynx: The voice box.

Laryngeal: Pertaining to the larynx.

Laryngeal block: During stuttering, the involuntary closure of the vocal cords.

Laryngeal prominence: Anterior projection of the thyroid cartilage, especially noticeable in some adult males; the "Adam's apple."

Laryngology: Medical speciality addressing the diseases and disorders of the larynx.

Laryngopharynx: The most inferior division of the pharynx lying between the oropharynx and the trachea.

Laryngoscopy: Observation of the interior of the larynx by any of several types of optic devices equipped with electrical lighting.

Lateral: In phonetics, a consonant produced by air pressure around one or both sides of the tongue.

Lax: In phonetics, sounds produced with reduced muscular tension; the opposite of tense.

Limbic system: A group of interconnected structures involving emotion, memory, and learning.

Lingua-alveolar: Relating to the tongue and the alveolar ridge.

Lingua-dental: Using the teeth and tongue in the production of a speech sound.

Lingual: In phonetics, a speech sound made with the tongue.

Lingual frenulum: Cord of tissue running from floor of the mouth to the middle of the undersurface of the tongue.

Lingua-palatal: Relating to the tongue and the hard palate (soft palate).

Lingua-velar: Relating to the tongue and the velum.

Lip rounding: In phonetics, production of a sound with the lips in a rounded position.

Liquid: A generic term for /l/ and /r/ sounds.

Listening: Thoughtful reception, perception, and association of acoustic events.

Localization: The identification of areas of the brain responsible for specific aspects of physical, mental, or emotional functioning. In neurology, the idea that all brain functions can be discovered and mapped.

Loft register: Falsetto.

Logorrhea: Continuous fluent incoherent production of words.

Lombard effect: Tendency to raise the level of speech loudness to compensate for background noise.

Long-term memory: Permanent memory of events what have been associated with other stored information and internalized; thought to involve permanent change in brain chemistry rather than a continuation of nervous energy.

Loudness: Psychological perception of amplitude or intensity of an acoustic signal.

Lung capacity: Potential amount of air contained by the lungs; also called respiratory capacity or forced inspiratory volume.

Lung volume: Actual space occupied by the air in the lungs at a given time; respiratory volume.

LVS: Laryngeal video stroboscopy.

M

Macroglossia: Abnormally large tongue compared with the oral cavity.

Magnetic resonance imaging: A scan of any part of the body where the patient is exposed to a magnetic field and a computer interprets movement of hydrogen ions into images.

Malleus: One of three bones in the ossicular chain; hammer.

Mandible: The lower jaw.

Manner of articulation: The characteristics of speech sound production by changes in air stream modulation and amount of vocal tract constriction.

Masking: Noise which interferes with the perception of another acoustic signal.

Mastoid process: Bony protuberance of the temporal bone behind and below the external ear.

Maxilla: The upper jaw.

Meningitis: Inflammation of the three membranes surrounding the surface of the central nervous system (dura mater, arachnoid mater, and pia mater).

Microbar: Unit of pressure; one-millionth of a bar.

Microglossia: Abnormally small tongue relative to the oral cavity.

Minimal contrasts: Bisyllables containing two vowels and slightly different acoustic features.

Minimal pair: Two words differing only by a single phoneme.

Mixed deafness: Combination of sensorineural and conductive hearing losses.

Mixed dysarthria: Two or more dysarthrias occurring concurrently or the changing of dysarthria type over time; multiple dysarthrias.

Modality: In language, any avenue or mode of communication.

Modulation: In voice, alteration of the voice quality and loudness during connected speech.

Moment of stuttering: The act of stuttering occurring at a point in time.

Monaural: Pertaining to one ear.

Monosyllable: Having one syllable.

Moro reflex: Sudden extension and abduction of the arms hands and fingers of an infant following loud auditory stimulation.

Morpheme: Smallest unit of meaning in language; minimal unit of speech that is meaningful.

Motor neuron: A nerve which passes from the central nervous system to a muscle and causes movement.

Motor strip: A term used to represent motor control areas in the precentral gyrus.

Motor speech disorders: Pertaining to disorders of motor tracts and muscles; apraxia of speech and the dysarthrias.

MRI: Magnetic resonance imaging.

Mutational falsetto: In males, the failure to change from the higher-pitched voice of a child to the lower-pitched voice of the adult male.

Mute: Inability to phonate and articulate.

Mutism: Completely without speech; inability to phonate and articulate.

Myofunctional: In speech, the action of a muscle or a muscle group in affecting oral development and structure.

N

Nasal: Pertaining to the nose; rhinal.

Nasal coupling: Lowering of the velum to allow airflow through the nasal passageway

Nasal emission: Air escape from the nose during speech, usually resulting from velopharyngeal incompetence or velopharyngeal insufficiency.

Nasal resonance: Coupling of the nasal to the oral cavities and the subsequent modification of the glottal tone by the nasal chambers.

Nasalance: Ratio of nasal resonance to oral resonance.

Nasality: Production of phonemes with the acoustic properties of excessive nasal resonance.

Nasalization: In phonetics, the quality of nasal resonance given to any phoneme when adjacent to a nasal sound; also called nasal assimilation.

Naso-oral: Pertaining to the nose and mouth.

Nasopharyngeal: Pertaining to the superior pharynx, between the choanae and the horizontal plane of the hard palate.

Neologism: A made-up or invented word. A conventional word used in an unconventional manner.

Nerve deafness: Deafness resulting from disease of the cochlea or auditory nerve.

Neurotransmitter: A chemical involved in presynaptic and postsynaptic activation.

NG: Nasogastric.

Nodule: A small node.

Noise: Any signal that competes with the perception of a stimulus; unwanted sound.

Nonfluency: Dysfluency or the absence of fluent speech. Speech produced with complications.

Non-nasal sound: Any sound not produced with the velum lowered.

O

OBD: Organic brain disease.

Obsessive-compulsive: Persistent adherence to thoughts and beliefs and the need to perform certain rituals to excess.

Obstruent: Consonants made with the vocal tract partially or completely occluded (fricatives, affricates, and plosives).

Omission: In articulation, the lack of a sound in a word where one would be expected.

Open head injury: Cerebral trauma of the penetrating variety which one or more cognitive functions are impaired or destroyed.

Open syllable: A syllable ending with a vowel.

Optimal pitch: The pitch level best suited to an individual that produces the voice with the least effort.

Oral apraxia: Loss of the ability to conceptualize, plan and sequence voluntary oral nonspeech movements due to a neurological disorder.

Organ of Corti: Part of the cochlea containing sensory receptors.

Organic: In medicine, the physical basis for a disorder.

Organic disorder: Any impairment resulting from structural defects, muscular weakness, genetic defects, biochemical irregularities, or illness.

Orientation: Awareness of time, place, person, and situation/predicament.

Oropharynx: Medial aspect of the pharynx.

Oscillator: Device for producing vibrations.

OSHA: Occupational Safety and Health Administration.

Ossicles: Bones of the middle ear.

Ostomy: A surgical procedure that creates a permanent opening between a hollow organ and the external environment.

Otitis: Inflammation of the ear.

Otolaryngology: Medical speciality concerned with diagnosis and treatment of disease and disorders of the ear and larynx.

Otology: Branch of medicine concerned with the diagnosis and treatment of diseases and disorders of the ear.

Otorhinolaryngology: Medical speciality concerned with diagnosis and treatment of disease and disorders of the ear, nose, and throat.

Otoscope: Device for visual examination of the external ear canal and tympanic membrane.

Overlearning: The practice of a speech motor skill beyond what is necessary for production, retention, or recall.

Overt features: Fully developed features of stuttering; those readily apparent.

P

Palatal-lift: A prosthetic device which elevates and extends the soft palate to help achieve closure.

Paraphasia: Aphasic naming disorder characterized by choosing the incorrect word which either rhymes (literal) or has a semantic relationship (verbal) to the correct one; literal and verbal paraphasias.

Pavlovian conditioning: A form of learning, especially emotional learning, where a previously learned neutral stimulus becomes a conditioned stimulus when presented repeatedly with an unconditioned stimulus. In stuttering, the way negative emotions are associated with dysfluent speech.

PB: Phonetically balanced.

Perception: Realizing the significance of sensory information; awareness and appreciation of the salient aspects of a stimulus. Organization and interpretation of incoming sensory information.

Perceptual-motor: The interaction between perception and motor activities.

Perseveration: The automatic continuation of a speaking or writing response seen in some patients with neurogenic communication disorders. Sensory and motor responses which persist for a longer duration than what the intensity and significance of the stimuli would warrant.

PET: Positron emission tomography.

Pharyngeal flap: A surgical procedure used to facilitate velopharyngeal closure.

PHLOTE: Primary home language other than English,

Phonation: Any voiced sound that occurs at the level of the vocal folds. Transformation of acoustic energy within the larynx by means of vocal fold vibration.

Phonatory apraxia: Loss of the ability to plan and sequence voluntary laryngeal movements due to a neurological disorder. Phonatory dyspraxia means that there remains some ability to make these voluntary movements.

Phoneme: A speech sound.

Phonemic fears: In stuttering, the fear of specific sounds or their positions in words.

Phonetic practice: Improvement of motor control and intelligibility by using sound repeatedly.

Phonetically balanced words: Lists of fifty monosyllabic words chosen so as to approximate the incidence of phonemes in English speech. Phonetically balanced words are used in speech discrimination testing.

Phonetics: The study of the acoustics, perception, classification, description, and production of speech sounds of a language.

Phonics: A method of teaching reading by addressing the phonetic pronunciation of letters.

Phonology: The study of the sounds of a language and the way they are combined into words. The study of the sound system of a language.

Pitch: Psychological perception of frequency of vibration.

Pitch range: In voice science, the distance between the lowest and highest glottal frequency, usually expressed in hertz or musical notes.

Place of articulation: The characteristics of speech sound production by contact or approximation in the oral tract of the articulators. The location of greatest vocal tract constriction brought about by approximation of the speech articulators.

Plosive: A consonant produced with complete cessation of the airflow and often occurring with an audible burst of air on release.

Pn: Pneumonia.

Polysyllable: Having multiple syllables.

Post linguistic deafness: Deafness occurring after the development of speech and language.

Practicum: Supervised clinical experience.

Pragmatic stuttering therapy: Stuttering therapy where the context, purpose, and environment is emphasized during fluency training.

Prelinguistic deafness: Deafness occurring before the complete development of speech and language.

Presbycusis: Age-related hearing loss.

Prevalence of a communication disorder: The total number of people having a communication disorder at a particular time.

Primary stuttering: Mild form of stuttering characterized by easy repetitions of words or syllable. The individual usually has no awareness or negativity associated with speech.

Prognosis: A prediction about how well a patient will recover from a disease, disorder, or disability.

Propositionality: The importance and significance of an utterance.

Prosody: Acoustic patterns of speech such as stress, intonation, rhythm, melody, pitch, and voice quality that extend across one or more segments. Includes fluency, cadence, inflection, and emphasis aspects of speech.

Psub: Pressure below the glottis.

Puberphonia: The voice of an adolescent.

Pure tone: Sound wave having only one frequency.

Q

Quality: In voice, the perceptual correlate of complexity of acoustic signals; the spectral characteristics of a sound.

R

Rarefaction: In acoustics, the separation of air particles in a sound wave from their neutral or resting positions.

Receptive aphasia: A neurologically based loss of the receptive components of language: auditory comprehension, reading, gesturing.

Receptive language: The decoding of phonemes, words, gestures, and graphemes into recognizable language patterns.

Recruitment: A disproportionate increase in the loudness of a particular sound.

Register: Pitch range and resonance properties of the voice.

Rehabilitation: Therapeutic restoration of a deficient function, such as communication, to normal or near normal levels.

Repetition: In stuttering, repeating a sound, syllable, word, or phrase.

Residual hearing: The amount of hearing remaining in an individual with a hearing loss.

Resonance: In speech, sympathetic vibration of vocal tract tissue and air columns in response to a vibrating source.

Resonance frequency: A system's natural frequency.

Resonator: In speech, a vocal tract cavity responsible for the amplification and damping of the fundamental vibrations produced at the level of the glottis.

Respiration: The act of breathing; inspiration and expiration.

Respiratory capacity: Potential contents of the lungs and airways leading to and from the them.

Respiratory tracts: Air passageways to and from the lungs.

Respiratory volume: Space occupied by the air in the lungs and the passages leading to and from them.

Retrocochlear: Neural structures of the auditory system beyond the cochlea.

Retrocochlear deafness: Deafness resulting from a lesion beyond the cochlea.

Retrograde amnesia: Amnesia for events prior to an illness, trauma, or injury to the brain.

Rhotic: An "r-colouring" of a vowel resonance, produced with a retroflexed lingual posture.

Rhythm effect: In stuttering, the observation that fluency is enhanced when speech is produced to a regular rhythm.

S

Saliva: A secretion from salivary and mucous glands of the mouth.

Schedules of reinforcement: The duration and frequency in which reinforcements are administered.

Schwa: A neutral vowel.

Screening: A gross measurement of a function to determine the need for additional testing; testing to detect the presence of a disorder.

Secondary stuttering: Stuttering associated with awareness of the disorder and subsequent escape and avoidance behaviors.

Seizure: A spontaneous excessive discharge of cortical neurons.

Semantic: Aspects of language concerned with word content rules and word meaning.

Semantic Theory of Stuttering: Also know as the Diagnosogenic Theory of Stuttering [Wendell Johnson]. Postulates that stuttering is caused by the misdiagnosis of normal dysfluencies in a child's speech usually by a lay person, frequently a parent.

Senility: Cognitive deterioration associated with pathological aging.

Sensorimotor: A combination of motor activity and sensations or feedback accompanying them.

Sensorineural deafness: Deafness resulting from cochlear or retrocochlear lesions.

Shimmer: In voice, the cycle-to-cycle variations in amplitude of a glottal sound; amplitude instability.

Short-term memory: The temporary storage of information limited in capacity; requires continual rehearsal.

Sibilant: High-pitched speech sounds produced by pushing air through a constricted area such as /s/ and /z/. A consonant produced with acoustic energy in the mid to high frequency ranges.

Sigh voice: In voice therapy, the uttering of words with deep audible expiration of breath.

Simple harmonic motion: Periodic oscillations of a body resulting in a sine wave.

Simple tone: Pure tone.

Simple wave: A sinusoidal wave.

Sine wave: The graphic record or waveform of simple harmonic motion or of a pure tone, having a constant period.

Situational fears: In stuttering, the communication environment or milieu possessing features which elicit anxiety and associated negative emotions in stutterers.

Sociocusis: Progressive loss of hearing due to aging, noise exposure, and/or disease.

Soft Palate: The soft part at the back of the roof of the mouth; velum.

Sonant: A phoneme produced with accompanying vocal fold vibration; a voiced phoneme.

Sound discrimination: The auditory ability to perceive the difference between two sounds, especially similar ones.

Sound field: Area into which sound is introduced through a loudspeaker.

Sound level meter: A device for measuring the amplitude of sound.

Sound pressure level: Decibel level relative to 0.0002 dyne/cm^2.

Spastic dysarthria: Neuromuscular speech disorder associated with bilateral upper motor lesions. Speech may be produced with harsh or hoarse voice quality, hypernasality, and indistinct sound production.

SPECT: Single photon tomography.

Spectrography: In voice, an instrument or computer program that analyzes the speech signal by passing it through a series of filters and graphically representing its frequency, duration, and intensity.

Speech audiometry: A hearing test measurement of speech awareness.

Speech act: The verbal expression of an intent; an act of propositional verbal communication.

Spirometer: A device used to record and measure air capacity of the lungs. Measurement of pulmonary volumes and capacities.

Spontaneous recovery: The period of time postonset where the brain naturally resolves part or all of the neurogenic disorder.

Stammering: Term used to describe stuttering in some countries outside the United States.

Stapes: One of three bones in the ossicular chain; stirrup.

Stimulability: The ability to produce a target speech sound by attending to visual, auditory proprioceptive, and kinesthetic feedback.

Stoma: In laryngectomy, the opening into the trachea.

Stop: In articulation, speech sounds made by momentarily ceasing completely the air stream and subsequent acoustic energy in the speech tract.

Strident: An affricate or fricative produced by directing the airstream against a hard articulator and creating high frequency acoustic energy.

Stroboscope: In voice, an instrument that provides intermittent light to be used to slow and illuminate the vibrating vocal folds.

Stroke: Sudden interruption of the flow of blood to the brain; cerebral vascular accident.

Stuttering: A word improperly patterned in time and the speaker's reaction thereto [Van Riper].

Subcortical: The areas of the brain below the cerebral cortex.

Subglottal air pressure: Pressure below the glottis.

Subglottic: Below the vocal folds.

Submucous cleft: A cleft in the posterior border of the hard palate due to failure of the maxillary palatine processes to fuse, but covered with tissue so as to appear normal.

Substitution: In speech articulation, replacing the correct sound with another one.

Supraglottic: Above the vocal folds.

Suprasegmental: Intonational, stress, and durational features of a language which extend across one or more segments; prosody.

Surd: A sound of a language produced without accompanying vocal fold vibration; voiceless.

Syndrome: A combination or cluster of symptoms usually occurring together.

Syntax: Linguistic rules for arranging morphemes into connected utterances. The grammatical structure of language, especially word order.

T

Tap: A speech sound resulting from brief contact between articulators, usually the tip of the tongue and the alveolar ridge.

TBI: Traumatic brain injury.

Telegraphic speech: Communication using a minimum of function words and using many content words; similar to a telegram.

Tempo: The rate or speed of speaking.

Tense: In phonetics, sounds produced with increased muscular tension; opposite of lax.

Thorax: The chest.

Threshold: The lowest stimulus amplitude that elicits a subject's responses over 50 percent of the total number of presentations.

Threshold shift: In audiology, the change in hearing sensitivity caused by exposure to noise.

TIA: Transient ischemic attack.

Timbre: The perceptual correlate of sound spectrum; also called quality.

Timing device: In stuttering, an activating behavior or response designed to compel utterances at a specific moment in time.

Tinnitus: Sensation of ringing, buzzing, or humming in the ear without an external source.

Total communication: Habilitative process consisting of oral, manual, and aural processes for patients with severe hearing loss.

Trachea: The windpipe.

Tracheotomy: A surgical procedure where an opening is made into the trachea and a tube inserted to help respiration.

Tract: Central nervous system axons having a common origin and destination; anatomically related parts of the central nervous system.

Transient ischemic attack: Like a stroke, but does not result in permanent damage to the brain and lasts fewer than 24 hours.

Transitional stuttering: Stage of stuttering development where the individual has increased awareness and engages in escape and avoidance behaviors.

Traumatic brain injury: Injury to the brain caused by a blunt force or a penetrating object.

Trigger posture: When a stutterer presets his or her articulators to activate speech; an attempt to prompt the speech act.

Trill: A speech sound produced by vibrating an articulator by the airstream.

Tripophonia: Three pitches produced simultaneously.

Tympanic membrane: Thin sensitive membrane found between the external and medial sections of the ear which transmits acoustic energy to the ossicles.

Tympanogram: A chart of the results of acoustic impedance audiometry depicting eardrum and middle ear compliance.

U

Ultrasonic: Frequency of vibrations not perceived as sound; above approximately 20,000 cycles per second.

Unvoiced: A sound produced with no vibration of the vocal folds.

Uvula: Small, midline muscular process hanging from the posterior border of the velum. The muscle that hangs down at the back of the soft palate.

V

Velar fricative: Audible friction or continuous noise produced at the velopharyngeal sphincter and associated with nasal air escape.

Velopharyngeal closure: The closing off of the nasal cavity by the actions of the velum and pharynx.

Velopharyngeal competence: Adequate separation of the nasal cavity from the oral cavity by the velum and pharynx to produce speech without nasalance.

Velopharyngeal incompetence: Inability to separate the nasal cavity from the oral cavity by the velum and pharynx.

Velopharyngeal insufficiency: Insufficient tissue or movement to effect closure of the velopharyngeal sphincter.

Velopharyngeal port: A sphincter formed by articulation of the pharynx and velum and allowing variable coupling of the oral and nasal cavities; also called velopharyngeal sphincter.

Velum: The soft palate.

Verbal jeopardy: Speaking with the knowledge that one's veracity is suspect.

Vertigo: Dizziness; sensation of spinning or falling caused by abnormalities of the vestibular system.

Vibrato: Rise and fall in pitch and loudness of the voice.

Vibratory cycle: One cycle of periodic acoustic or of vocal fold vibration.

Visual agnosia: Inability to appreciate the significance of written words or objects.

Vocal cords: Vocal folds.

Vocal fry: Low pitch, pulsating voice quality.

Voice: Sound produced by the vibration of the vocal folds. See Phonation.

Voiced: Sounds produced with simultaneous vibration of the vocal folds. See Sonant.

Voice onset time (VOT): The time between the release of an obstruent consonant and the start of voicing.

Voiceless: Sounds produced without vibration of the vocal folds.

Volume: The internal capacity of a closed space, usually measured in cubic meters or centimeters. In acoustics, the loudness of a sound.

Vowel: A voiced speech sound resulting from relatively unrestricted passage of the air stream though the vocal tract.

VPG: Velopharyngeal gap.

VPI: Velopharyngeal insufficiency.

VPO: Velopharyngeal opening.

VSS: Video swallowing study.

W

Waveform: In acoustics, the graphic representation of molecular displacement.

Wavelength: Distance a wave travels during each cycle of vibration.

Wernicke's area: The cortical receptive language center in the temporal-parietal area [Zemlin] of the dominant cerebral hemisphere. The part of the left side of the brain important for receptive communication (understanding).

White matter: The part of the brain that is white in appearance because it contains myelinated nerve fibers. A collection of axons lying just below the cerebral cortex.

White noise: Broad-band aperiodic sound with similar energy levels across the audible range of hearing.

Word fear: In stuttering, fear of specific words due to prior penalty, anxiety, and embarrassment associated with their dysfluent production.

Y

Yawn-sigh: In voice therapy, a method of obtaining soft glottal contacts and greater airflow to reduce vocal abuse.

Z

Zero hearing level: Minimum sound pressure level necessary to make any frequency audible.

Appendices

Appendix A

Quick Assessment Series for Neurogenic Communication Disorders: Aphasia, Apraxia of Speech, Dysarthria

Quick Assessment for Aphasia

by Dennis C. Tanner, Ph.D. and William Culbertson, Ph.D.

Please refer to the instruction booklet for explanations of individual items on this form.

Patient's Name: _____   Facility/Agency: _____

Age: _____   Patient's I.D. Number: _____

Physician: _____   Clinician:_____

Onset Date: _____   Assessment Date:_____

1. Diagnosis:

2. Mobility:

3. Medications:

4. Occupation:

5. Highest educational level completed:

6. Nature of family and/or social support:

7. Psychological adjustment to the communication disorder: Good   Fair   Poor

Instructions for the Scaled Items

The modified Likert scale to the right of items is arranged in discrete levels, from one to five. Five items are used to assess most of the skills on this form. With the exception of Item #31, the patient's score is determined by the number of responses that were judged to be correct or functional. Guidelines for scoring are described in the Administration Booklet.

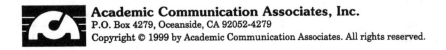

Academic Communication Associates, Inc.
P.O. Box 4279, Oceanside, CA 92052-4279

Peripheral Mechanism

8. Status of peripheral mechanism

Input	*Output*
Indicate unusual structure:	Indicate unusual structure:
Indicate unusual function:	Indicate unusual function:

9. Augmentative Devices:
   ___Corrective lenses
   ___Hearing amplification

   Augmentative Devices:
   ___Dentures
   ___Artificial larynx
   ___Alternative device (Specify):

| | **Clearly Abnormal or Nonfunctional** | | | | **Clearly Normal or Functional** | |

INPUT ASSESSMENT
Listening to Language

10. Follows one step directional commands	0	1	2	3	4	5
11. Follows two step directional commands	0	1	2	3	4	5
12. Points to objects when named	0	1	2	3	4	5
13. Points to body parts when named	0	1	2	3	4	5
14. Points to pictured objects when described	0	1	2	3	4	5
15. Answers "yes" or "no" correctly	0	1	2	3	4	5

Graphic (Reading)

16. Matches printed words	0	1	2	3	4	5
17. Matches written words with pictures	0	1	2	3	4	5
18. Reads single words aloud	0	1	2	3	4	5
19. Follows written instructions	0	1	2	3	4	5

	Clearly Abnormal or Nonfunctional				**Clearly Normal or Functional**	

OUTPUT ASSESSMENT

Speaking

20. Describes common objects   0   1   2   3   4   5

21. Names common nouns   0   1   2   3   4   5

22. Completes sentences   0   1   2   3   4   5

23. Imitates words   0   1   2   3   4   5

24. Imitates phrases   0   1   2   3   4   5

25. Gives opposites   0   1   2   3   4   5

26. Naming errors observed:
    Describe errors or give examples.

    ___Associations

    ___Approximations

    ___Random

    ___Jargon: Phonemic (Transcribe)/Semantic

Comments:

Graphic (Writing)

Note: Please note if there are any physical factors (e.g., paralysis) that may affect writing skills.

	Clearly Abnormal or Nonfunctional				Clearly Normal or Functional	
27. Writes sentences	0	1	2	3	4	5
28. Writes names of objects	0	1	2	3	4	5
29. Writes to dictation	0	1	2	3	4	5
30. Copies printed words	0	1	2	3	4	5
31. Signs name	0	1	2	3	4	5

Mathematical (Written)

32. Writes numbers from 1 to 5	0	1	2	3	4	5
33. Adds	0	1	2	3	4	5
34. Subtracts	0	1	2	3	4	5
35. Divides	0	1	2	3	4	5
36. Multiplies	0	1	2	3	4	5
37. Tells time	0	1	2	3	4	5
38. Gives change correctly	0	1	2	3	4	5

Comments and Recommendations:

Quick Assessment for Apraxia of Speech
by Dennis C. Tanner, Ph.D. and William Culbertson, Ph.D.

Please refer to the instruction booklet for explanations of individual items on this form.

Patient's Name: _____   Facility/Agency: _____

Age: _____   Patient's I.D. Number: _____

Physician: _____   Clinician:_____

Onset Date: _____   Assessment Date:_____

1. Diagnosis:

2. Mobility:

3. Medications:

4. Occupation:

5. Highest educational level completed:

6. Nature of family and/or social support:

7. Psychological adjustment to the communication disorder: Good   Fair   Poor

Instructions for the Remaining Items

The modified Likert scale to the right of the remaining items is arranged in discrete levels, from one to five. If the patient fails to respond satisfactorily to an item, mark the "0" at the left end of the scale. This would indicate that the patient was unable to perform that particular skill. If the patient responds correctly and without difficulty to the item, mark "5." This indicates clearly normal or functional behavior. The numbers between either extreme suggest some degree of abnormal function.

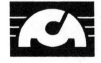

Academic Communication Associates, Inc.
P.O. Box 4279, Oceanside, CA 92052-4279

	Clearly Abnormal or Nonfunctional				Clearly Normal or Functional

Oral Apraxia

8. Oral

Blow air from your lungs.	0	1	2	3	4	5
Smile.	0	1	2	3	4	5
Bite your lower lip.	0	1	2	3	4	5
Pretend you are kissing a baby.	0	1	2	3	4	5
Puff out your cheeks.	0	1	2	3	4	5

9. Lingual

Lick your lips.	0	1	2	3	4	5
Move your tongue from side to side.	0	1	2	3	4	5
Stick your tongue out.	0	1	2	3	4	5
Try to make your tongue touch your chin.	0	1	2	3	4	5
Try to make your tongue touch your nose.	0	1	2	3	4	5

Apraxia of Speech

10. Vowels in isolation

i (as in *bit*)	0	1	2	3	4	5
ee (as in *tree*)	0	1	2	3	4	5
a (as in *had*)	0	1	2	3	4	5
o (as in *Bob*)	0	1	2	3	4	5
oo (as in *boot*)	0	1	2	3	4	5

11. Continuants

m (as in *man*)	0	1	2	3	4	5
v (as in *vase*)	0	1	2	3	4	5
l (as in *lady*)	0	1	2	3	4	5
w (as in *wife*)	0	1	2	3	4	5
sh (as in *shoe*)	0	1	2	3	4	5

12. Plosives /Affricates

t (as in *tiger*)	0	1	2	3	4	5
k (as in *kite*)	0	1	2	3	4	5
p (as in *pear*)	0	1	2	3	4	5
j (as in *judge*)	0	1	2	3	4	5
ch (as in *chair*)	0	1	2	3	4	5

	Clearly Abnormal or Nonfunctional				Clearly Normal or Functional	

13. **Diphthongs**

ie (as in *wife*)	0	1	2	3	4	5
ow (as in *fowl*)	0	1	2	3	4	5
oi (as in *boil*)	0	1	2	3	4	5
ay (as in *pay*)	0	1	2	3	4	5
ue (as in *fuel)*	0	1	2	3	4	5

14. **One syllable words**

pay	0	1	2	3	4	5
egg	0	1	2	3	4	5
cut	0	1	2	3	4	5
fall	0	1	2	3	4	5
sing	0	1	2	3	4	5

15. **Two syllable words**

bullet	0	1	2	3	4	5
flower	0	1	2	3	4	5
coffee	0	1	2	3	4	5
ocean	0	1	2	3	4	5
value	0	1	2	3	4	5

16. **Three syllable words**

basketball	0	1	2	3	4	5
recorder	0	1	2	3	4	5
educate	0	1	2	3	4	5
calendar	0	1	2	3	4	5
spaghetti	0	1	2	3	4	5

17. **Two words**

run up	0	1	2	3	4	5
can do	0	1	2	3	4	5
sing song	0	1	2	3	4	5
buy books	0	1	2	3	4	5
stop it	0	1	2	3	4	5

18. **Three words**

sky is blue	0	1	2	3	4	5
tree is tall	0	1	2	3	4	5
Can I go?	0	1	2	3	4	5
I ran home.	0	1	2	3	4	5
Climb the tree.	0	1	2	3	4	5

	Clearly Abnormal or Nonfunctional			Clearly Normal or Functional	

19. Multiple repetitions

aluminum	0	1	2	3	4	5
phenomena	0	1	2	3	4	5
specifically	0	1	2	3	4	5
supposedly	0	1	2	3	4	5
statistically	0	1	2	3	4	5

20. Progressively longer words

pen-penman-penmanship	0	1	2	3	4	5
state-statesman-statesmanship	0	1	2	3	4	5
friend-friendly-friendliness	0	1	2	3	4	5
truth-truthful-truthfulness	0	1	2	3	4	5
horse-horseman-horsemanship	0	1	2	3	4	5

21. Phrases

Do you have the movie ticket?	0	1	2	3	4	5
Fireworks filled the sky.	0	1	2	3	4	5
Did the police give you a ticket?	0	1	2	3	4	5
I rode the bus to the mall.	0	1	2	3	4	5
It is cold and windy outside.	0	1	2	3	4	5

22. Counting and serial tasks

Count to 10 by 2's	0	1	2	3	4	5
Say the alphabet.	0	1	2	3	4	5
Name the days of the week.	0	1	2	3	4	5
Name the months of the year.	0	1	2	3	4	5
Count to 10.	0	1	2	3	4	5

Other Observations

23. Struggles	0	1	2	3	4	5
24. Demonstrates an awareness of errors	0	1	2	3	4	5
25. Self-corrects	0	1	2	3	4	5

Comments and Recommendations:

Quick Assessment for Dysarthria
by Dennis C. Tanner, Ph.D. and William Culbertson, Ph.D.

Please refer to the instruction booklet for explanations of individual items on this form.

Patient's Name: _____   Facility/Agency: _____

Age: _____   Patient's I.D. Number: _____

Physician: _____   Clinician:_____

Onset Date: _____   Assessment Date:_____

1. Diagnosis:

2. Mobility:

3. Medications:

4. Occupation:

5. Highest educational level completed:

6. Nature of family and/or social support:

7. Psychological adjustment to the disorder: Good   Fair   Poor

Instructions for the Scaled Items

The modified Likert scale to the right of items is arranged in discrete levels, from one to five. If the patient fails to respond satisfactorily to an item, mark the "0" at the left end of the scale. This score indicates that the patient did not perform that particular skill. If the patient responds correctly and without difficulty to the item, mark "5." A score of "5" indicates behavior that is normal or functional. The numbers between either extreme suggest some degree of abnormal function.

Academic Communication Associates, Inc.
P.O. Box 4279, Oceanside, CA 92052-4279

Peripheral Mechanism

8. Status

Input	**Output**
Form:	Form:
Function:	Function:

9. Augmentative devices:
   ___Corrective lenses
   ___Dentures
   ___Hearing amplification

Augmentative devices:
   ___Artificial larynx
   ___Alternative device

Head and Neck Checklist

10. Physical or anatomical anomalies:

   ___facial asymmetry   ___tongue atrophy/fasciculations
   ___naso-labial fold   ___drooling
   ___velar sagging   ___contortions, tics, or grimaces
   ___lip drooping   ___flaccidity
   ___mouth breathing   ___spasticity
   ___tracheostomy

Assessment through Cranial Nerve Screening

	Clearly Abnormal or Nonfunctional				Clearly Normal or Functional	
OLFACTORY						
11. Ability to smell	0	1	2	3	4	5
OPTIC						
12. Ability to see	0	1	2	3	4	5
13. Accommodation reflex	0	1	2	3	4	5
14. Light reflex	0	1	2	3	4	5
15. Confrontation response	0	1	2	3	4	5
OCULOMOTOR, TROCHLEAR, and ABDUCENS						
16. Directed eye gaze	0	1	2	3	4	5

	Clearly Abnormal or Nonfunctional				Clearly Normal or Functional	

TRIGEMINAL

17. Responses to gross touch						
Right	0	1	2	3	4	5
Left	0	1	2	3	4	5
18. Ability to move mouth and jaw	0	1	2	3	4	5

FACIAL

19. Imitation of Various Facial Movements						
Smile (Voluntary)	0	1	2	3	4	5
Smile (Emotional)	0	1	2	3	4	5
Pucker	0	1	2	3	4	5
Sustaining Vowels /i/ and /u/	0	1	2	3	4	5

VESTIBULOCOCHLEAR

20. Responses to spoken input	0	1	2	3	4	5
21. Imitation of minimal pair words	0	1	2	3	4	5

GLOSSOPHARYNGEAL

22. Report of taste sense	0	1	2	3	4	5
23. Swallowing	0	1	2	3	4	5
24. Gag reflex	0	1	2	3	4	5

VAGUS and SPINAL ACCESSORY

25. Voice quality	0	1	2	3	4	5
26. Glottal closure	0	1	2	3	4	5
27. Ability to retain intraoral air	0	1	2	3	4	5
28. Laryngeal excursion on swallow	0	1	2	3	4	5

HYPOGLOSSAL

29. Tongue movement	0	1	2	3	4	5
30. Symmetry of tongue force against cheek	0	1	2	3	4	5
31. Speech diadochokinetic rate	0	1	2	3	4	5

| | Clearly Abnormal or Nonfunctional | | | Clearly Normal or Functional | |

Speech Task Assessment

Respiration

32. Create breath support for speech	0	1	2	3	4	5
33. Sustained vowel production	0	1	2	3	4	5

Phonation

34. Voice quality	0	1	2	3	4	5
35. Voice onset	0	1	2	3	4	5
36. Pitch range	0	1	2	3	4	5
37. Pitch control	0	1	2	3	4	5
38. Loudness	0	1	2	3	4	5

Articulation

39. Speech Intelligibility	0	1	2	3	4	5
40. Articulation at valve sites:						
bilabial	0	1	2	3	4	5
labio-dental	0	1	2	3	4	5
lingua-dental	0	1	2	3	4	5
alveolar	0	1	2	3	4	5
palatal	0	1	2	3	4	5
velar	0	1	2	3	4	5
glottal	0	1	2	3	4	5

41. Specific misarticulated sounds and
types of simplification errors:

Resonance

42. Nasality on isolated sounds	0	1	2	3	4	5
43. Nasality in connected speech	0	1	2	3	4	5
44. Nasal emissions	0	1	2	3	4	5

Prosody

45. Rate of speech	0	1	2	3	4	5
46. Rhythm	0	1	2	3	4	5

Comments/Recommendations:

Appendix B

Quick Assessment for Dysphagia

Quick Assessment for Dysphagia
by Dennis C. Tanner, Ph.D. and William Culbertson, Ph.D.

Please refer to the instruction booklet for explanations of individual items on this form.

Patient's Name: _____   Facility/Agency: _____

Age: _____   Patient's I.D. Number: _____

Physician: _____   Clinician:_____

Onset Date: _____   Assessment Date:_____

1. Diagnosis:

2. Mobility:

3. Medications:

4. Occupation:

5. Highest educational level completed:

6. Nature of family and/or social support:

7. Psychological adjustment to the disorder: Good   Fair   Poor

Instructions for the Remaining Items

The modified Likert scale to the right of the remaining items is arranged in discrete levels, from one to five. If the patient fails to respond satisfactorily to an item, mark the "0" at the left end of the scale. This score indicates that the patient did not perform that particular skill. If the patient responds correctly and without difficulty to the item, mark "5." This indicates behavior that is normal or functional.. The numbers between either extreme suggest some degree of abnormal function.

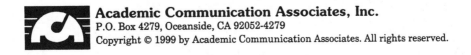

Academic Communication Associates, Inc.
P.O. Box 4279, Oceanside, CA 92052-4279

Oral Level	**Clearly Abnormal or Nonfunctional**				**Clearly Normal or Functional**	
8. Accept food and create bolus	0	1	2	3	4	5
9. Lip seal	0	1	2	3	4	5
10. Mastication	0	1	2	3	4	5
11. Dentition	0	1	2	3	4	5
12. Salivation	0	1	2	3	4	5
13. Pocketing	0	1	2	3	4	5
14. Tongue mobility	0	1	2	3	4	5
15. Mandibular movement	0	1	2	3	4	5
16. Propelling bolus along palatal vault	0	1	2	3	4	5
17. Impulsivity	0	1	2	3	4	5

Summary of Major Problems Observed:

Pharyngeal Level

	Clearly Abnormal or Nonfunctional				**Clearly Normal or Functional**	
18. Initiation of swallow reflex (purposeful, automatic)	0	1	2	3	4	5
19. Velopharyngeal closure	0	1	2	3	4	5
20. Gag reflex	0	1	2	3	4	5
21. Initiate pharyngeal peristalsis	0	1	2	3	4	5
22. Coordination with oral stage	0	1	2	3	4	5

Summary of Major Problems Observed:

Esophageal Level	**Clearly Abnormal or or Nonfunctional**				**Clearly Normal or Functional**	
23. Airway protection	0	1	2	3	4	5
24. Maintain velopharyngeal closure	0	1	2	3	4	5
25. Laryngeal elevation	0	1	2	3	4	5
26. Voice quality	0	1	2	3	4	5
27. Glottal valving	0	1	2	3	4	5
28. Cough reflex	0	1	2	3	4	5
29. Cough productivity	0	1	2	3	4	5
30. Delayed swallow reflex	0	1	2	3	4	5
31. Silent aspiration	0	1	2	3	4	5

32. Aspiration risk factors in neurogenic patients:

Dysphonia   Present:_____

Dysarthria   Present:_____

Abnormal volitional cough   Present:_____

Abnormal gag reflex   Present:_____

Abnormal cough reflex   Present:_____

Cough after swallow   Present:_____

Voice change   Present:_____

Summary of Major Problems Observed:

Primary concerns expressed by family members:

Comments and recommendations:

The Cognitive, Linguistic and Social-Communicative Scales (2nd ed)

THE COGNITIVE, LINGUISTIC AND SOCIAL-COMMUNICATIVE SCALES
Section I: Cognitive Development

Item No.	Level Definition	Clinical Description	Item Description	Example 1	Example 2	Age
1.1	Reflexive Behavior (28,35,46,52,66)*	The child's responses to objects, people and events in his world are determined entirely by his reflexes; he cries, grasps all objects placed in his hand, and sucks anything placed in his mouth.	The child reacts automatically to people and things; his reactions are the same no matter what the circumstances.	My child sucks on anything placed in his mouth, whether or not it is a nipple.	My child takes hold of anything placed in his hand.	birth to one month
1.2	Reflex Modification (28,35,46,52,66)	The child's responses to objects, people, and events in his world vary according to circumstances.	The child reacts differently to different people and things; his reactions change with the circumstances.	My child spits out an object which is not a nipple and turns his head in search of a real nipple.	My child spits out the nipple of an empty bottle and begins to fuss and search for a bottle.	
2.1	Primary Circular Reactions (28,35,46,52,66)	The child's behavior consists of simple patterns of movement of his head, arms and legs which are repeated.	The child moves his head, arms and legs. He repeats a movement several times.	My child bangs a toy against the side of his crib over and over.	My child kicks his feet up and down over and over while lying in his crib.	two to four months
2.2	Primary Intentionality (28,35,46,52,66)	The child develops elementary habits. He has the motor coordination necessary to bring his hand to his mouth voluntarily.	The child brings his hand to his mouth when he wants to.	My child sucks his thumb or fingers.	My child holds an object placed in his hand and puts it in his mouth or sucks on it.	
2.3	Visual Tracking & Coordination of Vision & Hearing (28,35,52)	The child follows moving objects across his field of vision and locates the source of sounds with his eyes.	The child follows an object with his eyes and turns to see what he hears.	My child moves his eyes to watch a toy swinging above his crib.	My child turns his head toward me when he hears me enter his room.	
2.4	Primary Object Permanence (28,35,46,52,66)	The child watches the spot where an object disappears.	The child stares at the place where he last saw an object as if he is waiting for it to return.	If I hide my child's rattle under a blanket while he watches, he looks at the blanket but does not lift it to find his toy.	If a toy rolls from my child's crib, he looks toward the side of the crib where he last saw it but does not reach out or move to it.	
2.5	Primary Anticipation (28,35,46,52,66)	The child's behavior indicates that he expects a common event to occur.	The child acts as if he knows something is about to happen.	My child begins to make sucking movements with his mouth as soon as he is picked up to be fed before I place a nipple in his mouth.	My child holds out his arms when he sees me coming to pick him up.	
3.1	Secondary Circular Reactions (28,35,46,52,66)	The child accidentally discovers interesting events and repeats the behaviors that produce the events.	The child accidentally discovers that he can make interesting things happen and repeats them several times.	If my child hits a toy hanging over his crib and finds that it rings a bell, he hits it over and over or ring the bell.	If my child discovers that pulling a string on a toy makes it move, he pulls it over and over.	five to eight months
3.2	Self-Imitation (28,35,36,46,52,66)	The child imitates his own and others' behavior as long as it is simple and familiar.	The child imitates simple, familiar sounds and movements.	If my child sees me clapping my hands, he claps his hands.	My child repeats sounds that he hears himself make.	

*The numbers in parentheses following Level Definitions refer to item sources found in the Reference section of the manual.

Item No.	Level Definition	Clinical Description	Item Description	Example 1	Example 2
3.3	Representing Action (28,35,46,52,66)	The child spontaneously resumes an activity following an interruption.	The child continues an activity after a brief interruption.	If my child is shaking his rattle and is interrupted by someone walking by, he begins to shake it again when the person is gone.	If my child is rolling a ball in his crib and is interrupted by the ball falling from the crib, he begins rolling it again when the toy is returned.
3.4	Object Permanence (28,35,46,52,66,69)	The child searches for and retrieves a partially hidden object.	The child looks for and finds something which is partially hidden.	My child pushes away an object which has been set on a toy he is playing with.	If my child watches me cover a doll's head with a cloth, he reaches over and uncovers it.
3.5	Anticipation (28,35,46,52,66)	The child visually anticipates what an object will do.	The child looks in the direction in which he expects to see something happen.	If my child drops a ball from his crib, he looks down to where he expects to see it hit the floor.	My child looks in the direction in which he expects a swinging object to swing after he hits it.
4.1	Coordination of Secondary Circular Reactions (28,35,46,52,66)	The child uses behaviors to attain goals.	The child does something to get what he wants or make something happen.	My child crawls or walks to get a ball which rolls out of his reach.	My child pushes my hand toward a toy that is out of his reach so I will get it for him.
4.2	Imitation of Novel Behavior (Unsuccessful) (28,35,46,52,66)	The child attempts to imitate others' behaviors which are new and difficult to perform.	The child tries to imitate unfamiliar sounds and movements.	My child tries to play games like "patty cake" with me, but he usually doesn't make the gestures quite right.	My child tries to say words which he hears me say, but he usually says them wrong.
4.3	Causality (28,35,46,52,66,69)	The child recognizes that objects themselves can be the causes of effects which he doesn't cause.	The child knows that something must be done to certain toys to make them work, but he doesn't know what to do.	My child pushes a wind-up toy instead of winding it to make it go.	My child shakes or bangs a talking toy instead of pulling the cord to make it talk.
4.4	Object Permanence (28,35,46,52,66,69)	The child retrieves an object which he watches being hidden, as long as it is hidden in the same place each time.	The child finds something which he watches being hidden as long as it is hidden in the same place each time.	If my child watches me hide a toy behind my back, he comes to me and looks for it.	If my child watches me hide his toy under a box, he goes to the box and uncovers it.
4.5	Anticipation (28,35,46,52,66)	The child infers from the actions of others that something is about to happen.	The child watches others' actions and acts as if he knows something is about to happen.	My child becomes upset or cries when he sees me get up to leave the room.	My child becomes upset or cries when I carry him into his room to put him to bed.
5.1	Tertiary Circular Reactions (28,35,46,52,66)	The child actively explores his world and discovers solutions to problems through trial and error experimentation.	The child experiments with things to figure out how to work them.	If my child is given a talking doll, he experiments with it (shakes it, squeezes it, etc.) until he discovers that by pulling the string he can make it talk.	My child experiments with a toy outside his playpen by turning in different ways until he figures out how to pull it into the playpen.
5.2	Imitation of Novel Behavior (28,35,46,52,66)	The child imitates a variety of behaviors which are unfamiliar and complex.	The child imitates many difficult sounds and actions.	My child is good at playing "patty cake" with me.	My child is good at imitating sounds and simple words he hears me say.
5.3	Causality (28,35,46,52,66,69)	The child relies on others to cause effects which he cannot cause.	The child relies on adults to work things which he can't do himself.	My child hands me a wind-up toy to wind for him.	My child puts my hand on the cord of a talking toy for me to pull for him.

nine to twelve months

thirteen to eighteen months

Item No.	Level Definition	Clinical Description	Item Description	Example 1	Example 2
5.4	Object Permanence (28,35,46,52,66,69)	The child follows an object through a series of hiding places as long as he watches it being hidden.	The child finds something that he has seen being hidden in several different places.	If my child watches me hide his toy in a box, then move it to a bag, and then put it under a pillow, he goes directly to the pillow to find his toy.	If my child watches me hide a toy in several different places, he goes directly to the last place he saw me hide his toy.
5.5	Object Concept: I (23,36,52)	The child believes that a change in some dimension of an object creates a completely new object. (a)	The child loses interest in something if it is changed in any way.	If my child is playing with a ball of clay and I flatten it into a pancake, he becomes upset or loses interest in the clay.	My child loses interest in a moving object when it stops moving.
6.1	Representation (28,35,46,52,66)	The child predicts solutions to simple problems without trial and error experimentation.	The child figures out how things work without having to experiment with them.	My child figures out how an unfamiliar toy works without having to experiment with it.	My child can turn on an appliance without previously having seen it operated.
6.2	Deferred Imitation (14,28,35,52,66)	The child imitates a complex series of behaviors of a model which he observed in the past but is no longer present.	The child imitates something which he has seen in the past.	My child pretends to talk on the telephone after having watched me talk on it.	My child imitates someone he has seen on T.V.
6.3	Causality (28,35,46,52,66,69)	The child recognizes that cause-effect relationships exist and is able to deduce causes from effects.	The child works toys that require winding or some other action to make them go.	My child winds a wind-up toy to make it go.	My child pulls a talking toy's cord to make it talk.
6.4	Object Permanence (28,35,46,52,66,69)	The child locates objects which he does not watch being hidden.	The child finds things which are hidden when he is not watching.	My child finds a toy which is hidden within several containers (a box within a box within a larger box).	If I place a candy in a small covered bowl, place that bowl in a larger covered bowl, and place that bowl in another bowl, my child immediately takes the bowls apart to find the candy.
6.5	Anticipation (28,35,46,52,66)	The child associates environmental cues that signal the future occurrence of events.	The child knows something is going to happen and acts appropriately.	My child holds out his hands if I pick up a ball and act as if I am going to throw it to him.	If my child sees a wind-up toy walking toward the edge of a table, he holds out his hands to catch it.
6.6	Alternative Means (28,35,46,52,66)	The child is aware of different means for attaining the same goal.	The child knows that there are different ways of getting the same thing.	My child climbs on a stool to reach a toy above his head and uses a stick or handle to reach a toy which he can't reach by climbing.	My child pushes a small object out of his way and climbs over, under or goes around a large object in his path.
6.7	Functional Categorization (28,36,48,59)	The child organizes objects according to functional relationships. (b)	The child forms groups of things according to how he uses them.	My child separates his cars from his other toys when he wants to play "race cars."	My child separates his animals from his other toys when he wants to play with them.
6.8	Symbolic Play (Imitative) (14,38,67)	The child acts out short scenes from events in his daily life.	The child acts out things he sees happening frequently at home.	My child plays "house" and pretends to be the mother for a while then plays the father.	My child plays with dolls, pretends to feed them or brush their hair.
7.1	Object Concept: II (23,36,52)	The child understands that an object can change in some dimension without becoming a completely new object. However, any change is bounded by two extremes, and he does not understand that there are intermediate states between the two extremes. (c)	The child does not understand the concepts "middle" or "some."	If my child is asked to put some water in a glass, he fills the glass completely; if asked to pour a little water out of the glass, he pours it all out.	If my child is shown three different size dolls, he calls the biggest one, "tall," and the smallest one, "not tall." He calls the middle sized one either, "tall" or "not tall."

nineteen to twenty-four months

Age	Item No.	Level Definition	Clinical Description	Item Description	Example 1	Example 2
twenty-five to thirty-six months	7.2	Primary Seriation (24,28)	The child divides rank-order items into two distinct categories. (d)	The child divides things into two "opposite" classes: either big or little.	My child divides a set of different sized dolls into a set of "big" ones and a set of "little" ones.	If given a set of successively sized sticks and asked to "put them into order," my child divides them into two groups "big" and "little" instead of arranging them in rank order.
	7.3	Symbolic Play (Spontaneous) (14,38,67)	The child acts out short scenes from infrequent events which are impressive or traumatic.	The child acts out things which were new or exciting for him.	My child plays "doctor" and pretends to be the doctor then the patient or nurse.	My child acts out a sequence of pretend events; he pretends to cook dinner, serve it, and wash the dishes.
thirty-seven to forty-eight months	8.1	Object Concept: III (23,36,52)	The child understands that there are intermediate points between two extremes. (e)	The child understands concepts like "middle," "some" and "half."	If shown three different sized balls of clay, my child calls the biggest one "big" and the smallest one "little" and the middle sized one "sort of big."	My child pours "some" water from a glass instead of dumping it all out and fills it "half way" if asked to do so.
	8.2	Categorization (28)	The child organizes according to personal associations rather than objective criteria. His sorted groups often represent something or have a theme. (f)	The child groups objects into pictures or scenes instead of separate categories.	If asked to sort a set of circles, squares and triangles, my child makes a picture with them instead of sorting them into different groups.	If given a set of toys and asked to sort them into groups that "go together," my child arranges them into a village or scene instead of sorting them into groups of people, animals, or cars.
	8.3	Symbolic Play (Object Representation) (14,38,67)	The child uses objects to represent other objects; he does not require realistic props in his play.	The child pretends that objects he sees or plays with are other things.	My child plays in a large box pretending it is a house or car.	My child uses blocks to build houses and fences for other toys and to build roads and bridges for cars.
forty-nine to sixty months	9.1	Object Concept: IV (23,36,52)	The child understands that there is is a continuum of change along any dimension. (g)	The child understands and uses words like "more," "less," "bigger."	My child uses words like "more," "less," "bigger," "faster," "taller," or "heavier" correctly in describing objects and events.	If shown three different sized dolls, my child labels the differences between them, "This one is taller than this one" or, "This one is shorter than this one."
	9.2	Transitional Seriation (24,28)	The child rank-orders items successfully only with trial and error experimentation. (h)	The child organizes things in a series only with much experimentation.	If given a set of different sized dolls, my child arranges them from smallest to largest after several attempts.	My child divides his toys into groups of "big" ones, "little" ones and "middle-sized" ones after several attempts.
	9.3	Symbolic Play (Personification, Compensation) (14,67)	The child gives personality to dolls and puppets and uses them as members of the pretend situation. The child acts out events he has experienced in the past but changes the outcomes to what he wished would have occurred.	The child uses dolls and puppets as playmates and makes up new endings for things he has done in the past.	My child names his dolls, talks to them and pretends that they talk to him.	My child sometimes makes up new endings when acting out things he has experienced or seen on T.V.

Item No.	Level Definition	Clinical Description	Item Description	Example 1	Example 2
10.1	Object Concept: V (23,36,52)	The child understands how a change along one dimension will cause a change along another dimension of an object. (i)	The child understands that changes will occur in two directions.	If shown a ball of clay and asked, "What will happen if I roll this into a hotdog?" my child says, "It will get longer and skinnier."	My child knows that the harder he throws his ball against a wall, the farther it will bounce back.
10.2	Categorization (Iconic) (28)	The child organizes objects into classes based on perceptual attributes: color, shape, size. (j)	The child groups things according to color, shape or size.	If given a set of circles, squares and triangles and asked to sort them into groups that "go together," my child sorts them according to color, size or shape.	My child separates a set of toy animals into groups of dogs, cats, horses, cows, etc.
10.3	Symbolic Play (Sequenced & Coordinated) (14,67)	The child plans a sequence of pretend events, hypothesizes events not experienced, and coordinates several play scenes at once.	The child plans his make-believe scenes in advance and can direct several activities at once.	My child plans out his make-believe scenes in advance and organizes the toys and other children which will be needed in the scenes.	My child plays "cops and robbers" and directs several make-believe scenes at once, such as the robbery, get-away and capture.
11.1	Object Concept: VI (23,36,52)	The child understands that the amount of change in one dimension is matched by an equal amount of change in another dimension. (k)	The child understands that change will occur in two directions and that the two changes are equal.	My child understands that pulling a curtain cord down a certain amount will cause the curtains to open the same amount.	My child understands that pulling a ball on one end of a pulley down four inches will cause the ball on the other end to move up four inches.
11.2	Class Inclusion (28)	The child understands the relationship between a class of objects and its members; he can explain how the members fit into the categories. (l)	The child understands how groups of things are alike and how categories are formed.	If shown a set of 5 red & 2 blue wooden beads, my child understands that there are more wooden beads than red beads because all of the beads are wooden.	If shown some apples and some grapes, my child answers correctly questions like: "How are these alike?" and "Are there more apples than fruit?"
11.3	Conservation of Quantity and Reversibility (23,35,46,52,66)	The child realizes that although the shape of an object is changed, the quantity remains the same unless something is added or taken away. (m)	The child understands that the shape of something can change while the quantity stays the same.	If my child is shown two equal sized balls of clay and one is rolled into a hotdog, he knows that the ball and the hotdog still have the same amount of clay although they are not the same shape.	If shown two equal sized rubber bands and then one is stretched, my child says that the rubber bands still have the same amount even though they are not the same shape.

sixty-one to seventy-two months

seventy-three months+

Section II: Linguistic Development

Item No.		Level Definition	Clinical Description	Item Description	Example 1	Example 2
1.1	birth to one month	Prelinguistic Undifferentiated (63)	The child's expressive behavior consists entirely of one pattern of crying.	The child has only one type of cry.	My child doesn't make any sounds except when he is crying and all his cries sound alike to me.	My child doesn't have different ways of crying; he cries the same way whether he is hungry, wet or just wants to be held.
1.2	birth to one month	Prelinguistic Differentiated (63)	The child's expressive behavior includes several patterns of crying which differ depending on his needs.	The child has several types of cries.	My child has a special cry which lets me know when he is hungry.	My child has a cry which lets me know when he is wet and one to let me know when he wants to be held.
2.1	two to four months	Vocal Play Vowel Production (19,68,63)	The child's expressive behavior includes random production of vowel sounds.	The child makes several types of vowel sounds; he coos.	My child plays with sounds and makes sounds like, "ah," "ee," "oh."	My child says, "oh" and "ah" when I am playing with him.
2.2	two to four months	Vocal Play Vowel Chains (19,68,63)	The child produces combinations of successive vowel sounds.	The child makes two vowel sounds together.	My child plays with sounds and puts two or three sounds together like, "ah, ee."	My child says, "e-e-e" or "o-o-o" when I am playing with him.
3.1	five to eight months	Syllable Production (19,68,63)	The child produces combinations of vowels and anterior consonants.	The child puts vowels and consonants together; he babbles.	My child plays with sounds and says things like, "ba ba."	My child talks to himself and says, "da da" when he is alone in his playpen.
3.2	five to eight months	Pseudo-Vocabulary (19,68,63)	During vocal play the child produces sound combinations that resemble words.	The child makes sounds that sound like words.	My child often says things that sound like words although he is just playing with sounds.	My child sometimes seems to say, "Hi" when he is playing with sounds by himself.
4.1	nine to twelve months	Multiple Unit Vocalization (19,68,63)	The child produces syllable combinations in succession in sentence-like utterances without using true words.	The child babbles in long strings of syllables that sound like sentences.	My child often talks using long strings of his made-up words.	My child says, "da-da-no-ba."
4.2	nine to twelve months	Single Word Utterances (19,68,63)	The child's expressive behavior includes use of single words which function as sentences.	The child uses one word which serves as a whole sentence.	My child says the name of one or two people or toys.	My child says, "mama" when he sees me and, "ba" when playing with his ball.
4.3	nine to twelve months	Receptive Vocabulary: Name, Negatives, Greetings (70,63)	The child responds appropriately to verbal stimuli including his name, negative commands and greetings.	The child knows his name, the words "no," "hi," and "bye."	My child stops what he is doing if I say, "no no" to him.	My child turns and looks at me or comes to me if I call his name.
5.1		Nominals: General & Specific (9,10,19,41,46,68)	The child labels objects in his environment and uses the proper names of familiar persons and pets.	The child uses the names of several toys and people which he knows well.	My child names one or two of his toys; he says, "ball" and "car."	My child says the names of his brother and sister and our dog.
5.2		Overextension (19,68)	The child uses one word for several loosely related referents.	The child uses one word to refer to several different things.	My child points to cats and says, "doggie."	My child uses one word to name several different things; he calls anything he's given to drink, "milk."

Item No.	Level Definition	Clinical Description	Item Description	Example 1	Example 2
5.3	Rejection (6,11,29)	The child uses the word "no" to refuse an object or action.	The child uses the word "no."	My child says, "no," when I am feeding him something that he doesn't like.	My child says, "no," to tell me to stop doing something or to tell me that he doesn't want something.
5.4	Notice (6,11,29)	The child acknowledges the presence of a person or object by using a greeting.	The child uses the word "hi" or a word for "hi" to greet people.	My child says, "hi" when I come in to his room.	My child says, "aha" when someone comes in; this is his word for "hello."
5.5	Action (6,11,29,49)	The child uses verbs to request actions from others.	The child uses verbs to ask others to do something for him.	My child says, "up" when he wants to be picked up.	My child says, "go" when he wants to go outside.
5.6	Expressive Vocabulary: Ten Words (70,63)	The child uses ten or more words consistently.	The child uses ten or more words regularly.	My child often uses the words "mama, baby, doggie, keys, papa, car, no, up, go and ball."	My child uses at least ten different words.
5.7	Receptive Vocabulary: Body Parts (70)	The child responds appropriately to requests for a pointing response to a body part (show me your eyes.)	The child knows the names of body parts such as nose, eyes and hair.	My child points to his nose when I say, "Show me your nose."	My child points to his eyes when I say, "Where are your eyes?"
5.8	Comprehension of Direct Commands (70)	The child responds appropriately to simple instructions or requests.	The child follows simple instructions.	My child understands and follows directions like, "Go get the book."	My child understands and follows directions like, "Put the book on the table."
6.1	Two Word Utterances (6,11)	The child produces two word combinations which function as sentences.	The child uses two-word sentences.	My child says, "Mommy up" when he wants to be picked up.	My child uses two-word sentences to ask for or tell me something.
6.2	Agent-Object (6,11)	The child comments on the performer of an action and the thing that received the action.	The child talks about someone and what he is working on.	My child says, "Mommy bottle" when he sees me filling a bottle.	My child says, "Doggie ball" when he sees our dog carrying a ball.
6.3	Agent-Action (6,11)	The child comments on the performer of an action and the action itself.	The child talks about someone and what he is doing.	My child says, "Ball roll" when he sees his ball roll across the floor.	My child says, "Baby cry" when he sees his baby brother crying.
6.4	Action-Object (6,11)	The child comments on the action and the receiver of the action.	The child talks about what someone is doing and what he is doing it to.	My child says, "Read book" when he sees me reading a book.	My child says, "Push car" as he pushes his toy car around the room
6.5	Action/Entity-Locative (6,11)	The child comments on the location of an object or action.	The child talks about the place where something is or where something is happening.	My child says, "Fall down" when he sees his toy fall off the table.	My child says, "Daddy home" when he sees his father's car drive up.
6.6	Recurrence (6,11)	The child comments on or requests the recurrence of an action or object.	The child talks about something happening again.	My child says, "More milk" when he wants me to give him some more milk.	My child says, "Play again" when he wants me to play a game with him again.
6.7	Existence (6,11)	The child comments on the presence of objects to point them out to others. (b)	The child talks about things he sees; he uses the words "there" or "here" to point out things.	My child says, "There ball" to show me where his toy is.	My child says, "Here toys, here books, here bed" to show me things in his room.
6.8	Cessation (6,11)	The child comments on the ending of an action. (c)	The child talks about the ending of something.	My child says, "Car stop" when his wind-up car stops moving.	My child says, "Music off" when I turn off the radio.

thirteen to eighteen months

nineteen to twenty-four months

Item No.	Level Definition	Clinical Description	Item Description	Example 1	Example 2
6.9	Disappearance/ Non-Existence (6,11)	The child comments on the disappearance of an object which had been present and on the non-existence of an object which he expects to be present. (d)	The child talks about things which he sees leave or which are missing.	My child says, "Doggie all gone" when he sees our dog leave the yard.	My child says, "Daddy away" when his father goes to work.
6.10	Possession (6,11)	The child comments on the possession or ownership of objects. (e)	The child talks about things which belong to him or to others.	My child says, "My car" when his brother starts to play with his car.	My child says, "Mommy book" to tell someone who this book belongs to.
6.11	Locative (6,11)	The child comments on spatial locations of objects or actions. (f)	The child talks about where things are or where he is going.	My child says, "Go home" to tell me that he is going home.	My child says, "Toys box" to tell me that his toys are in the toy box.
6.12	Nominative (6,11)	The child comments on or points out a specific object through use of a demonstrative. (g)	The child talks about a specific person or thing; he uses the word "that" or "this."	My child says, "That ball" to show me which particular ball he wants.	My child says, "This kind" to show me which kind of candy he wants.
6.13	Attributive (6,11)	The child comments on perceptual attributes of objects or actions. (h)	The child uses adjectives to describe how things look.	My child says, "Big dog" when he sees our neighbor's German Shepard.	My child says, "Fast car" when he plays with his race cars.
6.14	Receptive Vocabulary: Familiar Pictures (70)	The child correctly identifies at least five pictures of common objects in response to "Show me the . . . ."	The child knows the names of familiar things which he sees in pictures.	My child points to a picture of a dog if I say, "Show me the dog."	My child points to a picture of a car if I say, "Show me the car."
7.1	Three-Four Word Utterances (6,11)	The child uses simple sentences consisting of three or four words.	The child uses three and four word sentences.	My child says, "Mommy spill milk" when he sees me spill a glass of milk.	My child says, "Milk all gone" when he is done with his milk.
7.2	Agent-Action Object (6,11)	The child comments on the performer of an action, the action performed and the receiver of the action.	The child talks about someone, what he is doing and what he is doing it to.	My child says, "Mommy drop glass" when he sees me drop a glass.	My child says, "Billy push car" when he sees his brother pushing the toy car.
7.3	Agent-Action Locative (6,11)	The child comments on the performer of an action, the action performed, and the location of the action.	The child talks about someone, what he is doing and where he is doing it.	My child says, "Mommy go kitchen" when he sees me going into the kitchen.	My child says, "Doggie run home" when he sees me chase a dog from our yard.
7.4	Action-Object Locative (6,11)	The child comments on an action, the receiver of the action and the location of the action.	The child talks about what someone is doing, what he is doing it to and where he is doing it.	My child says, "Push car here" when he is pushing his toy car around the room.	My child says, "Put baby down" when he sees me putting his sister in bed.
7.5	Agent-Object Locative (6,11)	The child comments on the performer of an action, the receiver of the action and location of the action.	The child talks about someone, what he is working on and where he is working.	My child says, "Doggie ball chair" when he sees our dog drop his ball on a chair.	My child says, "Kris bottle floor" when he sees his brother drop his bottle on the floor.
7.6	Present Progressive (11)	The child uses present progressive (ing) verb forms to indicate a present or ongoing action or event.	The child uses -ing verbs.	My child says, "Doggie running" when he sees our dog playing in the yard.	My child says, "Baby crying" to tell me that his sister is crying.
7.7	Prepositions: In and On (11)	The child uses the prepositions "in" and "on" to indicate spatial relationships.	The child uses the words "on" and "in."	My child says, "Doll on bed" to tell me where his toy is.	My child says, "Ball in box" to tell me where his toy is.
7.8	Plural (5,11)	The child adds -s or -es to nouns to indicate plurality.	The child talks about several things by adding -s or -es to the noun.	My child says, "Billy play blocks" to tell me what he is doing.	My child says, "Mommy see doggies" to point out his friend's dogs to me.

twenty-five to thirty-six months

Item No.	Level Definition	Clinical Description	Item Description	Example 1	Example 2
7.9	Past Irregular (5,11)	The child uses past tense forms of irregular verbs.	The child uses past tense verbs like "went," "had" or "did."	My child says, "Daddy came home" to tell me about something that happened when I was not present.	My child says, "Baby fell down" to tell me what happened to his sister.
7.10	Possessive (5,11)	The child adds 's to nouns to indicate ownership or possession.	The child talks about things that belong to someone by adding 's to the noun.	My child says, "Mommy's dress" to tell someone who this dress belongs to.	My child says, "Kay's truck" to tell me who this truck belongs to.
7.11	Uncontractible Copula (11)	The child uses forms of the verb "be" as a main verb to indicate a state of being. (i)	The child uses the words "is," "am" or "are."	My child says, "Daddy is tall" when telling his friends about his dad.	My child says, "Cars are broke" to tell me what happened to his toy cars.
7.12	Articles: A and The (11)	The child uses "a" and "the" in indicating specific or nonspecific referents.	The child uses the words "a" and "the."	My child says, "I want the ball" to tell me which toy he wants.	My child says, "Here is a car" when showing me what he is playing with.
7.13	Negation (34)	The child uses the negative elements "can't," "don't and won't" as single morphemes in coding negation.	The child uses the words "can't," "don't" or "won't."	My child says, "I can't reach" to tell me that he is unable to get a toy off the counter.	My child says, "Billy don't take toys" to tell his brother to stop taking his toys.
7.14	Receptive Vocabulary: Action, Prepositions (70)	The child identifies action pictures from present progressive verbs and follows directional commands involving spatial relationships.	The child knows the names of different actions and follows instructions like, "Put this beside the book."	My child points to a picture of a man running if I say, "Show me running."	My child follows directions like, "Put this under the box."
8.1	Past Regular (5,11,34)	The child uses the past tense of regular verb forms: adds -ed or -d to the verb.	The child uses -ed and -d to make past tense verbs.	My child says, "Billy spilled the milk" to tell me about something that happened when I was not present.	My child says, "Daddy played with me" to tell me about playing with his dad when I was not there.
8.2	Third Person Regular and Irregular (5,11,34)	The child uses the third person tense of regular and irregular verb forms: adds -s to the verb.	The child adds -s to verbs to talk about what someone else does.	My child says, "He works in the store" to tell his friend what his dad does.	My child says, "He sleeps here" when showing a friend where his brother sleeps.
8.3	Uncontractible Auxiliary (11,34)	The child uses forms of the "be" verb as an auxiliary (helping) verb. (j)	The child uses the verbs "is," "am" or "are" along with other action verbs.	My child says, "I am playing" to tell me what he is doing.	My child says, "Tammy is eating" to tell me what his sister is doing.
8.4	Contractible Copula and Auxiliary (11,34)	The child uses contracted forms of the verb "be." (k)	The child uses contractions like "here's," "I'm" and "they're."	My child says, "Daddy's tall" to tell me about his dad.	My child says, "I'm playing cars" to tell me what he is doing.
8.5	Personal Pronouns (34)	The child uses first, second and third person singular pronouns. (l)	The child uses words like "I," "me," "you," "he" and "she."	My child says, "I want to go out."	My child says, "You go away."
8.6	Dimensional Terms (67)	The child refers to perceptual attributes using terms to indicate size, shape, color, texture and spatial relationship.	The child talks about the size, shape, color or texture of things.	My child says, "I want the big red crayon."	My child says, "See the big circle that I made."
8.7	Future Tense (34)	The child refers to events that are anticipated.	The child talks about future events.	My child says, "I'm gonna be four."	My child says, "Billy's gonna come play."

Item No.	Level Definition	Clinical Description	Item Description	Example 1	Example 2
8.8	Receptive Vocabulary: Colors, Comparison (70)	The child identifies colors and differentiates objects based on verbal comparison of perceptual dimensions.	The child knows the names of most colors and understands words like "long" and "short."	My child points to something red if I say, "Show me red."	My child points to the longer of two objects if I say, "Show me the long one."
9.1	Metalinguistic Language (19)	The child uses language to talk about language. (m)	The child talks about things he has heard others say.	My child says, "Daddy said I can."	My child corrects his little brother's speech; he says, "Don't say 'me go,' say, 'I go.'"
9.2	Modals (34)	The child uses the modals (can, may, might, must, will, would, shall, should) to vary and clarify main verbs.	The child uses words like "can," "may," "might," "must," "would," "could," "shall" or "should."	My child says, "I can get my cars."	My child says, "I might want some."
9.3	Conjunctions (34)	The child uses conjunctions to relate subjects, actions and ideas. (n)	The child uses words like "and," "if" or "because" to connect ideas.	My child says, "I went home and he took my toys."	My child says, "I want that one because it's mine."
9.4	Plural Pronouns (34)	The child uses first, second and third person plural pronouns. (o)	The child uses words like "you," "we," "us," "they" or "them."	My child says, "We went to the zoo."	My child says, "They took our toys."
9.5	Receptive Vocabulary: Action Agents (70)	The child identifies objects given the function of the object.	The child knows the function of objects.	My child points to a clock if I say, "Show me which one tells time."	My child points to a car if I ask, "Which do we drive in?"
10.1	Relational Terms (67)	The child refers to temporal relationships. (p)	The child uses words like "first," "last," "after," "before" or "next."	My child says, "I want to play first."	My child says, "I get cookies after lunch."
10.2	Derived Adjectives (5)	The child produces and uses adjectival derivations. (q)	The child uses words like "furry" or "hairy."	My child sees a cat covered with spots, he says, "See the spotty cat."	My child sees a dog covered with fur, he says, "See the furry dog."
10.3	Comparative/Superlative (5)	The child produces and uses the comparative (-er) and superlative (-est) forms of adjectives.	The child uses -er and -est forms of adjectives as in bigger and biggest.	My child says, "My dog is bigger than yours."	My child says, "I have the biggest house."
10.4	Reflexive Pronouns (34)	The child uses pronouns as direct objects of reflexive verbs. (r)	The child uses words like "myself," "himself" or "itself."	My child says, "I dressed myself."	My child says, "You get it yourself."
10.5	Receptive Vocabulary: Multiple Degree Commands (70)	The child follows directional commands involving two or more directions given at once.	The child follows directions even when several are given at once.	My child follows directions like, "Raise your hand, then touch your nose, then sit down."	My child follows directions like, "Go get the book and put it on the table next to the phone."
11.1	Diminutive (5)	The child produces and uses derived suffixes that denote smallness. (s)	The child uses -let suffixes to describe very small objects.	My child sees a small book, he says, "See the booklet."	My child sees a small pig, he says, "See the piglet."
11.2	Agentive (5)	The child produces and uses agentive derivations. (t)	The child uses words like "runner," "player" or "drummer"; he adds -er to verbs.	If asked, "What do you call someone who runs?" my child says, "A runner."	If asked, "What do you call someone who plays?" my child says, "A player."
11.3	Passive Voice (34)	The child uses passive verb forms to indicate that the subject is the object of the action or effect of the verb. (u)	The child uses phrases like "was broken" or "has taken."	My child says, "My train was broken."	My child says, "The picture was taken by Daddy."

forty-nine to sixty months

sixty-one to seventy-two months

seventy-three months +

Section III: Social-Communicative Development

Item No.		Level Definition	Clinical Description	Item Description	Example 1	Example 2
1.1	birth to one month	Perlocutionary Acts: Differentiated Crying (3,4,63)	The child's expressive behavior consists of different patterns of crying from which the listener must infer his needs.	The child has several different types of cries for each of his different needs.	My child has a special cry which lets me know he is hungry.	My child has a special cry which lets me know when he is uncomfortable or wants to be held.
2.1	two to four months	Perlocutionary Acts: Smiling and Laughing (3,4,63)	The child's expressive behavior includes vocal and visual signs of pleasure.	The child smiles and laughs.	My child smiles at me when he is happy and comfortable.	My child laughs while being played with.
3.1	five to eight months	Reciprocal Imitation (12,63)	The child repeats his vocalizations when imitated by an adult.	The child repeats sounds he makes when he is imitated by someone else.	If I repeat a sound I have heard my child make, he tries to make the same sound.	If my child says, "oh oh" and I repeat it, he says, "oh oh" again.
3.2		Nonverbal Greeting (3,4)	The child expresses recognition or acknowledges the presence of a person with gestures or vocalizations subsequent to the person's entrance.	The child uses gestures or sounds to greet someone he recognizes.	When someone enters my child's room, he makes sounds as if to say, "Hi" to them.	My child reaches out to me and turns to look at me when he hears me enter his room.
4.1	nine to twelve months	Illocutionary Acts: Nonverbal Requesting and Rejecting (3,4,63)	The child uses nonverbal means of communication by pointing, pushing and showing objects to others.	The child points at things, holds them up to show others and pushes away things he doesn't want.	My child points at something he wants me to look at.	My child pushes my hand away when I try to feed him something that he doesn't want.
4.2		Performatives: Indicative and Volitional (29)	The child accompanies nonverbal communication with vocalization, neologism or labeling.	The child uses sounds or made-up words while pointing or reaching out for something.	My child says, "Ba" while reaching out for his ball.	My child says, "Ada" while pointing at a dog that he wants me to see.
4.3		Verbal Turn Taking (7,12,36)	The child engages in reciprocal exchanges of vocalizations and responds to speech by vocalizing.	The child makes sounds when he is spoken to.	My child and I take turns making funny sounds and words, and when I talk to my child, he tries to talk back by making sounds of his own.	If I say, "Hi baby" to my child, he makes sounds or says, "Ma ma."
4.4		Instrumental Function: Requesting Action/Object (20,30)	The child uses one word utterances to satisfy his material needs in terms of goods or services. (a)	The child uses one word sentences to ask for something.	My child says, "Mip" to say, "I want some milk."	My child says, "Aba" to say, "Give me that ball."
4.5		Regulatory: Calling, Protesting (20,30)	The child uses one word utterances to exert control over the behavior of others. (b)	The child uses one word sentences to tell others to do something.	My child says, "Ma ma" when he wants me to come to him.	My child says, "Ee" when he wants me to do something.
4.6		Routine Games (7,12)	The child participates in imitative gestural and verbal games.	The child plays imitative games.	My child plays games that involve imitating my gestures or sounds.	My child plays "patty cake" with me and tries to imitate both the gestures and words of the game.

Item No.	Level Definition	Clinical Description	Item Description	Example 1	Example 2
5.1	Interactional: Greeting (20,30)	The child uses one word utterances to get attention and to interact with others. (c)	The child uses one word sentences to get someone's attention.	My child says, "Hi" and "Bye bye" to people.	My child calls his sister's name to get her attention.
5.2	Personal (30)	The child uses one word utterances to express his personality, his likes and dislikes. (d)	The child uses one word sentences to tell about things he likes and dislikes.	My child says, "Um um" to tell me that he likes something.	My child says, "Nap" or, "Sleepy" to tell me that he is tired.
5.3	Heuristic: Labeling, Requesting Answer (20,30)	The child uses one word utterances to ask about things in the environment. (e)	The child uses one word sentences to ask about things he sees and hears.	My child says, "Da" when he sees something new as if to ask, "What is that?"	My child says, "That" and points to something when he wants me to tell him the name of it.
5.4	Imaginative (30)	The child uses vocalizations to create a pretend environment. (f)	The child makes sounds to enhance his make believe play.	My child makes motor noises when playing with his cars.	My child says, "Woof woof" while playing with his toy dog.
5.5	Practice: Repetition (36,51)	The child repeats his own utterances and those of others for pleasure. (g)	The child repeats words and sounds which he hears several times.	My child repeats, "Baby," as if to practice saying it.	If my child hears me say, "Hi" he says, "Hi" a couple of times as if to practice saying it.
5.6	Rejection (20)	The child uses words like "no," "not" or "uh uh" to reject an object or action.	The child uses words like "no," "not" or "uh uh" to reject something.	My child says, "Uh uh" and turns his head when I try to feed him something he doesn't like.	My child says, "Not," if I give him a ball when he wants his car.
6.1	Pragmatic (30)	The child uses language to satisfy his needs and to control and interact with others. (h)	The child uses two word phrases to ask for something and to tell others to do something at the same time.	My child says, "Mommy, milk," to ask me to give him some milk.	My child says, "Help tie" to ask me to help him tie his shoes.
6.2	Mathetic (30)	The child uses language to learn about the environment. (i)	The child uses two word phrases to tell about things he sees and hears.	My child says, "Big dog" to describe a dog he sees.	My child says, "Two block" to tell me he has two blocks.
6.3	Informative (30)	The child uses language as a means of sharing information. (j)	The child uses two word phrases to share information.	My child says, "Train broke" to tell me that his train is broken.	My child says, "Doggie bite" to tell me he has seen a dog bite someone.
6.4	Monologue: Self-Directing (51,36,64)	The child uses language to direct, control and plan his own actions. (k)	The child talks to himself about his thoughts and actions.	My child often talks to himself about what he is doing and what he is thinking.	My child describes his actions while he is playing; "Here block, car go, throw ball."
6.5	Answering (20)	The child responds to simple questions which call for a label or location of an object.	The child answers simple questions.	My child says, "Ball" if I point to a ball and ask, "What's this?"	My child says, "There ball" if I ask him, "Where is the ball?"
6.6	Collective Monologue (51,48,64)	The child talks in the presence of others and takes turns talking with others but no real information exchange takes place and anyone can serve as an audience. (l)	The child talks to himself while others are present and takes turns talking but doesn't seem to care whether or not he is listened to.	My child talks to me about what he is doing but it doesn't matter to him whether I respond to his comments or just talk about what I am doing.	Tom: "My car's going here." Bill: "Here big house." Tom: "Go race car." Bill: "Man live here."
6.7	Solitary Play (67)	The child plays in the presence of others but with separate toys and materials and without interacting with the others.	The child plays in the same room as other children but does not share toys or play with the others.	When my child is with a group of children he usually plays by himself and uses toys different from those used by the others.	My child prefers to play alone with his blocks rather than building a block tower with other children.

thirteen to eighteen months (rows 5.1–5.6)

nineteen to twenty-four months (rows 6.1–6.7)

Item No.	Level Definition	Clinical Description	Item Description	Example 1	Example 2
7.1	Textual (30)	The child organizes his utterances into contextual phrases and structures conversation for different listeners and settings. (m)	The child organizes words and sentences into conversations appropriate for different people he speaks to.	My child puts two or three words together into sentences that are easily understood by most people that he speaks to.	My child says, "Doggie bite baby" to tell me that a dog has bitten the baby.
7.2	Interpersonal (30)	The child uses language to express his own involvement in the speech situation; roles, judgements, attitudes, wishes and feelings are expressed to exert certain effects on listeners. (n)	The child talks about his feelings, attitudes and wishes.	My child tells me how he feels about things, what he likes, and what he wants.	My child says, "Don't like Billy" or, "Billy is bad" when he is angry with his friend.
7.3	Ideational (30)	The child uses language to express his knowledge and ideas about the world and his experiences. (o)	The child talks about his ideas and experiences.	My child says, "Billy go" when he sees Billy ride the bicycle.	My child points to a pool and says, "Fall in get wet."
7.4	Dialogue (36,51)	The child talks about the topic of another's comment. (p)	The child responds appropriately to someone else's comment.	If I say, "I am hungry," my child says, "I am really hungry."	Tom: "I have a big dog." Bill: "My dog is bigger."
7.5	Contingent Query: Response (27,54)	The child responds appropriately to requests for revisions or repetitions to clarify a comment he has made.	The child responds appropriately to wh- questions.	My child repeats or changes something he has said if someone asks, "What?" or doesn't understand what he has said.	If my child says, "Billy hit me," and I ask, "Who hit you?" he repeats, "Billy hit me."
7.6	Topic Change (7,31)	The child maintains a conversational topic for only 3-4 successive utterances.	The child maintains a conversational topic for only 3-4 sentences.	My child's conversations are very short, and he changes the subject often.	Mom: "You went to the zoo?" Child: "I saw animals." Mom: "Were there lions?" Child: "See my picture."
7.7	Parallel Play (67)	The child's play is of a companionable nature with similar materials and activities but with no personal interaction or cooperation with other children.	The child plays with other children but little cooperation or interaction takes place between them.	When my child is with a group of children, they usually play with the same kinds of toys and do similar things, but they don't share toys or activities.	My child and his friend prefer to each build a separate block tower with their own sets of blocks rather than building one tower together.
8.1	Contingent Query: Use (27)	The child uses wh- questions to make requests for clarification or for additional information about another's comments.	The child uses wh-questions to ask for more information from someone.	My child asks questions like "what, when, where or why."	My child asks, "Who's coming?" if he misunderstands me when I say, "Billy's coming over to play."
8.2	Topic Maintenance (7,31)	The child sustains the topic of conversation over several successive utterances.	The child maintains a conversational topic for several sentences.	My child and I talk about one subject for several minutes before changing to a new subject.	My child holds a conversation for 3-5 minutes about what he did at preschool today.
8.3	Form Adjustment (19,68)	The child modifies his speech as a function of the age of the listener.	The child changes his speech according to the age of his listener.	When my child speaks to a younger child, he uses shorter, simpler sentences than when he speaks to an adult.	My child says, "This is my dog Ralph," to an adult but says, "See doggie; he's Ralph" to his little sister.
8.4	Subjective Role-taking (36,48,58)	The child temporarily assumes another's perspective.	The child pretends to be someone else for a brief period.	My child "role-plays" or pretends to be another person for a short time.	My child pretends to be "mommy" while playing house.

twenty-five to thirty-six months

thirty-seven to forty-eight months

Item No.	Level Definition	Clinical Description	Item Description	Example 1	Example 2
8.5	Associative Play (67)	The child interacts with other children in loosely organized activities; materials and interests are shared, but there is little group cooperation or shared goals.	The child plays in loosely organized activities with other children.	When my child is with a group of children, they share toys, talk about what they are doing, and play together in a group activity.	My child shares his cars with his friends, and they play "race track."
9.1	Indirectives (22)	The child uses hints and indirect means of communicating requests.	The child uses hints and indirect means of asking for something.	My child hints around about something he wants instead of asking for it directly.	My child says, "I like cookies" or, "Mrs. Smith always gives us cookies" rather than saying, "Can I have a cookie?"
9.2	Metalinguistic Awareness (19)	The child is aware of language as a distinct entity; there is an awareness of component sounds, word-meaning correspondence and rules of grammar. Language is used to think about language and to comment on it.	The child uses language to think about language and to comment on it.	My child knows the first letter in his name.	My child corrects my speech; if I say, "Two dog," he will say, "No, two dogs."
9.3	Cooperative Play (67)	The child's play involves long complex sequences with different roles, common goals and cooperation with a leader.	The child plays with other children in organized, planned out activities; there is group cooperation.	When my child is with a group of children, they usually plan in advance what they are going to play, and one child becomes the leader who directs the other children's activities.	When my child plays with his friends, he says, "We'll play house, I'll be the dad, you be the mom, and I'll fix this car while you cook dinner."
9.4	Game (67)	The child participates in rule governed game activities and demonstrates an understanding of the rules.	The child plays organized games and makes up new games.	My child follows the rules of an organized game and makes up rules for games he invents.	My child plays "hide and seek" and simple card games like "Old Maid."
9.5	Directing (64)	The child uses language in controlling, instructing and directing others' activities.	The child uses language to control and direct others' activities and to tell someone how to do something.	My child gives another child instructions on how to do something.	My child teaches his brother how to build a block house: "First you have to put the big ones down; then put the bricks on top for the sides . . ."
10.1	Relating (64)	The child uses language in expressing needs and interests and in justifying his actions to others.	The child uses language to express his needs and interests and to justify his actions.	My child gives logical reasons for his wanting to do something.	My child says, "I want the big paper because I need more room for my picture than you do."
10.2	Reasoning (64)	The child uses language in expressing recognition of cause-effect relationships and demonstrating knowledge of a principle.	The child uses language to express understanding of cause-effect relationships and to tell about something he knows.	My child correctly answers, "What happens if?" questions. ("What happens if I drop this glass?" "It will break.")	My child says, "The popsicles melted because we forgot to put them in the freezer."
10.3	Predicting (64)	The child uses language in forecasting events and anticipating consequences of his actions.	The child tells about future events and consequences.	My child tells me about things that are going to happen in the future.	My child says, "We're going to the zoo next week if I'm a good boy all week."
10.4	Empathizing (64)	The child uses language in understanding and sharing others' emotions and attitudes.	The child uses language to share feelings and attitudes with others.	My child talks about how others feel and can give reasons for their feelings.	My child says, "Sue is sad cause Bill was teasing her and she didn't like it."
10.5	Imagining (64)	The child uses language in creating pretend situations and characters.	The child uses language to create make-believe situations and characters.	My child has imaginary friends and pets which he talks to and tells me about frequently.	My child has a make-believe playmate "Bob" that he talks to and plays with.

forty-nine to sixty months — *sixty-one to seventy-two months*

Item No.	Level Definition	Clinical Description	Item Description	Example 1	Example 2
11.1	Communicative Competence (54)	The child demonstrates the ability to operate as an effective communicator of needs, desires, feelings and ideas.	The child is an effective communicator.	My child participates in "Show and Tell" at school and has no problem in telling his story or in being understood by the teacher or other children.	My child uses speech and language which is easily understood and appropriate for most situations.

seventy-three months +

Index